Fostering a Community of Success for Neurodivergent Collegiate Students

Carol Rogers-Shaw
University of Dayton, USA

Tulare Williams Park
Commonwealth University of Pennsylvania, USA

Kayla D. Mohney
Commonwealth University of Pennsylvania, USA

Kari Sheward
University of Dayton, USA

IGI Global
Scientific Publishing
Publishing Tomorrow's Research Today

Vice President of Editorial Melissa Wagner
Director of Acquisitions Mikaela Felty
Director of Book Development Jocelynn Hessler
Production Manager Mike Brehm
Cover Design Jose Rosado

Published in the United States of America by
IGI Global Scientific Publishing
701 East Chocolate Avenue
Hershey, PA, 17033, USA
Tel: 717-533-8845
Fax: 717-533-7115
Website: https://www.igi-global.com E-mail: cust@igi-global.com

Library of Congress Cataloging-in-Publication Data

Names: Rogers-Shaw, Carol, 1959- editor. | Park, Tulare Williams, 1975- editor. | Mohney, Kayla, 1982- editor. | Sheward, Kari, 1968- editor.
Title: Fostering a community of success for neurodivergent collegiate students / edited by: Carol Rogers-Shaw, Tulare Park, Kayla Mohney, Kari Sheward.
Description: Hershey, PA : IGI Global Scientific Publishing, [2026] | Includes bibliographical references and index. | Summary: "This book aims to explore various aspects of neurodiversity on college campuses, with a focus on collaborative initiatives that promote inclusivity, foster community engagement, and support the successful transition to college and the workplace for neurodivergent individuals"-- Provided by publisher.
Identifiers: LCCN 2024059673 (print) | LCCN 2024059674 (ebook) | ISBN 9798369389201 (hardcover) | ISBN 9798369389218 (paperback) | ISBN 9798369389225 (ebook)
Subjects: LCSH: Neurodivergent people--Education (Higher) | People with disabilities in higher education. | College students with disabilities.
Classification: LCC LC4818.38 .C65 2025 (print) | LCC LC4818.38 (ebook) | DDC 378.0087--dc23/eng/20250326
LC record available at https://lccn.loc.gov/2024059673
LC ebook record available at https://lccn.loc.gov/2024059674

British Cataloguing in Publication Data
A Cataloguing in Publication record for this book is available from the British Library.

Table of Contents

Detailed Table of Contents

There is a growing recognition of the diverse range of neurodifferences among college students. This acknowledgment has paved the way for a shift towards fostering inclusive environments that support the academic success and holistic wellbeing of Neurodivergent students. This chapter defines neurodivergence and outlines the transition process Neurodivergent students must navigate. It seeks to prepare campus faculty, staff, students, and administrators with knowledge they need to effectively promote inclusivity, foster community engagement, and support the successful transition to college for Neurodivergent individuals. Foundations in K12 special education that form the basis for Neurodivergent student transition to postsecondary education, legal and procedural differences between K12 and college, and challenges Neurodivergent students face during the transition process are shared. The focus is the need for campus stakeholders to adopt a mindset shift and apply a new framework to come together effectively to build community, avoid ableism, and support Neurodivergent students.

This chapter explores how Malcolm Knowles' (1990) principles of andragogy can be effectively applied to support Neurodivergent students in higher education settings and demonstrates how andragogical strategies, focusing on the self-directed, experiential, and relevant learning needs of adults, can be adapted to create inclusive and supportive learning environments for Neurodivergent individuals, including

Preface

In 2019, a collaborative research group was developed between Carol, Tulare, and Kayla. At that time, Carol and Tulare were doctoral students at Pennsylvania State University and Kayla had recently completed her doctoral degree in 2017. Tulare and Kayla were working at Lock Haven University where Tulare served in the role of Director of Disability Resources and Kayla was an Assistant Professor. As special education department colleagues, Kayla approached Tulare with the idea of submitting a conference proposal together. Tulare then reached out to Carol, and later that same year, the trio presented together at the annual Pennsylvania Training and Technical Assistance Network (PaTTAN) conference. This presentation was titled *Identifying the Gaps to Higher Education: Parent, Professor, & Disability Services Perspectives,* with each of us providing our view of Neurodivergent student transition to college based on our roles at the time. During the presentation, the questions and comments came fast and furiously for over an hour and a half, and when it was over, we realized parents and professionals in the field were searching for this knowledge. What followed was a series of five additional (refined and focused) presentations and an academic paper that we tried to have published. The manuscript was rejected time and again either because the focus did not specify enough strategies for families and secondary schools or higher education publications were not interested in what happened in high school.

When Carol and Kari met as professor and doctoral student at the University of Dayton and shared stories of parenting Neurodivergent children, we all began writing together on transition issues and tips for faculty members working with Neurodivergent students. It seemed we always went back to that transition article and decided to publish a book where we could finally share the information that was so needed and desired by others, but that we couldn't publish elsewhere. That article became Chapter 1 of this text. As parents of Neurodivergent individuals, professors of Neurodivergent students, teacher educators, Neurodivergent center professionals, and researchers, we knew we had valuable expertise to share and that our own collaborations could be models for improved campus collaboration.

In recent years, there has been a growing recognition of the diverse range of neurocognitive and developmental differences within the college student population. This increased awareness has prompted a critical shift toward fostering intentionally inclusive environments that affirm and support the academic success, personal agency, and holistic wellbeing of *all* students including Neurodivergent learners. Central to this shift is an explicit commitment to anti-ableism—a rejection of practices, policies, and attitudes that marginalize or devalue individuals based on perceived cognitive or behavioral differences. This book aims to equip campus faculty, staff, students, and administrators with the knowledge and tools necessary to build inclusive, accessible, and affirming postsecondary environments. It defines neurodivergence through a strengths-based lens and outlines the complex transition process Neurodivergent students experience as they move from K–12 into higher education. Rather than placing the responsibility of adaptation solely on the students, this book emphasizes the obligation of institutions to engage in a mindset shift—centering an anti-ableism framework. It calls on all campus stakeholders to actively challenge deficit-based narratives, foster authentic community engagement, and co-create learning environments where Neurodivergent students are not only accommodated, but truly valued and empowered. Ultimately, it emphasizes the importance of a mindset shift among campus stakeholders, encouraging them to adopt new frameworks that build community, prevent ableism, and provide comprehensive support for Neurodivergent students.

The inspiration behind this endeavor is the people we know and love who are part of the neurodiversity community. We have been encouraged to take on this project through our work with and study of amazing and successful Neurodivergent individuals in our lives and in the stories told throughout the world. Neurodiversity is important to us, and we are proud that our authors, 61% of whom represent countries other than our home base in the United States, have shared the amazing work being done around the globe. Research on neurodiversity must include the perspectives of Neurodivergent individuals; some of our contributors have chosen to disclose that they are Neurodivergent or have a family member who is Neurodivergent. We value their voices, ideas, and accomplishments, and we know our readers will appreciate the contributions of all of our authors. We hope this text is the first step in creating a world-wide collaborative community of researchers and practitioners who can come together on future projects that support the educational and social success of Neurodivergent individuals

The use of language choices is highly personal, complicated, and ever changing. We have made our choices for this book based on our own preferences, discussions with Neurodivergent family members and friends, colleagues (both Neurodivergent and neuromajority) in the field, and responses from authors and editors we have worked with. We consulted with the chapter authors to make sure the language choices reflected their preferences. We acknowledge the importance of individual choices regarding person first or identity first language. The decision of self-identification may not fall within either person first or identity first. It can also be fluid or conditional. We made language choices based on this awareness, and our goal is to be respectful and inclusive of all individuals no matter what language decisions they make for themselves.

We use Neurodivergent to describe individuals and neurodiverse to describe a group, a project, a concept, or research. We have edited the book to reflect the use of the terms as described by Abbott (2022): "Neurodiversity is a recognition that not all brains think or feel the same way, and that these differences are natural variations in the human genome. A group of people are neurodiverse, an individual is not. Neurodivergent refers to an individual who has a less typical cognitive variation such as Autism, ADHD, dyslexia, dyspraxia etc." The term Neurodivergent is also more identity based rather than medically founded on diagnosis labels that can reinforce the idea of neurodivergence as a disorder or deficit to be cured or remediated rather than accepted as human variation.

We also adhere to the American Psychological Association (APA) 7th edition style guide in using the pronoun choice they/their rather than he/his or she/her when the pronoun choice of an individual is not known or when it is a generic reference like an instructor or an advisor. If the chosen pronouns of an individual were known, those pronouns were used. We chose to capitalize Neurodivergent and Autistic when referring to individuals, thereby acknowledging neurodivergence and autistic as a cultural/identity marker. This is similar to speaking of a Black student, a Jewish student, and/or a Cisgender student. We followed the same process for neurodiverse and autism, which do not refer to an individual and are not capitalized. We eliminated the acronym ND (neurodivergent) as we would not use letters for other cultural/identity markers; for example, we would not use BLK for Black or CG for Cisgender.

"Disability" is the legal term that includes neurodivergence so it is used in the chapter when referring to legalities, yet we recognize the importance of focusing positively on difference rather than deficit or disorder in terms of Neurodivergent students. We used "neuromajority" rather than "neurotypical" due to the more positive association with the word "majority." With "neuromajority," it becomes about the size of the group rather than one group being "better" than the other. We do not capitalize neuromajority as it is not viewed as a cultural/identity group. We avoided words like "condition" that implies a negative element of a Neurodivergent student's being and reflects the medical model of disability that requires "curing." We replaced it with a reference like "presentation" (how something might arise and be seen) or neurodivergences, neurodifferences, differences, traits, or characteristics. We used "multiply neurodiverse" or "co-occurring challenges/differences/traits" rather than "comorbidity." We made these decisions keeping in mind that being respectful of personal choice and using affirming terminology is an important way to show others a welcoming perspective and an example of inclusion of *all* individuals.

The terms postsecondary education, higher education, tertiary education, college, community college, and university are often used interchangeably in the United States, although a community college is a 2-year institution and a college or university refers to one with a 4-year undergraduate program. The chapters use the words the authors choose, and they might refer to a similar type of institution by multiple identifiers. The acronym HEI refers to Higher Education Institutions and includes any postsecondary education or training institution. There are many different names for campus offices that refer to departments that support Neurodivergent students in attaining accommodations such as the Disability Resources Office, Accessibility Services, Student Disability Services, or the Disability Resource Center that are used interchangeably. We refer to these departments by the names and acronyms chosen by the authors.

The contents of this text offers a wide range of topics reflecting the expertise and context of our authors. Chapter 1 identifies significant differences in Neurodivergent student academic and social support between secondary and postsecondary education that can affect their college experiences. Obtaining this knowledge is vital for campus entities if they are to understand how a student's elementary and high school experiences shape their expectations of and reactions to supports available in college. With this comprehension, university stakeholders can better support Neurodivergent students.

Chapter 2 applies the adult education theory of andragogy to practices supporting Neurodivergent college students. Focusing on the self-directed, experiential, and relevant learning needs of adults, the authors argue that changing the pedagogical approach on campus can enhance Neurodivergent students' campus experiences and increase their persistence.

Chapter 3 uses Phenomenological Variant of Ecological Systems Theory (PVEST) to improve Neurodivergent student outcomes. The authors examine the impact of Neurodivergent students' context and coping mechanisms through participatory approaches.

Chapter 4 recognizes the roles of social workers on campus and analyzes how the application of the principles of social work can be adopted to improve Neurodivergent student support. The related ideas include person-in-environment and ecological perspectives, a strengths-based approach, advocacy, and allyship.

Chapter 5 offers a model program that has designed inclusive university experiences for learners with intellectual disabilities (ID) in Ireland. Through the lens of Bronfenbrenner's bio-ecological systems theory (1979, 1989), the chapter examines how social and environmental systems impact the experiences, development, and outcomes of students with ID in higher education.

Chapter 6 addresses systemic barriers to success faced by international and female Neurodivergent students in universities in the United Kingdom. Using the tenets of sociocultural theory, it examines financial structures, cultural expectations, and institutional policies that foster disengagement and learned helplessness among Neurodivergent students.

Chapter 7 reviews the importance of self-advocacy and self-determination in student success. The study presented highlights the implementation of the Think College Standards for Inclusive Higher Education.

Chapter 8 connects the collective capacities and capabilities of Neurodivergent individuals as crucial to the socio-economic development of society. It identifies cultural, economic, and location based barriers to the implementation of inclusive policies and practices at universities in Pakistan.

Chapter 9 highlights the development of a faculty and staff training program created in partnership with Neurodivergent students and guided by the Universal Design for Learning (UDL) and Students as Partners (SaP) frameworks. It recommends ways to develop and sustain neurodiversity campus-wide training for faculty and staff.

Editing this book has been a journey that we are thrilled to have taken as we learned about the editing process and acquired new knowledge of neurodiversity from our talented and expert authors. We hope readers will expand their own understanding of neurodiversity and find strategies to implement collaborative practices on their own campuses to better support Neurodivergent learners.

REFERENCE

Abbott, L. (2022). Neurodiversity & Neurodivergent: What do they mean and how do they impact me as a PGR. *University of Glasgow PGR Blog*. https://uofgpgrblog.com/pgrblog/2021/3/24/neurodiversity#:~:text=A%20group%20of%20people%20are,%2C%20and%20intellectual%2Fcognitive%20functioning

Acknowledgement

The journey to publication has been an adventure filled with friendship and scholarship as the editors and chapter authors all contributed their best work with the goal of enhancing understanding and empathy of Neurodivergent college students. We all want to make a positive difference in our worlds. I am grateful for the experiences encountered and the relationships developed along the way. As always, I am extremely appreciative of the support of my husband and daughters who have always been there for me.

– Carol Rogers-Shaw

I'm incredibly thankful to have worked with my amazing co-editors on this project and am grateful for the fantastic authors who have contributed their voices, stories, and time to it. I also thank my family for their love and support.

– Tulare Williams Park

Life presents us with countless paths, and I'm grateful I chose this one with Tulare, Carol, and Kari. This project has been a truly enriching experience. To everyone who contributed their time, effort, and encouragement, I offer my sincere thanks - your support has been essential in bringing this book to life. Finally, I would be remiss if I didn't express my deepest appreciation to my husband, your unwavering support means more to me than words can ever express.

– Kayla D. Mohney

I am grateful for the opportunity to collaborate and learn from this wonderful group of co-editors. Their expertise in the field, combined with their experience in writing and publishing, was essential to this project. I appreciate all of the author's contributions as well. Additionally, I would like to thank my family for their unwavering support and encouragement.

– Kari Sheward

Tulare, Kayla, & Kari want to acknowledge Carol as the driving force and recognize her unwavering dedication to bringing this project to fruition. We are eternally grateful for her positivity, encouraging spirit, tenacity, humor, and brilliance. Since we've started this project, we've all had our own ways that life has thrown things at us. Carol has always been the one to pick up the load for all of us, even in the midst of her own storms. We couldn't have imagined all that would happen during this process. We've all supported each other, but Carol really has been that constant presence and support. She's truly a remarkable woman who we are all fortunate to call our friend.

Chapter 1
The Starting Point:
Establishing a Framework for an Inclusive College Community

Carol Rogers-Shaw
https://orcid.org/0000-0003-0550-290X
University of Dayton, USA

Tulare Williams Park
https://orcid.org/0000-0002-9092-5968
Commonwealth University of Pennsylvania, USA

Kayla D. Mohney
https://orcid.org/0000-0003-4264-8318
Commonwealth University of Pennsylvania, USA

Kari L. Sheward
https://orcid.org/0009-0003-8800-8727
University of Dayton, USA

ABSTRACT

There is a growing recognition of the diverse range of neurodifferences among college students. This acknowledgment has paved the way for a shift towards fostering inclusive environments that support the academic success and holistic wellbeing of Neurodivergent students. This chapter defines neurodivergence and outlines the transition process Neurodivergent students must navigate. It seeks to prepare campus faculty, staff, students, and administrators with knowledge they need to effectively promote inclusivity, foster community engagement, and support the successful transition to college for Neurodivergent individuals. Foundations in K12 special education that form the basis for Neurodivergent student transition to postsecondary education, legal and procedural differences between K12 and

DOI: 10.4018/979-8-3693-8920-1.ch001

college, and challenges Neurodivergent students face during the transition process are shared. The focus is the need for campus stakeholders to adopt a mindset shift and apply a new framework to come together effectively to build community, avoid ableism, and support Neurodivergent students.

INTRODUCTION

Special education can be said to have a turbulent past (Florian, 2007; Thomas & Loxley, 2022); however, improved K12 special education and transition services over time have provided current Neurodivergent learners greater opportunities to attend college, increasing the demand for collegiate based services (Jaird, 2022; Leake & Stodden, 2014). Research has revealed growing numbers of Neurodivergent learners are enrolled in postsecondary education, and when they receive appropriate support, they can often be academically successful and socially engaged (Kuder et al., 2023). Although while colleges and universities have increased the resources devoted to Neurodivergent learners, higher numbers of Neurodivergent learners fail to graduate than their neuromajority peers (Dwyer et al., 2023; Santhanam & Wilson, 2024; Schaefer & Sanchez, 2024). To create an inclusive environment that effectively supports *all* students, including those who are neurodivergent, members of the campus community must create a framework of inclusivity and shed ableist perspectives. The framework includes gaining knowledge of neurodiversity, recognizing the changes needed, valuing Neurodivergent students by acknowledging what they can do, and leading with a strength-based perspective rather than focusing on challenges. Making sure the college community is appropriately and continuously trained so that everyone adopts this mindset shift is crucial.

Students are classified as Neurodivergent learners after they have received a diagnosis or have identified themselves as having symptoms of a particular neurodifference including but not limited to Autism Spectrum Disorder (ASD), Attention Deficit Hyperactivity Disorder (ADHD), learning disabilities (LD) (i.e., dyslexia, dyspraxia, dyscalculia, dysgraphia), Tourette Syndrome, and other neurological and/or developmental delays (McDowall & Kiseleva, 2024). Neurodivergent learners are often not trusted to make decisions about their learning and are frequently counseled to follow paths contrary to their own desires (Dwyer, 2024; Gragoudas, 2014; Westby, 2023). Thus, among these learners, a need for self-advocacy, clear communication, independence, and recognition of new and different types of instructional practices at the college level that are different from high school cannot be understated. Bridging to college through the Disability Resource Office (DRO), in the college classroom, and during social activities (Rogers-Shaw et al., 2023) often presents a complicated set of obstacles for Neurodivergent students.

Some of the difficulties experienced by Neurodivergent students in educational settings may be related to ableist attitudes. Ableism is defined as:

discrimination of and social prejudice against people with disabilities based on the belief that typical abilities are superior. At its heart, ableism is rooted in the assumption that disabled people require 'fixing' and defines people by their disability. Like racism and sexism, ableism classifies entire groups of people as 'less than,' and includes harmful stereotypes, misconceptions, and generalizations of people with disabilities. (Eisenmenger, 2019, para. 2)

Dolmage (2017) described how the educational system privileges "able-bodiedness and able-mindedness," which creates ableist practices (p. 70). Ableism is often unintentional (e.g., holding meetings in locations that are not accessible, offering help without asking if it is needed, or making assumptions about a person's capabilities based on diagnoses) and often stems from a lack of understanding of neurodiversity and/or lacking a strength-based thought process. This is why the framework presented in this chapter and this book is so critical for higher education faculty, staff, and administrators; moving away from ableism requires that we learn from each other and work together.

Functional collaboration across campus to create a suitable support system can only be achieved when all university stakeholders clearly understand that Neurodivergent learners need to possess an additional set of skills and knowledge to successfully transition to college. Furthermore, regardless of institutional systems, Neurodivergent learners must also employ a strong sense of resilience and perseverance, as both institution and individual are essential in meeting these learners' academic and social goals. This requires faculty, staff, and administrators to more effectively communicate, prepare for, and collaboratively spread an intentional mindset shift away from ableist attitudes and toward inclusion. By coming together, the community can utilize the framework to accomplish this goal.

Unless college administrators, faculty, and staff have previous experience with special education services in the K12 setting, it is unlikely that they know about the methods of support which Neurodivergent learners received during elementary, middle, and high school, or know the corresponding legal mandates that K12 institutions follow, and the process of transition planning for college. Collegiate instructors, residential, support and ancillary staff, program directors, and DRO staff across campuses can benefit from a deeper understanding of learner backgrounds, a comprehension of Universal Design, and a mindset shift away from ableist attitudes. This knowledge supports compliance with legally mandated accommodations, as well as the creation of inclusive environments, adaptable instructional strategies, course designs, and assessments that meet the needs of all students, including Neurodivergent learners (Ross-Gordon & Procknow, 2021).

Unfortunately, neither clear avenues nor requirements have been developed for campus stakeholders to gain that knowledge. Individuals on campus may provide support for Neurodivergent college students, but the siloed nature of their work limits the impact. Positive aid could be exponentially increased if university personnel were well-versed in K12 special education regulations and support provisions, and best practices across campus collaboration to assist Neurodivergent learners in achieving success. This chapter aims to fill these knowledge gaps and offers a place to begin the journey to effectively supporting Neurodivergent students in postsecondary settings.

K12 SPECIAL EDUCATION & ITS COMPONENTS

Individuals with disabilities have always been a part of society. However, specialized teaching techniques did not arise until the late 18th century (Hallahan et al., 2022). Prior to this time, asylums were commonly used to house those with mental, physical, sensory, or intellectual differences without regard to their disability or attention to their individual needs (Conrad, 2020). With the establishment of specialized residential schools for those who were deaf by Thomas Gallaudet in 1817, and those who were blind by Samuel Howe in 1829, a focus on the treatment of individuals with other types of disabilities arose in the early 19th century. Most scholars believe that European physicians were the first to attempt to educate individuals with disabilities, the work of Jean-Marc-Gaspard Itard in the early 19th century frequently being cited as establishing the first individualized, systematic instructional techniques (Francisco et al., 2020; Richards & Hulewicz, 2024).

The use of such techniques was expanded throughout Europe and into the United States leading to the institutionalization movement of the 19th century. Although such facilities were established to house and educate individuals with disabilities and remedy issues affecting them, residents of these institutions endured horrific conditions due to underfunding, lack of training for staff, and gross overpopulation. The deinstitutionalization movement of the 1960's and 1970's brought about social justice reform and legislative action to protect vulnerable members of the disability community (Conrad, 2020; Hallahan et al., 2022). In 1975, the United States passed its first legislation to include provisions for learners with disabilities in K12 education, the Education for All Handicapped Children Act (PL 94-142), which granted some disabled learners access to a public education.

Special education is commonly defined as specifically designed instruction that meets the needs of individuals with disabilities who require special materials, teaching techniques, and/or equipment in order to meet their full potential (Hallahan et al., 2022). At that time, not all learners with disabilities were permitted to attend schools; those with the most severe disabilities were still excluded due to a lack of ability to provide services. The passing of the Individuals with Disabilities Education Act (IDEA) in 1990 provided a pivotal change in special education with the provision of "free appropriate public education" (FAPE) for all students (IDEA, 2004). IDEA has undergone many revisions and improvements, including altering the original language to require support to all learners with disabilities in K12 education. The major provisions of IDEA include identification procedures, nondiscriminatory evaluation methods, parent/guardian participation, least restrictive environment, and individualized education programs (IEP). The history of special education provides a glimpse into the differences between K12 and postsecondary education and the need for attention to the transition process. Gaining a better understanding of the complex system of public special education can be beneficial to campus stakeholders. This knowledge can explain student expectations that often surprise faculty and staff members and offer practical strategies for teaching Neurodivergent students while encouraging collaboration with campus colleagues to better support these learners. This vital information can guide postsecondary professionals in moving away from ableist perspectives to embrace inclusive communities.

Figure 1 outlines the factors that affect students' successful transition from K12 special education to the college environment.

Figure 1. Factors Affecting Neurodivergent Student Transition to Postsecondary Education

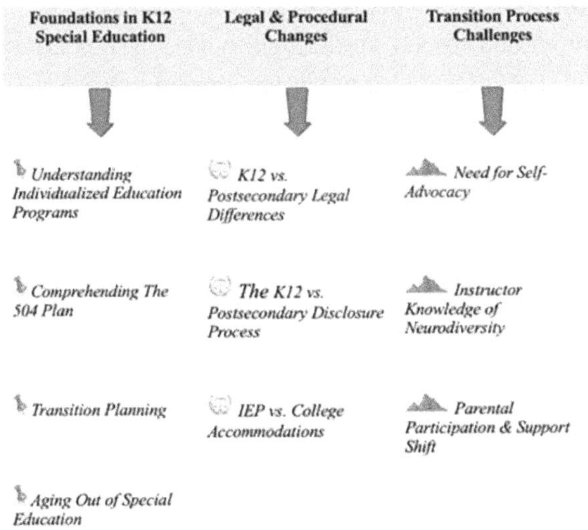

Note. This figure identifies the transition topics discussed in this chapter that are essential for campus and community stakeholders to understand to effectively support Neurodivergent college students.

Understanding Individualized Education Programs

According to IDEA (2004), an Individualized Education Program (IEP) is a legal document developed by the IEP team that is specifically designed to meet the unique learning needs of a K12 student with a diagnosed disability and their documented needs for specially designed instruction to meet age/grade level skills. To receive IEP, students must meet both criteria. The IEP team must consist of a parent/guardian of the child, at least one regular education teacher of the child, a special education teacher, an individual who can interpret the results of evaluations, a representative of the school/district who (a) is qualified to provide, or supervise the provision of specially designed instruction, (b) is knowledgeable about general education curricula, and (c) is aware of the availability of resources of the school/district, and other individuals requested by a parent/guardian. When appropriate, the child with the disability under the age of 16 can participate, and participation is mandated at 16 years of age. School personnel who have direct contact with the student are all familiar with the details of that student's K12 plan, but this is not true of postsecondary education unless the student discloses their disability.

The year in which the student turns 16 years of age is critical because at that point the law requires that the student be invited to participate in the IEP process to discuss transition planning (IDEA, 2004). Students' participation while in high school can provide a strong foundation for self-advocacy in college, but not all students are actively involved in the decision-making process. If IEP teams are to make appropriate recommendations for student supports, they need to consider learner traits and individual student learning needs and preferences while following relevant laws. Implementing the supports is a complex process (Gupta et al., 2023; Strunk et al., 2022). It is important to note the size and skills of the IEP team that supports an individual student is significant as the loss of this personalized network of assistance and expertise can make transitioning to postsecondary education challenging.

IEPs are comprehensive documents which must be updated yearly (IDEA, 2004). The IEP must include:

- a student's present levels of academic and functional performance which are used to develop goals;
- a description of specially designed instruction, related services (e.g. occupational therapy, physical therapy, speech therapy, etc.), and supplemental aids (e.g. adapted equipment, assistive technology, and accommodations and modifications) that will be provided to the child to meet those goals;
- the transition services to be provided in the areas of postsecondary education and training, employment, and independent living skills; and
- a transfer of rights at the age of majority (typically 18) (IDEA, 2004).

All services terminate upon graduation from K12 education. It is critical to recognize the complexity of the IEP itself to understand the individualized nature of the programming provided, the amount of collaboration that exists amongst the IEP team, and the various types and levels of supports students with disabilities have access to in the K12 setting (Amend et al., 2024; Dillon et al., 2021) in contrast to supports they can receive in college.

One cohesive support team with the level of expertise of the IEP team is not duplicated in postsecondary education, and, therefore, there is a need for postsecondary community stakeholders to collaborate across campus to effectively meet the needs of Neurodivergent learners. The change in concentrated support skills and knowledge can create transition challenges for Neurodivergent learners who are accustomed to this type of support. This highly structured, adult-led, individualized programming that students with disabilities had received in K12 can lead to students having unrealistic expectations when they begin college. They may infer that they will have the same level of support and services in college.

Despite research showing Neurodivergent students can meaningfully participate in IEP and transition planning meetings and effectively build self-determination skills (McNaught et al., 2024; Sanderson et al., 2021), the lack of required input from the learner before the age of 16 can lead students to become reliant on adults. Self-disclosure of a disability does not become the responsibility of the student until they begin postsecondary education (Cox et al., 2017; Kerschbaum et al., 2017; Sapir & Banai, 2024). The IEP, as outlined by IDEA, is not the only legislation that contributes to the support of Neurodivergent learners.

The 504 Plan

High school students with disabilities identified as *not* requiring special education services under IDEA but who are still in need of accommodations can receive them under a separate non-discrimination statute, the Rehabilitation Act of 1973 Section 504 (29 U.S.C. § 794) that provides non-discrimination protections to learners with disabilities in both the K12 and higher education settings. Section 504 is a federal law which prohibits discrimination within all programs and activities that are federally funded including healthcare, public education, and transportation; it applies to service availability, accessibility, delivery, employment, and administrative activities and responsibilities. No qualified individual with a disability can be excluded from, denied benefits of, or be discriminated against in any program or activity that receives federal financial assistance (Section 504 29 U.S.C. § 794). According to Section 504, K12 school districts are not required to provide transition planning (Dragoo & Cole, 2019). For example, a student with an injury (e.g. broken leg or concussion) may receive temporary accommodation through a Section 504 plan in the K12 setting (e.g. use of the school elevator) and on the higher education campus (e.g. the student may receive consideration for additional time to arrive to classes). Campus stakeholders must understand the legal ramifications of Section 504 as it pertains to student support in postsecondary education. In addition, students with a 504 plan may be under the false impression that parents/guardians are still in charge of their education information, and they may not understand the need to disclose to the DRO to continue 504 accommodations.

A major challenge with the process of transition to postsecondary life for students with 504 plans is that they may not have had as much involvement with or understanding of the support process of planning, communicating, and self-advocating, so they may not be well-prepared to do so on their own in college. Just as Neurodivergent students benefit from participating in IEP meetings, students can become better acquainted with their strengths, weaknesses, and needs by taking part in 504 meetings. While a useful resource for students, 504 plans are not common in many schools across the United States, often due to a lack of awareness and understanding of the process, thus limiting the supports available (Burke et al., 2024; Rodriguez et al., 2021; Zirkel & Gullo, 2024). Collegiate stakeholders need to be aware of this deficiency in knowledge to better understand and support Neurodivergent learners through the transition process, as well as to proactively make the learning environment accessible and inclusive. Neurodivergent students may lack sufficient self-advocacy and self-determination skills needed in college if they do not practice advocating for themselves and making educational decisions while in high school.

Transition Planning

Transition plans are a coordinated set of services that focus on improving the academic and functional achievement of students with disabilities for their move from high school to post-school activities in three areas: employment, postsecondary education and training, and as needed, independent living (IDEA, 2004). The transition plan includes goals in each area, a description of the services and/or activities to be completed, the courses that support the goal, and service or activity locations, frequency, projected dates, and individuals responsible for facilitating the plan. These complimentary areas are designed to meet the goal of the student becoming an independent, gainfully employed adult. Sheward et al. (2022) identified additional transition challenges surrounding executive functioning and relationship building. These areas can be added to a transition plan to demonstrate a need for additional training for success on a college campus.

Transition planning includes actions that can be taken before a student graduates from high school such as researching appropriate postsecondary options which include four-year universities and two-year community colleges (with or without Inclusive

Postsecondary Education (IPSE) programs), vocational schools, and online programs. This exploration can be accomplished through campus visits or websites such as Think College, the College Autism Network (CAN) database, the Neurodiversity Hub, and the National Center for College Students with Disabilities clearinghouse. Connecting with college and university admissions counselors can offer students the chance to understand the admissions process and ask questions about campus support if they choose to disclose during the admissions process. Becoming familiar with the DRO on campus, taking a college course while still attending high school, or participating in a pre-college program during the summer can also be beneficial (Clayburn, 2023; Connor, 2012; Educational Advocates, 2024).

The goals, activities, and actions within the transition plan are driven by the IEP team, as students are still largely supported by adults. Developed self-advocacy skills are vital for Neurodivergent learners as they work to identify personal goals by evaluating their strengths and challenges. Helping learners with disabilities to increase self-knowledge, take risks, embrace opportunities, and practice reflection is essential. It is crucial that the groundwork is laid early for students to become self-advocates and take ownership of their college academic and social experiences (McNaught et al., 2024; Rogers-Shaw et. al, 2023; Ross-Gordon & Procknow, 2021; Santhanam & Wilson, 2024). Bal et al. (2015) studied the importance of daily living skills on independence as individuals transition to different settings. The ability to learn the skills to live independently–managing money, taking care of personal hygiene, and preparing food–may take more time for some individuals than others, particularly when the new environment provides additional challenges, thus highlighting the need for a strengths-based inclusive environment that campus professionals can develop and implement. Skill-building should begin in primary education and progress through secondary education where the familiar environment and consistent supports can be leveraged. The preparation for life on a college campus is a team effort involving all stakeholders in the student's life (Elias & White, 2018).

Aging Out of the Special Education System

Notification from the K12 school to the student and their parents/guardians that the education rights of the student will transfer from the parents/guardians to the student must take place the year prior to the student reaching the age of majority. This Transfer of Rights, as well as IDEA (2004), both state that students must be awarded legal control of their education including placement, records, eligibility, evaluations, programming, and any mediation or due process needed to resolve disputes. Students are permitted to appoint their parents/guardians as representatives to continue to make education decisions on their behalf through secondary school graduation. University faculty and staff may find being familiar with the law can provide educators with the confidence to work with the student without parental/guardian interference, yet they should also recognize the significant role of parents/guardians in K12 special education and how the loss of this support can present challenges for students. With increased confidence and self-advocacy skills, students are likely to be better prepared to take ownership of their educational rights. They may come to rely less on their parents/guardians. Similarly, students who have been involved in their IEP process may be more prepared for postsecondary transition planning.

Americans with Disabilities Act

The Americans with Disabilities Act of 1990 (42 U.S.C. § 12101) is a civil rights law that protects persons with disabilities from discrimination in employment settings and schools and requires public accommodations for accessibility, transportation, and communication. Amended in 2008 (ADA Amendments Act, 42 U.S.C. 12101 et seq), it is now more inclusive of persons with a variety of disabilities. The ADA "ensures the right of individuals with disabilities to nondiscriminatory treatment in other aspects of their lives; it provides protections of civil rights in the specific areas of employment, transportation, public accommodations, state and local government, and telecommunications" (Hallahan et. al., 2022, p. 14). The provision of accessibility to facilities and the allowance of reasonable accommodations in the ADA applies in collegiate settings. Accommodations can be provided to those students who disclose that they are a student with a disability and provide evidence of a disability to the institution's DRO or disability services representative (Lee, 2024).

Table 1 illustrates the contrasting supports offered in the K12 setting versus accommodations available in postsecondary education. Universities do not provide the same tightly controlled, well-defined, individualized structure of supports controlled by K12 school professionals and parents/guardians. However, Neurodivergent learners who disclose their disabilities are offered appropriate accommodations which can be effective if they are understood and supported through cross campus collaboration.

Table 1. Comparison of Supports for Neurodivergent Learners

K–12 Support	Postsecondary Support	College Collaborative Support
IDEA facilitates success.	ADA facilitates access.	Administrators, faculty, and the DRO can collaborate to ensure that a sample syllabus statement about the disclosure process is provided to faculty for inclusion on all course syllabi and that course materials are provided in accessible formats.
Testing, diagnosis, and accommodation implementation are school responsibilities.	Disclosure is the student's responsibility through self-advocacy.	The DRO, admissions office, and orientation staff can collaborate on bringing awareness to incoming students about how to disclose and request support/information.
Modified assessments (e.g., no multiple choice) are allowed.	Accommodations such as extended time on tests or taking tests in a quiet space is permitted, but there is no modification of test format.	Professors, DRO, tutoring center, and peer mentors can work together with students on improving test-taking skills.
Class materials are provided in accessible formats if a student has an IEP requiring it.	Course materials are provided in accessible formats if the student requests it through the DRO, and it is determined that this is needed as a reasonable accommodation.	Administrators, faculty, and DRO staff can work with library, instructional design, and information technology staff to proactively prepare accessible course materials to be available in multiple modalities.
When academic or personal challenges arise, parents/ guardians and school personnel control the process of resolution; the student may or may not be able to self-advocate.	Students are required to reach out to university personnel for help as needed for academic and personal challenges; they must locate resources on their own.	Administrators, student affairs staff, academic affairs staff, and health/ wellness staff can collaborate to develop student success centers, care teams, and wellness resources, and inform the campus community through coordinated messaging campaigns.
Related Services (e.g. speech and language therapy, occupational and/or physical therapy, counseling, and transportation) are available through the school district.	Students are responsible for connecting with medical and/or mental health service providers to receive continuation of treatment.	DRO, student affairs, success centers, admissions counselors, and peer support programs on campus can provide students with guidance and lists of providers in the area.

Note: The National Technical Assistance Center on Transition (n.d.) provides resources and toolkits for transition, including an explanation of The Differences Between Secondary and Postsecondary Education compiled by Holzberg (2017).

Students' early involvement and participation gives them the opportunity to practice educational and vocational decision-making and promotes ownership of their choices which contributes to their self-determination and independence. "Students need to be the decision-makers in their lives" (Rogers-Shaw et. al. 2023), and campus faculty and staff can support a student's development of independence through participation in a variety of activities, organizations, and programming. When parents and/or IEP team members do not expect students to be involved, or when they are only minimally involved, transition to college can pose additional challenges as they are used to being told what to do and how to do it. Collegiate expectations are more student-driven, requiring the learner to be independent in reading coursework, completing assignments, and requesting assistance when needed. Campus stakeholders need to understand the importance of transition activities and education that can bridge the gap between student self-determination begun in high school and its full development in college. Moreover, during the admissions process, counselors can work together with the DRO and residential life staff to inform prospective students about available support services on campus. Connecting students to tutoring centers, health facilities, and mentoring programs can also have a meaningful impact. Orientation planning should also involve student affairs, student organizations, and academic departments to ensure that first-week activities are neurodiversity sensitive.

TRANSITIONS WITHIN THE LEGAL SYSTEM

The differences between high school and college are significant for Neurodivergent learners particularly because their educational situation falls under different laws. IDEA covers students in K12 education, while students in postsecondary education fall under the Americans with Disabilities Act (ADA) of 1990. However, Section 504 of the Rehabilitation Act of 1973 (29 U.S.C. § 794) prevents discrimination at both levels.

High School & College Legislative Differences

Legally, IDEA facilitates success while ADA facilitates access, with the responsibility for success moving to the student once they are in college (Dragoo & Cole, 2019; Holzberg, 2017). Thus, if Neurodivergent learners are not provided with appropriate assistance transitioning from coverage under IDEA to ADA, the progression becomes more difficult than the transition for neuromajority learners (Getzel & Thoma, 2008; Heiman & Shemesh, 2012). When students are made explicitly aware of the differences between the IDEA and ADA before they arrive on campus, there are fewer obstacles to a smooth transition. Postsecondary community stakeholders need to be aware that Neurodivergent learners might not have this knowledge. Faculty and staff should increase their own understanding of these legal differences so they can help students to make the transition successfully. Students who understand the impact of these differences can prepare for the changes.

Many Neurodivergent students successfully master the responsibilities of college life. There are also postsecondary instructors who embrace their responsibility to support Neurodivergent student success through implementing DRO approved accommodations and keeping disability information confidential. Educators who want their students to learn and flourish can include teaching practices that are inclusive of *all* learners such as providing a range of assessment types, offering materials that can be accessed in a variety of forms, and sharing campus resources like tutoring centers and mentoring programs (Martin et al., 2019; Picault, 2021; Shaewitz & Crandall, 2020). Admissions counselors, DRO staff, residence life personnel, and academic advisors can serve an important role in ensuring students are aware of the changes between K12 and higher education laws and their responsibilities. After a student has disclosed their disability status to the DRO, individual and group meetings, training, online resources, and other supportive measures can be provided to students to encourage informed decision-making.

Colleges and universities are required by the ADA to provide academic accommodations to students with disabilities, but it is the responsibility of the student to initiate the process by self-identifying and requesting adjustments. These accommodations are individualized to the student's specific needs and functional limitations (U.S. Department Of Education [USDOE], 2011b) and include "auxiliary aids and services" such as quiet environments for exams, course material formatted for screen-readers, and early course registration (USDOE, 2011a, para. 12).

Changes in Disclosure Procedures

When a Neurodivergent student begins college, the choice to disclose their neurodifferences is theirs alone. Neither a specific procedure nor a written format mandated by the ADA exists for determination or implementation of accommodations. A college or university can create its own process, paperwork, and documentation requirements (Gould et al., 2019). Most postsecondary institutions designate a DRO to receive student self-disclosure and determine/implement accommodations. However, some colleges instead designate other personnel to manage the process, such as a Dean or ADA coordinator.

Prospective college students should contact the university to inquire about the required procedure for disclosure and requesting accommodations. The student's choice must be respected even if supporters disagree. If the student chooses not to disclose at first, but later decides to disclose at any point during their college experience, they can do so. Furthermore, faculty and advisors must be aware of their institution's policies and procedures related to student disability disclosure and request for accommodations. Should a student disclose to a faculty member or academic advisor that they have a disability and need accommodations, the faculty member should aid the student in connecting with the appropriate office or staff member in a timely manner (Kerschbaum et al., 2017; Sapir & Banai, 2024).

High school IEPs and Section 504 Plans, based on evaluations conducted by and at the expense of school districts, document the eligibility of K12 students for services. Once identified, these students are supported by school personnel and family members. The responsibility lies solely on the school to provide appropriate accommodations. On the postsecondary level, each disability category requires specific documentation on students' functional limitations and necessary accommodations. This material must be provided by students, and if students are unable to transfer evaluation results, they may be responsible for arranging and paying for testing (Dragoo & Cole, 2019; Holzberg, 2017).

The Individualized Education Program Supports versus College Accommodations

Accommodations and *modifications* are both used to aid K12 students (University of Washington, 2025). Understanding the differences between these terms is important for students and their families, but also for university faculty, staff, and administrators. Accommodations are changes made to the presentation of materials, the physical environment, or equipment used in educational settings to allow a student to learn the same material as their peers. The purpose of accommodations is to level the playing field for students and do not indicate changes to the curriculum or learning expectations of students. For example, if the class is assigned to read a novel, an audio version of the novel would be an accommodation, or a student may be permitted to type their responses on a computer in lieu of writing information out by hand. Common accommodations in higher education include preferential seating, note taker, extended time on exams, distraction free environments for exams, assistive technology use in the classroom, and early course registration (LDAA, 2024). Many assistive technologies are available at postsecondary institutions and can often be found on university websites like *Assistive Technology Resources* at the University of Michigan, *Assistive Technology* at the Purchase College Office of Disability Resources, and *Assistive Technology for Online Learning* at Stanford University. Searching for this information on university websites is a valuable activity as students transition from IEPs to ADA accommodations. In postsecondary education, neither the university nor individual faculty members have the responsibility for reaching out to students and arranging accommodations. Students must manage their own time and use of support services (Holzberg, 2017).

Modifications are changes which constitute alterations to the curriculum or expectations of the learner, and they create a new playing field for learners by outlining what will be taught and/or what a student must demonstrate in terms of achievement. An example of a modification could be to assign a different book or project in lieu of reading the assigned novel or a student may be permitted to use a calculator when completing mathematics equations instead of being required to memorize multiplication facts. Modifications to curricula or learning expectations in college could reduce the level of rigor within a program, invalidating assurances postsecondary institutions have made to their accrediting bodies; it can also result in individuals graduating from programs and not being truly ready for the expectations of the field. Therefore, students will not receive modifications after high school, although they might arrive on campus expecting them (Holzberg, 2017; LDAA, 2024). Collegiate stakeholders need to be aware of these differences so they can explain why modifications cannot be provided. This can improve relationships with students who may expect to receive modifications.

When instructors understand the differences between accommodations and modifications, they can make appropriate adjustments to course assignments, presentation of materials, and expectations through Universal Design for Learning (UDL) (CAST, 2024b) while maintaining the rigor of the course and protecting the course content. This practice makes the course environment more inclusive for all learners, including Neurodivergent students and those with other learning challenges. Understanding the difference between accommodations and modifications is paramount for faculty as they may be reluctant to comply with accommodation requests thinking that students are not expected to meet the same level of rigor as their neuromajority peers, which is not the case. Accommodations do not change the content or expectations of the learner (Holzberg, 2017; LDAA, 2024; Smith & Myers, 2024).

TRANSITION CHALLENGES

A lack of fully developed student self-advocacy skills, limited faculty knowledge of neurodiversity, and changes in parental support can negatively affect student success. Mental health challenges and finding a place on campus to feel a sense of belonging can present Neurodivergent learners with unique obstacles to overcome.

Self-Advocacy

Transition to postsecondary schools is often more difficult for Neurodivergent learners, not only due to neurodiverse characteristics, but also due to increased self-management and self-advocacy requirements and more strenuous coursework (Getzel & Thoma, 2008). Self-advocacy becomes important as the student bears the responsibility to self-disclose a disability and request accommodations. Another significant issue for postsecondary Neurodivergent learners is non-disclosure because they fear stigmatization, and unfortunately, non-disclosure can lead to failure due to a lack of accommodations (Kerschbaum et al., 2017; Kranke et al., 2013; Rogers-Shaw et al., 2023). Students frequently do not recognize the formal accommodation process where instructors do not automatically implement accommodations without official notification from the DRO. After registering with the DRO, students must choose to provide permission for instructors to be notified of their disability and must continue to collaborate with instructors to have accommodation needs met. Typically, students are strongly recommended to schedule a meeting with each instructor to review the content of the accommodation letter and how the requested accommodations apply to the course.

Students, faculty, and DRO staff must have effective communication during the development and implementation of accommodations. Rogers-Shaw et. al (2023) noted that students must become proficient communicators to manage interactions with professors, allowing them to speak openly about the need for support, clarification, and direction. Students can feel more confident in advocating for themselves if they understand their legal rights. The USDOE (2011a) offers a pamphlet on student rights: *Students with Disabilities Preparing for Postsecondary Education: Know Your Rights and Responsibilities*. The Learning Disability Association of America also offers information on *Rights and Responsibilities of College Students with Learning Disabilities (LD)* on their website.

Student Self-Awareness and Instructor Knowledge

New college students are familiar with the level of support, accommodations, and modifications afforded to them previously through IDEA. As noted previously, these same options may not be provided through ADA which in turn may cause significant challenges for the student and their instructors. In high school, curriculum and assignments can be changed to meet the specific needs of Neurodivergent learners. Additionally, individual and group tutoring may be provided within the structured school day (Holzberg, 2017; Madaus & Shaw, 2010). However, these options are not available in the same way in college. Thus, students need to understand their disability and know what accommodations are most effective for them (Rogers-Shaw et. al. 2023) to successfully communicate with the DRO and subsequently, their instructors.

Understanding one's disability and having the capacity to self-monitor the use of accommodations can greatly increase a person's self-determination not only in completing their academic program, but also in self-advocating for accommodations in future employment. Neurodivergent learners in college must develop their own achievement strategies, as universities often only concentrate on providing an open door (Holzberg, 2017). When students are actively engaged in the self-monitoring process, they are more likely to be able to self-advocate for accommodations that they need and seek out support, particularly from their professors. The counseling center, DRO, academic advisors, or career and professional development offices should encourage the student to carefully monitor their progress. By sharing their personal knowledge of neurodiversity, students can help educate professors about neurodiversity and the applicability of accommodations.

Without this collaborative communication, instructors may become frustrated with student expectations for support. There is often little, or no training provided to instructors about these issues (Holzberg, 2017; LDAA, 2024; Park et al., 2023; Rogers-Shaw et al., 2023). There are stakeholders on college campuses such as DRO staff members, teaching and learning center personnel, individuals involved in specialized programming, and faculty members who understand neurodiversity. Unfortunately the majority of instructors and college staff with whom Neurodivergent students interact lack this information. Through collaboration with Neurodivergent students, faculty gain valuable knowledge.

Although making a specific accommodation request is the responsibility of the student, instructors' knowledge of more proactive curriculum and instructional design methods can lessen the need for accommodations and create a more inclusive learning environment. Instructors who avoid ableist biases and design courses that are inclusive of *all* learners, can effectively support Neurodivergent students. According to CAST Universal Design for Learning (UDL) guidelines, "in virtually every report of research on instruction or intervention, individual differences are not only evident in the findings; they are prominent" (CAST, 2024a). One example of a UDL strategy is to offer options that meet the learning goal from which students can choose to complete an assignment, such as writing a paper, recording a presentation, or completing an exam. CAST has long recommended that instructors anticipate and plan instruction for a wide variety of students to reduce barriers in the learning environment. *All* learners can benefit from courses where UDL strategies have been implemented to enhance accessibility, inclusivity, equity, and challenge (CAST, 2024b). Employing UDL techniques can decrease the need for additional individual accommodations as the course materials are already accessible to all learners.

Parent/Guardian Participation and Support

The parental role changes during the student's transition to college. While their student is enrolled in K12 education, parents/guardians have access to student records and have a voice in determining what services will be offered (IDEA, 2004). In postsecondary education, the parental role is limited by law, and it is a worthwhile goal for parents/guardians to limit their involvement, so students become more independent. The aforementioned changes are mandated by the Family Educational

Rights and Privacy Act [FERPA] (Holzberg, 2017; U.S. Department of Education [USDOE], 2020).

College students must provide written consent for their parents/guardians to have access to their records and foregoing that permission can lessen family support for struggling Neurodivergent learners (Holzberg, 2017; Madaus & Shaw, 2010; USDOE, 2020). Without written permission, parents/guardians are not entitled to information about a student's grades, levels of support, or other previously accessible information, limiting their ability to support their student as they may have done throughout primary and secondary school. For those seeking more resources, Jane Jarrow, the mother of a college student with a disability offered her advice in *An Open Letter to Parents of Students with Disabilities About to Enter College.* David J. Connor's (2012) article "Helping Students with Disabilities Transition to College: 21 Tips for Students with LD and/or ADD/ADHD" in *Teaching Exceptional Children* provides useful ideas. Elizabeth Hamblet's book, *Seven Steps to College Success: A Pathway for Students with Disabilities* (3rd edition) published in 2023 is also beneficial.

Parental Involvement at the College Level Across Campus

The transition to college is an evolution and beginning of a new era in the parent/young adult relationship. To prepare students to be successful, parents/guardians should concentrate on "encouraging students to be advocates, fostering students' academic competency, showing moral support and high expectations, and providing opportunities for students to make decisions" (Zeng et al., 2023) rather than remaining in control of decision-making processes. For example, parents/guardians of successful college students do not attend meetings and do not contact professors directly. For students who are used to others advocating on their behalf, this can be a difficult shift to manage and stress-inducing for parents/guardians. College professionals from various areas of campus can assist with reducing parental stress and understanding how to most effectively support their child from behind the scenes.

Admissions and orientation staff coordinate online and in-person events for prospective and admitted students several times each year. During these events, a wide range of student support office personnel provide information, such as the counseling center, learning/tutoring center, academic advisors, specialized student success programs, and faculty representatives from various majors.

A helpful tactic for parents/guardians is to foster an awareness of available support services, enabling them to encourage their students to use them if needed. After their student begins college, parents/guardians understanding the confidentiality-based boundaries of the DRO, academic advisors, faculty, and all other campus staff is critical. While these offices can provide general information about their services to parents/guardians during phone calls or via email, they cannot give student-specific details unless the student has signed a document permitting disclosure (APA, 2024; Spindler, 2008). Although it is not always easy, it is advisable for parents/guardians to be open with their child if concerns arise. They can then suggest to their child who to contact for help as well as practice what to say when reaching out for help. Residence life, student success, and academic advising center webpages are valuable sources of information for parents/guardians to learn about their child's support resources and effective strategies for communicating with their child about concerns. In the event of an emergent concern, these offices also can help parents/guardians and students get immediate assistance.

The Disability Resource Office is an excellent resource to provide information for parents/guardians, particularly during their child's admission and orientation process. DRO staff frequently hold information sessions or brief talks during orientation events and are generally available to answer questions. In addition, the college's DRO web page often contains resources giving guidance for supporting their students in college yet establishing appropriate boundaries.

Continuation of Mental Healthcare

For Neurodivergent students receiving mental healthcare as a child and/or adolescent, transition planning is essential not only from secondary school to postsecondary education, but also from childhood and adolescent mental healthcare to adult mental healthcare. Children and youth are typically referred for mental health services by an adult, whereas adults must seek out mental health services independently. A disruption in services between previous providers in a student's hometown and new providers in their college community may not be smooth. Securing the appropriate level of care (intensive or occasional), location of care (in-person or online), and type of care (one-on-one or group therapy) that matches their level of need might not only be difficult but also change as they experience higher levels of stress on campus (Appleton et al., 2019).

Due to FERPA requirements (Holzberg, 2017; USDOE, 2020), Neurodivergent students can struggle with advocating for mental health services and arranging for new assessments of their need for care. Neurodivergent students may be accustomed to their parents being the decision-makers regarding healthcare. Availability of mental health services may be varied both on college campuses and within the surrounding community depending on its rural, suburban, or urban settings. When there is a need for specialists due to multiple neurodivergent characteristics, complications may arise (Appleton et al., 2019; Paul et al., 2015; Wenzler & Keeley, 2024).

The stigma of receiving mental health support can prevent Neurodivergent college students from accessing care (Davis et al., 2023; Paul et al., 2015; Wenzler

& Keeley, 2024), just as students often avoid disability disclosure due to stigma. Students and parents need to work with providers prior to the transition to college to prepare a smooth transfer in mental healthcare services. Research has revealed that student mental healthcare facilities can be more welcoming if there is capacity to meet student demand, social media is used to reach out to students, and working with students reduces the stigma from receiving mental health services (Davis et al., 2023). University stakeholders can encourage mental healthcare facilities to specialize in the mental health issues frequently visible in college students, advertise their campus location and access procedures, provide staff modeling of self care, and create an inclusive and friendly environment (Davis et al., 2023). While more complex diagnoses and a lack of acknowledgement of multiple issues can inhibit the process, effective collaboration with clinicians and sufficient parental support is more likely to increase the success of the mental healthcare transition process (Swift et al., 2013).

Building Social Skills and Community

In addition to having available support services, new college students have a better, more successful transition and overall college experience when they are able to build community within their new environment (Manett, 2022). A critical option for students to begin connecting with others and building their social experiences and skills in college is through visiting universities for open houses, programs for accepted students, and orientation events (Nachman, 2020). Opportunities to visit campus allow connections with others to be forged early. Incoming students can meet other students attending the event, as well as student leaders who are staffing the event. For example, a student orientation leader can provide extensive information about campus experiences, such as potential peer mentoring programs, and academic, social, and identity-based organizations (Nachman, 2020). This advanced knowledge is helpful for students so they can consider their interests, plan how to participate in the future, and envision themselves following through to become more socially integrated within campus life.

Visiting campus can also help Neurodivergent students gain awareness of student support offices. Their staff and students are generally present and offer information at open house and orientation events. Specific transition programs for Neurodivergent learners, for example, will likely be recruiting new students who self-disclose their interest in the program. Meeting the program's staff and fellow Neurodivergent student leaders can potentially reduce some of the trepidation a new student might experience as they navigate their transition to college and increase their willingness to engage with the program.

BRINGING THE COLLEGE COMMUNITY TOGETHER

A framework for bringing together the college community in support of Neurodivergent learners' success begins with an open mind and welcoming attitude on the part of faculty, staff, administrators, and peers. Next, we refer back to Table 1, which offers guidance about specific steps for collaboration:

- Administrators, faculty, and the DRO can collaborate to ensure that a sample syllabus statement about the disclosure process is provided to faculty for inclusion on all course syllabi, and that course materials are provided in accessible formats.
- Administrators, the DRO, and other faculty/staff can collaborate to provide training to new faculty/staff about the disclosure process, legal requirements, effective communication, and how to refer students to support offices on campus. Update/refresher trainings should be provided at least annually.
- The DRO, admissions office, and orientation staff can collaborate on bringing awareness to incoming students about how to disclose and request support/information.
- Professors, DRO, tutoring center, and peer mentors can work together with Neurodivergent students on improving test-taking skills, in addition to providing requested academic accommodations.
- Administrators, faculty, and DRO staff can work with library, instructional design, and information technology staff to proactively prepare accessible course materials to be available in multiple modalities. This should include a training process.
- Administrators, student affairs staff, academic affairs staff, and health/wellness staff can collaborate to develop student success centers, care teams, and wellness resources, and inform the campus community through coordinated messaging campaigns.
- DRO, student affairs, success centers, admissions counselors, and peer support programs on campus can provide students with guidance and lists of medical and/or mental health service providers on campus and in the area.

This framework offers a broad perspective on ways that collaboration and community can be built in postsecondary education settings to increase understanding of neurodiversity and effectively provide support and guidance to Neurodivergent learners as they transition to college. With this framework in mind, we encourage personnel in higher education to talk with each other and build partnerships as they use these principles to create their policies and procedures for supporting students.

CONCLUSION

The transition to post-secondary education is a comprehensive process that requires active engagement from K12 educators and staff, parents/guardians and the Neurodivergent student. Collegiate faculty and staff, in collaboration with the Neurodivergent college student, should work together to identify a student's interests, needs, and goals. For a student to thrive in the higher education environment, collaboration is essential. It is also crucial for the college community to have plans in place for this collaboration to occur. Creating an inclusive environment requires applying the framework for consultation, referrals, and training for faculty and staff.

The differences between K12 and postsecondary educational settings include not only different legal requirements for supporting learners with disabilities, but also changes in the types of accommodations available, the process of obtaining support, the individuals responsible for planning and managing supports, and the decision-making power of students. To both students and their families, this often seems like an abrupt change unless transition planning is in place and includes gradual work toward building learners' capacity for managing these changes. Once in college, tension can arise when college personnel and Neurodivergent students both believe the other party should be doing more to ensure student success. Thus, due to the reduced level of immediate assistance, self-determination becomes a key factor in learners' successful transition to postsecondary education. Anti-ableist attitudes on the part of college professionals is also crucial. An inclusive collegiate environment which has implemented UDL practices and networks of support can ease challenges and make it a more successful transition as students find their way and build their skills for self-determination.

Recognizing the differences between K12 and higher education, as well as emphasizing the importance of collaboration, can lead to successful experiences for all stakeholders. The resources mentioned in this chapter, as well as the following suggested readings and case studies, illustrate a variety of options that students and their supporters can learn about and draw upon to make decisions about Neurodivergent students' postsecondary journeys. Connection and collaboration among Neurodivergent students and university personnel across campuses offers great promise for creating more inclusive learning environments where students can grow and thrive.

CASE STUDIES AND DISCUSSION QUESTIONS

Case Study 1: Sam's Story

Sam is a first-year college student with ADHD and dyslexia. He was reluctant to request accommodations in college because he did not want to be viewed as different from his peers, and he wanted more independence as an emerging adult. He did not recall what was discussed in his high school IEP meetings where his parents and teachers did most of the talking. In high school, Sam received daily reminders of upcoming assignment deadlines and was able to return to his classrooms or go to the school counselor's office during lunch or study periods to finish a test if he needed more time. During the summer before starting college, Sam's parents called the DRO at his college to inquire about accommodations, but Sam was not involved in the call. When his mother later mentioned it to him, he said that he would think about emailing the DRO once he arrived on campus. A few weeks into his first semester of college, Sam began to struggle with the significantly increased amount of reading required for each class and found it difficult to concentrate while reading in his residence hall room. Sam felt overwhelmed and wasn't sure how to study or what to study. He felt embarrassed to ask questions or tell his professors or friends that he needed help. He was aware that the professor would meet with students during office hours, but he did not know what to say and did not attend them. By the fourth week of the semester, Sam received low grades for two in-class quizzes and an exam. He began to worry about his ability to pass all of his classes, and he called his mother in a panic. His mother contacted the DRO to ask for guidance. The DRO encouraged her to give their contact information to Sam so that he could contact the DRO for support.

Questions

1. What steps can Sam take now to connect with campus support people and make improvements?
2. In what ways can the DRO work with campus partners to provide support for Sam?
3. How can the DRO provide information/education to faculty and staff across campus about neurodiversity to prepare them more effectively for working with Neurodivergent students?

Case Study 2: Shae's Story

Shae is an Autistic high school student in the beginning of her senior year who also experiences moderate anxiety. She had a 504 plan in middle school which provided her supports to aid her in managing her anxiety, but she did not want to have any formal support in high school. Shae has been able to find a few minutes in between her high school classes to talk with favorite teachers when she feels anxious, and she has some close friends upon whom she relies as well. Shae wants to go to college but is undecided about a career path. Shae's school counselor has been encouraging students to meet with college representatives when they visit the high school and to schedule some college tours, but Shae is reluctant to do so because she feels so unsure of which major to pick. In October, Shae's friends decide to attend an information session and tour a state university not far from their town, so she decides to go with them. At the information session, Shae learns about the wide variety of majors available, as well as the option to begin college without choosing a major and explore options. On the tour of campus, Shae is introduced to various student support offices she previously did not know were available, such as the learning center, the academic advising office, the disability resources office, the wellness/counseling center, and the career center. She was surprised to learn that there is a support network available to students outside of the classroom. Shae decides to talk with her mother upon returning home to schedule visits at some other colleges before she makes a decision.

Questions

1. What steps would you advise Shae to take to further investigate the best fit or best choice of college?
2. If Shae did not have a 504 plan in high school, how could she go about getting information about potential options for support in college? How might she be eligible for accommodations?
3. If Shae experiences challenges with anxiety during her first semester, to whom can she speak with to get support?

REFERENCES

ADA Amendments Act, Pub. L. No. 110-325, 42 U.S.C. 12101 et seq. (2008).

Amend, D. J., Lein, A. E., Taylor, A. J., & Dinkins, E. G. (2024). Collaborative inclusion: IEP team perspectives on supporting students with extensive needs and the implications for teacher preparation programs. *Kentucky Teacher Education Journal: The Journal of the Teacher Education Division of the Kentucky Council for Exceptional Children, 11*(2), 6. DOI: 10.61611/2995-5904.1062

American Psychological Association. (2024). *For parents: Adjusting to college - a brief guide and frequently asked questions for parents of students with disabilities.* https://www.apa.org/pi/disability/resources/parent-college-guide

Americans with Disabilities Act, 42 U.S.C. § 12101 et seq. (1990).

Appleton, R., Connell, C., Fairclough, E., Tuomainem, H., & Singh, S. P. (2019). Outcomes of young people who reach the transition boundary of child and adolescent mental health services: A systematic review. *European Child & Adolescent Psychiatry, 2019*(28), 1431–1446. DOI: 10.1007/s00787-019-01307-7 PMID: 30850925

Bal, V. H., Kim, S. H., Cheong, D., & Lord, C. (2015). Daily living skills in individuals with autism spectrum disorder from 2 to 21 years of age. *Autism, 19*(7), 774–784. DOI: 10.1177/1362361315575840 PMID: 25922445

Burke, M. M., Mercer, C., Ramos-Torres, S., Lindsay, R., & Burakov, I. (2024). Frequently asked questions and answers for supporting students with Section 504 plans. *Intervention in School and Clinic, 60*(4), 214–219. DOI: 10.1177/10534512241297322

CAST. (2024a). *Research evidence*. Universal Design for Learning Guidelines version 3.0. https://udlguidelines.cast.org/more/research-evidence/

CAST. (2024b). *The UDL Guidelines*. Universal Design for Learning Guidelines version 3.0. https://udlguidelines.cast.org

Clayburn, C. (2023, November 14). How to navigate college admissions with a learning disability. *U. S. News & World Report.* https://www.usnews.com/education/articles/how-to-navigate-college-as-a-neurodivergent-student

College Autism Network (CAN). (2025). *College Autism Network advocacy, research, training.* https://collegeautismnetwork.org

Connor, D. J. (2012). Helping students with disabilities transition to college: 21 tips for students with LD and/or ADD/ADHD. *Teaching Exceptional Children, 44*(5), 16–25. DOI: 10.1177/004005991204400502

Conrad, J. A. (2020). On intellectual and developmental disabilities in the United States: A historical perspective. *Journal of Intellectual Disabilities*, *24*(1), 85–101. DOI: 10.1177/1744629518767001 PMID: 29621909

Cox, B. E., Mintz, A., Locks, T., Thompson, K., Anderson, A., Morgan, L., Edelstein, J., & Wolz, A. (2017). Academic experiences for college students with autism: Identity, disclosure, and accommodations. *Journal of College Student Development*, *58*(1), 71–87. DOI: 10.1353/csd.2017.0004

Davis, R. A., Wolfe, J., & Heiman, N. (2023). Increasing utilization of student mental health services on a college campus: Eight actionable tips. *Journal of American College Health*, *71*(3), 655–659. DOI: 10.1080/07448481.2021.1909035 PMID: 33891531

Dillon, S., Armstrong, E., Goudy, L., Reynolds, H., & Scurry, S. (2021). Improving special education service delivery through interdisciplinary collaboration. *Teaching Exceptional Children*, *54*(1), 36–43. DOI: 10.1177/00400599211029671

Dolmage, J. (2017). *Academic ableism: Disability and higher education*. University of Michigan Press. https://muse.jhu.edu/book/57058

Dragoo, K. E., & Cole, J. P. (2019). *Laws affecting students with disabilities:Preschool through postsecondary education*. Congressional Research Service, Rep. No. R45595. https://files.eric.ed.gov/fulltext/ED597875.pdf

Dwyer, P. (2024). Autonomy and inclusion. In Halder, S., Goldstein, T., & Caudel, D. (Eds.), *Inclusion and Autism* (pp. 39–59). Routledge. DOI: 10.4324/9781003559276-3

Dwyer, P., Mineo, E., Mifsud, K., Lindholm, C., Gurba, A., & Waisman, T. C. (2023). Building neurodiversity-inclusive postsecondary campuses: Recommendations for leaders in higher education. *Autism in Adulthood: Challenges and Management*, *5*(1), 1–14. https://www.liebertpub.com/doi/pdf/10.1089/aut.2021.0042 PMID: 36941859

Education For All Handicapped Children Act, Public Law 142, U.S. Statutes at Large 89 (1975): 773-796.

Educational Advocates. (2024). *Learning Disabilities and the College Process: Navigating Admissions and Support Services*. https://educationaladvocates.com/college-student-with-learning-disabilities/

Eisenmenger, A. (2019, December 12). *Ableism 101*. Access Living. https://www.accessliving.org/newsroom/blog/ableism-101/

Elias, R., & White, S. W. (2018). Autism goes to college: Understanding the needs of a student population on the rise. *Journal of Autism and Developmental Disorders*, *48*(3), 732–746. DOI: 10.1007/s10803-017-3075-7 PMID: 28255760

Florian, L. (2007). *The SAGE handbook of special education*. SAGE., DOI: 10.4135/9781848607989

Francisco, M. P. B., Hartman, M., & Wang, Y. (2020). Inclusion and special education. *Education Sciences*, *10*(9), 238. https://www.mdpi.com/2227-7102/10/9/238. DOI: 10.3390/educsci10090238

Getzel, E. E., & Thoma, C. A. (2008). Experiences of college students with disabilities and the importance of self-determination in higher education settings. *Career Development for Exceptional Individuals*, *31*(2), 77–84. DOI: 10.1177/0885728808317658

Gould, R., Harris, S. P., & Mullin, C. (2019). Higher education and the ADA: An ADA knowledge translation center research brief. *ADA National Network*. https://adata.org/research_brief/higher-education-and-ada

Gragoudas, S. (2014). Preparing students with disabilities to transition from school to work through self-determination training. *Work (Reading, Mass.)*, *48*(3), 407–411. DOI: 10.3233/WOR-131782 PMID: 24284673

Gupta, A., Chaplot, I., Detamore, B., Thakkar, S., Nguyen, K., Camilli, S., & Nguyen, D. (2023). Individualized Education Program (IEP) under examination: A literature review of systemic flaws in education for students with disabilities. *Social Science Research Network*. DOI: 10.2139/ssrn.4508281

Hallahan, D. P., Kauffman, J. M., & Pullen, P. (2022). *Exceptional Learners: An introduction to special education* (15th ed.). Pearson Publishing.

Hamblet, E. C. (2023). *Seven steps to college success: A pathway for students with disabilities* (3rd ed.). Rowman & Littlefield Publishers., https://www.ldadvisory.com/high-school-to-college/ DOI: 10.5771/9781475864458

Heiman, T., & Shemesh, D. O. (2012). Students with LD in higher education: Use and contribution of assistive technology and website courses and their correlation to students' hope and well-being. *Journal of Learning Disabilities*, *45*(4), 308–318. DOI: 10.1177/0022219410392047 PMID: 21252373

Holzberg, D. (2017). Differences between secondary and postsecondary education. *National Technical Assistance Center on Transition*. https://transitionta.org/wp-content/uploads/docs/Highschool_vs_College_list.pdf

Individuals with Disabilities Education Act, 20 U.S.C. § 1400 et seq. (2004). https://sites.ed.gov/idea/statute-chapter-33/subchapter-i/1400

Jaird, M. A. (2022). Mapping out student support: An exploration of student disability programs and practices at selective higher education institutions. University of Vermont. *Graduate College Dissertations and Theses*. 1506. https://scholarworks.uvm.edu/graddis/1506

Jarrow, J. (2022). *An open letter to parents of students with disabilities about to enter college*. https://daisclasses.com/wp-content/uploads/2022/01/OpenLetterParents.pdf

Kerschbaum, S., Eisenman, L., & Jones, J. (Eds.). (2017). *Negotiating disability: Disclosure and higher education*. University of Michigan Press. DOI: 10.3998/mpub.9426902

Kranke, D., Jackson, S. E., Taylor, D. A., Anderson-Fye, E., & Floersch, J. (2013). College student disclosure of non-apparent disabilities to receive classroom accommodations. *Journal of Postsecondary Education and Disability*, *26*(1), 35–51. https://eric.ed.gov/?Id=EJ1026808

Kuder, S. J., Accardo, A., & Woodruff, J. (2023). *College success for students on the autism spectrum: A neurodiversity perspective*. Taylor & Francis. DOI: 10.4324/9781003443452-2

Leake, D. W., & Stodden, R. A. (2014). Higher education and disability: Past and future of underrepresented populations. *Journal of Postsecondary Education and Disability*, *27*(4), 399–408. https://files.eric.ed.gov/fulltext/EJ1059990.pdf

Learning Disabilities Association of America (LDAA). (2024, December 12). *Modifications vs. accommodations: High school vs. college*. LDAAmerica.org. https://ldaamerica.org/lda_today/modifications-vs-accommodations-high-school-vs-college/

Lee, A. M. I. (2024). *Accommodations: What they are and how they work*. Understood.org. https://www.understood.org/en/articles/accommodations-what-they-are-and-how-they-work

Madaus, J., & Shaw, S. (2010). College as a realistic option for students with learning disabilities. *InfoSheets*. Council for Learning Disabilities. http://www.council-for-learning-disabilities.org/wp-content/uploads/2013/11/College-Realistic-Option-for-Students-with-Learning-Disabilities.pdf

Manett, J. (2022). The Social Association for Students with Autism: Principles and practices of a social group for university students with ASD. *Social Work with Groups*, *45*(2), 157–171. DOI: 10.1080/01609513.2021.1994511

Martin, F., Budhrani, K., Kumar, S., & Ritzhaupt, A. (2019). Award-winning faculty online teaching practices: Roles and competencies. *Online Learning : the Official Journal of the Online Learning Consortium*, *23*(1), 184–205. https://eric.ed.gov/?id=EJ1211042. DOI: 10.24059/olj.v23i1.1329

McDowall, A., & Kiseleva, M. (2024). A rapid review of supports for neurodivergent students in higher education. Implications for research and practice. *Neurodiversity*, *2*, 27546330241291769. Advance online publication. DOI: 10.1177/27546330241291769

McNaught, J., Biegun, D., & Swartzentruber, K. (2024). Student-led Individualized Education Programs: A gateway to self-determination. *Language, Speech, and Hearing Services in Schools*, *55*(2), 276–302. DOI: 10.1044/2023_LSHSS-23-00079 PMID: 38266231

Nachman, B. R. (2020). Enhancing transition programming for college students with autism: A systematic literature review. *Journal of Postsecondary Education and Disability*, *33*(1), 81–95. https://eric.ed.gov/?id=EJ1273654

National Center for College Students with Disabilities. (n.d.). *Future College Students.* University of Minnesota. https://nccsd.ici.umn.edu/clearinghouse/audience-specific-resources/future-college-students

National Technical Assistance Center on Transition, & the The Collaborative. (NTACT:C). (2024). *Differences between high school and postsecondary education.* https://transitionta.org/differences-between-hs-postsecondary-education/

Neurodiversity Hub. (n.d.). *Changing the narrative about autism and neurodiversity through awareness, education, and engagement.* https://www.neurodiversityhub.org/

Park, T. W., Sheward, K. L., & Rogers-Shaw, C. (2023). Tips for supporting students with social skill, mental health, and communication disabilities in digital settings. *eLearn, 2023*(2023). DOI: 10.1145/3596691.3596515

Paul, M., Street, C., Wheeler, N., & Singh, S. P. (2015). Transition to adult services for young people with mental health needs: A systematic review. *Clinical Child Psychology and Psychiatry*, *20*(3), 436–457. DOI: 10.1177/1359104514526603 PMID: 24711585

Picault, J. (2021). Structure, flexibility, and consistency: A dynamic learning approach for an online asynchronous course. *Applied Economics Teaching Resources (AETR), 3*(4), 30-43. https://ageconsearch.umn.edu/record/316503/?v=pdf

Purchase College. (n.d.). *Assistive technology.* Office of Disability Resources. https://www.purchase.edu/offices/disability-resources/assistive-technology/

Richards, S. B., & Hulewicz, R. (2024). Historical concepts and perspectives. In Richards, S. B., Brady, M. P., & Taylor, R. L. (Eds.), *Understanding Intellectual Disabilities: Historical perspectives, current practices, and future directions* (3rd ed., pp. 3–37). Routledge. DOI: 10.4324/9781003345602-2

Rodriguez, D. D., Menchaca, V. D., & Padilla, G. (2021). Social justice: School administrative staff perceptions of strengths, challenges, and training needs in Section 504-only services. *Journal of Leadership, Accountability and Ethics, 18*(1), 89–101. http://www.na-businesspress.com/JLAE/JLAE18-1/7_MenchacaFinal.pdf

Rogers-Shaw, C., Park, T. W., & Mohney, K. D. (2023). Strategies for supporting learners with disabilities in postsecondary education. *New Horizons in Adult Education and Human Resource Development, 35*(4), 199–207. DOI: 10.1177/19394225231189136

Ross-Gordon, J. M., & Procknow, G. (2021). Adult education and disability. In Rocco, T. S., Smith, M. C., Mizzi, R. C., Merriweather, L. R., & Hawley, J. D. (Eds.), *Handbook of adult and continuing education* (pp. 392–400). Stylus.

Sanderson, K. A., Goldman, S. E., & Rojas, A. (2021). A review and analysis of single-case research examining adolescent participation in IEP Meetings. *The Journal of Special Education, 56*(2), 97–109. DOI: 10.1177/00224669211047232

Santhanam, S. P., & Wilson, K. (2024). A comparison of autistic and non-autistic college students' perceived challenges and engagement in self-advocacy. *American Journal of Speech-Language Pathology, 33*(3), 1471–1484. DOI: 10.1044/2024_AJSLP-22-00381 PMID: 38470839

Sapir, A., & Banai, A. (2024). Balancing attendance and disclosure: Identity work of students with invisible disabilities. *Disability & Society, 39*(8), 2032–2052. DOI: 10.1080/09687599.2023.2181765

Schaefer, J., & Sanchez, A. (2024). *Shining a light on neurodiversity in higher ed.* University of Wisconsin-Madison School of Education. https://education.wisc.edu/news/shining-a-light-on-neurodiversity-in-higher-ed/

Section 504 of the Rehabilitation Act of 1973 (29 U.S.C. § 794).

Shaewitz, D., & Crandall, J. R. (2020, October 19). Higher education's challenge: Disability inclusion on campus. *Higher Education Today.* https://www.higheredtoday.org/2020/10/19/higher-educations-challenge-disability-inclusion-campus/

Sheward, K., Rogers-Shaw, C., & Park, T. W. (2022). *Creating connection by design: Supporting adult learners by building inclusive online academic communities.* Proceedings of the Adult Education Research Conference, Virtual. https://newprairiepress.org/aerc/2022/papers/27

Smith, P. S., & Myers, B. (2024). Instructor experiences providing accommodations and modifications for students with intellectual disability in inclusive higher education. *International Journal of Inclusive Education*, •••, 1–14. DOI: 10.1080/13603116.2024.2305653

Spindler, C. M. (2008, March). You, me, and mom makes three: How academic advisors can capitalize on parental involvement. *Academic Advising Today, 31*(1). https://nacada.ksu.edu/Resources/Academic-Advising-Today/View-Articles/You-Me-and-Mom-Makes-Three-How-Academic-Advisors-Can-Capitalize-on-Parental-Involvement.aspx

Stanford University. (n.d.). *Assistive technology for online learning*. Office of Accessible Education. https://oae.stanford.edu/students/remote-learning-coping-during-covid-19/assistive-technology-online-learning

Strunk, K., Hinkle, A. R., & Thurlow, M. L. (2022). Supporting IEP team decisions. *Journal of Special Education Leadership*, *35*(2), 73–85. https://files.eric.ed.gov/fulltext/EJ1370360.pdf

Swift, K. D., Hall, C. L., Marimuttu, V., Redstone, L., & Hollis, C. (2013). Transition to adult mental health services for young people with Attention Deficit/Hyperactivity Disorder (ADHD): A qualitative analysis of their experiences. *BMC Psychiatry*, *13*(74), 1–11. DOI: 10.1186/1471-244X-13-74 PMID: 23497082

Think College. (2025). *College search*. Institute for Community Inclusion. University of Massachusetts Boston. https://thinkcollege.net/college-search

Thomas, G., & Loxley, A. (2022). *Deconstructing special education and constructing inclusion*. McGraw-Hill Education.

University of Michigan. (n.d.). *Assistive technology resources*. Services for Students with Disabilities. https://ssd.umich.edu/article/assistive-technology-resources

University of Washington. (2025). *What is the difference between accommodation and modification for a student with a disability?* Disabilities, Opportunities, Internetworking, and Technology (DO-IT). https://doit.uw.edu/knowledge-base/what-is-the-difference-between-accommodation-and-modification-for-a-student-with-a-disability/

U.S. Department of Education. (2011a, September). *Students with disabilities preparing for postsecondary education: Know your rights and responsibilities*. https://www.ed.gov/higher-education/students-with-disabilities-preparing-for-postsecondary-education

U.S. Department of Education. (2011b, March). *Transition of students with disabilities to postsecondary education: A guide for high school educators.* https://www.ed.gov/teaching-and-administration/supporting-students/transition-of-students-with-disabilities-to-postsecondary-education-a-guide-for-high-school-educators

U.S. Department of Education. (2020, April). *The Family Educational Rights and Privacy Act: Guidance for parents.* https://studentprivacy.ed.gov/sites/default/files/resource_document/file/FERPAGuidanceForParents.pdf

Wenzler, S., & Keeley, J. (2024). The initiation or continuation of mental health services in the transition to college. *Journal of American College Health*, *72*(6), 1768–1777. DOI: 10.1080/07448481.2022.2089851 PMID: 35728259

Westby, C. (2023). Promoting self-determination. *Word of Mouth, 34*(5), 13-15. https://journals.sagepub.com/doi/abs/10.1177/10483950231161474d

Zeng, W., Ju, S., & Hord, C. (2023). Parental influences on student self-determination: Perspectives of college students with learning disabilities. *Learning Disability Quarterly*, *46*(3), 180–190. DOI: 10.1177/07319487221107890

Zirkel, P. A., & Gullo, G. (2024). Public school rates of Section 504-only students: The latest update. *West's Education Law Reporter*, 420, 1–13. https://perryzirkel.com/wp-content/uploads/2018/07/zirkel-and-huang-state-by-state-504-only-rates-article-061118.pdf

ADDITIONAL READING

Clare, E. (2017). *Brilliant imperfection: Grappling with cure.* Duke University Press.

Combs, D. (2023). *Supporting Neurodivergent and Autistic people for their transition into adulthood: Blueprints for education, training, and employment.* Taylor & Francis. DOI: 10.4324/9781003353959

Garcia, E. (2021). *We're not broken: Changing the autism conversation.* Houghton Mifflin.

Goodley, D. (2014). *Dis/ability studies: Theorising disablism and ableism.* Routledge. DOI: 10.4324/9780203366974

Park, T. W., Sheward, K., & Rogers-Shaw, C. (2023, May). Tips for supporting students with social skill, mental health, and communication disabilities in digital settings. *eLearn Magazine.* https://elearnmag.acm.org/archive.cfm?aid=3596515

Prizant, B. M., & Fields-Meyer, T. (2022). *Uniquely human: Updated and expanded: A different way of seeing autism*. Simon and Schuster.

Shakespeare, T. (2014). *Disability rights and wrongs revisited*. Routledge.

Siegel, B. (2018). *The politics of autism*. Oxford University Press.

Silberman, S. (2015). *Neurotribes: The legacy of autism and the future of neurodiversity*. Penguin.

Vogler-Elias, D., & Jamanis, S. (Eds.). (2024). *Autism, neurodiversity, and equity in professional preparation programs*. IGI Global Publishing.

Chapter 2
Supporting Neurodivergent Learners in Higher Education by Applying the Assumptions of Andragogy

Adrienne Taylor
https://orcid.org/0009-0009-1400-1403
Texas State University, USA

Joellen E. Coryell
https://orcid.org/0000-0003-3182-4486
Texas State University, USA

ABSTRACT

This chapter explores how Malcolm Knowles' (1990) principles of andragogy can be effectively applied to support Neurodivergent students in higher education settings and demonstrates how andragogical strategies, focusing on the self-directed, experiential, and relevant learning needs of adults, can be adapted to create inclusive and supportive learning environments for Neurodivergent individuals, including those with autism, ADHD, dyslexia, and other cognitive variations. The objectives of the chapter are to highlight the unique needs of Neurodivergent learners, to show how andragogical principles can address these needs, and to provide practical recommendations for educators and institutions. Key arguments include the need for educators to reassess their current pedagogical assumptions and practices, the

DOI: 10.4018/979-8-3693-8920-1.ch002

alignment between andragogical assumptions and Neurodivergent learners' needs, and the transformative potential of tailored instructional strategies for both learner and educator.

INTRODUCTION

Andragogy, "the art and science of helping adults learn" (Knowles, 1980, p. 43) that Knowles introduced to the field of adult learning in the United States in the late 1960s, has had a lasting impact on the way scholars, theorists, and practitioners of adult education view the role of the adult learner and those who teach them (Feuer & Geber, 1988; Grace, 1996; Milligan, 1995; Rachal, 2014). Andragogy initially encouraged us to consider that adults learn differently from the ways children learn and further provided a set of assumptions about adult learners to inform research and practice. These assumptions include that adults are self-directed learners who take ownership of and responsibility for their own learning, want to understand why they need to learn something, rely on their life experiences as influence on their learning, inhabit social roles that affect their readiness to learn, tend to be intrinsically motivated, and prefer to engage in learning to solve problems rather than solely for content knowledge (Knowles, 1980, 1990). Andragogy also promotes individual development and self-fulfillment (Pratt, 1993). Additionally, andragogy encourages the creation of comfortable physical and emotionally safe spaces that include an environment of mutual trust, respect, support, authenticity, and collaboration (Tipton & Wideman, 2021).

Andragogy is not without its critiques. These include that the assumption that adults and children learn very differently may incorrectly posit education is value neutral and apolitical, disregard the inherent linkage between individual and community/society, and ignore cultural and positional ways of knowing that can generate inequalities (Sandlin, 2005). Despite its criticisms, andragogy has persisted as a dominant adult learning theory in Western and global north societies. Nafukho et al. (2005) posited that andragogy's principles offer important insights into adult education's goals and professional identity in Africa, while Moll (2024) asserted the theory continues to gain purchase around the world. Moll recently argued that Knowles' theory of andragogy, though, should not be juxtaposed with children's learning processes. Andragogy isn't the opposite of pedagogy but rather describes the learning needs of adults, encompassing the spontaneous learning that occurs throughout life and beyond formal instructional settings (Moll, 2024). While learning across the lifespan has similarities in terms of motivations and needs, andragogy's set of assumptions help educators and perhaps society at large acknowledge that learning doesn't stop after childhood, and that the learning needs, motivations, and expectations of adults, as modeled, are important to consider for planning adult educative experiences.

With the number of Neurodivergent students entering higher education (HE) steadily on the rise (Dwyer et al., 2023; Evans et al., 2023; Friedman & Nash-Luckenbach, 2024; Henning et al., 2022), this means that more Neurodivergent students than ever are attempting to complete their studies despite the challenges they encounter on campus and in the classroom. There are myriad theories and strategies on teaching and learning from which HE instructors can choose, but those that stress self-directed learning and acknowledge learner autonomy show promise for the success of Neurodivergent learners (Friedman & Nash-Luckenbach, 2024). As instructors, administrators, and institutions look to improve student success and engagement while simultaneously maintaining healthy student enrollment and retention rates, a focus on the learner and their needs has the potential to meaningfully engage Neurodivergent students using instructional attitudes and practices traditionally leveraged specifically for adults. In doing this, it may be possible to expand on the principles of andragogy in pursuit of more effective methods of planning for and engaging with Neurodivergent learners in HE.

CHAPTER OBJECTIVES

The goals of this chapter are to examine the assumptions of andragogy and their relevance to today's Neurodivergent HE learners and to present strategies that promote cross-campus collaboration to support them. First is a definition and brief historical overview of the concepts of neurodivergence and neurodiversity and their role for HE students. Next is a detailed description of the assumptions of andragogy, followed by an explanation of the ways in which Neurodivergent students can be better served by instructional practices aligned to each of the assumptions. Practical recommendations for implementing andragogy in HE, including advice for addressing challenges, bring the chapter to a close.

UNDERSTANDING NEURODIVERGENCE

Neurodivergence and neurodiversity are two terms used almost interchangeably to refer to a broad range of neurodevelopmental presentations including Autism Spectrum Disorder (ASD), Attention-Deficit/Hyperactivity Disorder (ADHD), dyslexia, dyscalculia, dysgraphia, intellectual disabilities, epilepsy, and traumatic brain injuries (Grummt, 2024; Sidjaja, 2024; Spaeth & Pearson, 2023). However, there is additional nuance to the concept that describes the individuals who identify as members of the neurodiverse community. From a socio-political perspective, neurodiversity focuses on affirming the experiences of individuals who view their neurodifference(s) as influencing the way they experience life and thus inseparable from their personalities or sense of self. Singer introduced the term in 1997 (Miclea, 2024), which contributed to the shift to use of an umbrella term that frames neurodevelopmental presentations as possible and necessary variations along a spectrum of being (Miclea, 2024) and not medical problems in need of cure or therapy (Clouder et al., 2020; Grummt, 2024; Sidjaja, 2024). Neurodivergence describes how "one's ways of thinking, perceiving and acting deviate from a dominant social standard" (Grummt, 2024, p. 3) without casting judgment on their appropriateness or similarity to the majority. In this way, both terms are used to promote acceptance of individuals who experience them.

Neurodiversity in HE

Neurodiversity within HE settings is an emerging research topic (Accardo et al., 2024). What has been established is that Neurodivergent students have both academic and nonacademic challenges that intensify the stress of transitioning into postsecondary education which has an impact on their academic performance (Evans et al., 2023) and eventual employment outcomes (Hamilton & Petty, 2024). Academic accommodations meant to ease this adjustment may fall short. Faculty's perspectives on the state of education for Neurodivergent students point to frustration with the limitations of "pre-determined, pre-approved accommodations" (Nash-Luckenbach & Friedman, 2024, p. 606) that are insufficiently customized to students' needs. Faculty and students agree that faculty need additional professional development to help them teach and interact effectively with Neurodivergent students (Accardo et al., 2024; Sarrett, 2018).

Neurodivergent students also struggle with creating and maintaining a community of collaborative peers and supportive mentors. Difficulties related to nonacademic, social-emotional elements such as forming social relationships and resulting feelings of isolation and loneliness (Butcher & Lane, 2024; Evans et al., 2023; Hamilton & Petty, 2024; Sarrett, 2018) are common. Furthermore, students express conflict over disclosing their neurodiversity to others based on the negative social consequences they anticipate (Accardo et al., 2024; Evans et al., 2023). Those fears may be reasonable. A recent study showed that while neuromajority students who do not know a lot about neurodiversity are generally accepting of Neurodivergent students, they tend to mistakenly view neurodifferences like autism as an illness or problem needing to be cured (Hotez et al., 2023). Perhaps due to these social challenges, students describe a need for digital and physical neurodiverse spaces to avoid or recover from social or sensory overstimulation and to gather with other

Neurodivergent students (Accardo et al., 2024; Brandsen et al., 2024; Sarrett, 2018; Seelmeyer, 2024). Reconciling students' needs for likeminded neurodiverse communities as well as more positive interactions with neuromajority peers presents a unique challenge to educators in creating an inclusive space for learning. However, this delicate balance becomes difficult to achieve when Neurodivergent students are treated differently from their peers for exhibiting behaviors that diverge from neuromajority expectations.

Neuromajority Pedagogy and its Consequences: Author's Experience

As a child, I thought of myself as a good student. I enjoyed learning and received high marks in all my classes. I decided that I wanted to be a writer when I was 7 years old, and my English Language Arts teacher led our class in authoring short works of fiction by starting a "writing workshop" that included a special chair each of us would sit in and read our work to our peers. At that age, the opportunity to sit in front of the class in the fancy, comfortable upholstered chair was viewed as a treat. The time we spent learning how to create a story and share it with others was special. Our teacher explained that, once we had all finished our stories, she would choose several students to represent our school at a conference for young authors from around the state. I was chosen as one of those students and participating ended up being a formative event in my life that influenced my perception of my strengths and weaknesses, led me to pursue writing professionally, and had a profound lifelong impact on my career.

One might assume the experience of writing and learning from my teacher would be a highlight, a treasured memory of the person who inspired me to become who I am today. But decades later, my memories of that time are clouded in shame and a general sense that I had done something wrong. The teacher who rewarded my writing abilities during our writing workshops often reminded me rather impatiently to talk less, tamper my enthusiasm, and fade more into the background. As a good student I did my best to comply, but this was an incredibly difficult task for a 7-year-old with undiagnosed and untreated ADHD. Consequently, I became more focused on avoiding being the target of my teacher's discipline than on learning, without much success. I did not know how to stop being bad, and that made me think I failed to learn whatever lesson about my character or my personality that she had been trying to teach me.

This personal vignette is meant to illustrate the detrimental effects that neuromajority pedagogy can have on Neurodivergent learners. Neuromajority pedagogy, also referred to as Neurotypical pedagogy, is a term used to describe the system of instruction used to enforce desirable behaviors based on neuromajority pathology that dominates the United States public educational system (Sullivan, 2024). Neurodivergent students enter this system unaware of the assumptions and expectations of educators, which are largely based around neuromajority patterns of behavior and interaction.

Consequently, Neurodivergent students are measured by their abilities to adhere to neuromajority behaviors of obedience and conformity in group settings. When students are unable to mimic actions like sitting still for long periods of time, making eye contact, or suppressing their emotions, educators can misinterpret it as a refusal to follow classroom rules or demonstrate listening skills. "There is a tendency ... to incorrectly assume that there is a set of definable social norms and rules that exist for people to follow" (Milton, 2012, p. 884) that leads to conflict between neuromajority and Neurodivergent people, known as the double-empathy problem (Milton, 2012). The problem states that the inherent difference in the ways that neuromajority and Neurodivergent people process thoughts and emotions makes it difficult for either group to accurately interpret the intentions of the other; that is, a neuromajority person is likely to misattribute neuromajority causes to neurodivergent behaviors.

The double-empathy problem is mostly documented in adult social (Cheang et al., 2024; Jones et al., 2024) and workplace interactions (Drader-Mazza et al., 2024), but it also affects instructor-student relationships (Spaeth & Pearson, 2023). For example, a student who refuses to make eye contact is seen as rude or bored, and a learner who abruptly leaves the room in the middle of a lecture as storming off in anger or being overly emotional. Instructors might frame the student who loudly interrupts them to complain as acting aggressive. The student with consistently poor spelling and transposed letters may be viewed as lazy or unprofessional. An educator's misperceptions of a student's neurodivergence can have effects on the quality of their relationship and the student's experience with learning (Franz et al., 2023; Röhm et al., 2022) and has the potential to alienate Neurodivergent students, decreasing the quality of their education (Butcher & Lane, 2024; Hamilton & Petty, 2024). A neuromajority pedagogy is one that reinforces sameness and punishes deviation based on erroneous assumptions about student behavior and motivations (Cook, 2024). It works to wear down Neurodivergent students emotionally and intellectually (Shepherd et al., 2024), leaving them ill-equipped to persevere.

A NEW PERSPECTIVE

In contrast to neuromajority pedagogy's objective to squeeze all students into a single "good student" mold, andragogy describes the common motivations and preferences that adults express about what and how to learn, and tit highlights the psychological importance of allowing learners to demonstrate choice in their learning to derive personal meaning and satisfaction (Moll, 2024). In higher education, instructors may find andragogical principles helpful for learning for nontraditional students aged 25 and older. However, traditional students can and often do share characteristics with adult learners. Legally, college students are adults with the same rights as older individuals, including the right to make their own decisions. Many also juggle adult responsibilities—such as work and caregiving—alongside their education. Due to these factors, their learning needs are more similar to those of adults than children. Andragogy, when applied to Neurodivergent learners, emphasizes social-emotional growth and academic development. This learner-centered theory supports the importance of creating learning environments where Neurodivergent adults of all ages can thrive by focusing on their unique emotional, social, and sensory needs.

For Neurodivergent university students, andragogical approaches emphasize a sense of belonging, self-confidence, and self-advocacy, which are crucial for adult learning. These students often benefit from teaching methods that prioritize self-direction, emotional safety, and experiential learning. By differentiating between formal (structured) and nonformal (flexible or applied) environments, andragogy can create space for Neurodivergent students to engage with materials in ways that feel meaningful to them (Moll, 2024). In formal settings like universities, for instance, Neurodivergent learners might benefit from opportunities to process information at their own pace, explore content that aligns with their interests, and practice self-directed inquiry.

Nonformal educational settings allow for more relaxed, adaptive learning structures that can accommodate the sensory and emotional needs that may otherwise be overwhelming in rigid traditional environments. Recognizing these needs helps Neurodivergent learners to build social-emotional skills, fostering confidence and resilience as they embody adult roles and responsibilities. By adapting educational environments to meet Neurodivergent students where they are, andragogy can empower learners for both personal and academic growth.

Andragogy

In the late 1800s in Europe, andragogy became the predominant descriptor of the practice of teaching adults and inspiring both individual and social change (Note et al., 2021). Knowles (1990) cemented its meaning in history in North America when he borrowed the term for his personal theory of adult learning (Loeng, 2018). Based on the research and writings of Eduard Lindeman (1926), this model was meant to serve as a single unifying theory of adult education (Feuer & Geber, 1988; Rachal, 2014; Taylor & Kroth, 2009). But whereas European scholars were interested in the potential for social change and community development implicit in adult education,

American democratic values made for a comparatively more individualistic philosophy (Grace, 1996; Loeng, 2018). This viewpoint on andragogy favored the development of individuals to achieve independence and enlightenment (McGrath, 2009). Unlike the traditional teacher-student paradigm based on obedience and conformity to standards, teachers of adults serve as facilitators or enablers of learning, experts on content, or providers of information (Galbraith & Jones, 2008), but not authorities.

Knowles (1970) initially defined andragogy as being markedly different from the pedagogical theory used in K-12 school systems in the United States, although over time he acknowledged that the differences might not be as age-dependent as he first posited. He contrasted learning with the rigid, formal instructional strategies used to educate children and denounced its use for adults (Moll, 2024). His view states that there are six basic assumptions of adult learning which we explain here. Those six assumptions concern the learner's self-concept, experience, readiness to learn, orientation to learning, motivation, and need to know (Knowles, 1990). We also offer more contemporary nuances and views of these assumptions that are helpful for teaching diverse learners. The six assumptions Knowles derived from these characteristics form a basis for learning that puts the educator into a new supportive position of guiding – but not dictating – what and how students learn (Taylor & Kroth, 2009). What follows is an expanded definition of each assumption.

Self-Concept

An adult's self-concept – how they perceive themselves, their strengths, and their weaknesses – directs the course of their learning (Knowles, 1990). Knowles theorized adult learners as progressing through a common set of developmental milestones that influence their need for learning, ultimately leading them to be more self-directed and to assume ownership of their learning processes as they mature. Contemporary interpretations of this assumption acknowledge that adults possess multiple overlapping and sometimes contradictory identities and roles, needs, and obligations to themselves and the communities in which they participate.

These complex personal circumstances can have an effect on a learner's view of themselves and their capacity to learn in different ways. For example, learners who enroll in higher or continuing education courses can be motivated to do so due to their self-concepts. Lanford (2021) indicated that adults use education to improve their perception of themselves as role models and prioritize respect from their instructors and peers as part of the experience. Conversely, negative experiences with instructors who fail to demonstrate respect can also cause an adult learner to question their ability to learn and succeed as learners (Lanford, 2021). In exploring the experiences of learners from diverse backgrounds, Ross-Gordon et al. (2017) indicated that one of the major obstacles for adult students is a poor academic self-concept. For students transitioning into a university environment, this self-concept is especially fragile and deserves attention. Higher education is a place where students develop their identities independently and begin to exercise greater responsibility and self-regulation of their learning, which affects their confidence and feelings of competency (Gavín-Chocano et al., 2024). A comprehensive understanding of learning requires considering the multitude of self-concepts that learners bring with them and their myriad origins, as these varied identities dynamically influence their confidence in navigating their own educational paths.

Experience

Adults accumulate a wealth of experiences throughout their lifetimes that they call upon when in learning situations (Knowles, 1990). These experiences can be valuable learning resources and may lead to enriching discussions with others. Details of an experience may also affect a learner's self-concept or motivation to learn (Merriam & Bierema, 2014). Foote (2015) emphasized that while learners bring valuable prior experiences to their educational journeys, they may not always recognize how to apply these experiences in meaningful ways. To maximize the benefits of experiential learning, learners require guidance in identifying relevant aspects of their past experiences and strategically integrating them into new learning contexts. This process necessitates both critical thinking and reflection, enabling learners to analyze past situations, extract key insights, and apply them effectively to new challenges.

Additionally, McGrath (2009) maintained that a new experience has the possibility to impede a learner in developing understandings that might conflict with their previously held beliefs: "Some students may not be ready for their beliefs to be challenged and as a result they may feel threatened and not participate in future classes or… they cannot accept that their previous beliefs are wrong" (p. 107). Providing experiential learning activities with guided reflection and critical thinking skills can help learners develop the emotional distance they need to evaluate their experiences objectively. One suggested strategy is narrative writing activities that challenge learners to explore their prior learning from a new perspective (Foote, 2015).

Another strategy encourages adults to practice critical thinking to consider not just their isolated individual experiences, but those that have made them feel connected to a community or group. Note et al. (2021) described experiences that build a sense of interconnectedness as being a valuable form of learning and recommend using andragogical principles to encourage learners to recognize and appreciate when these experiences naturally occur in their daily lives.

Readiness to Learn

Adults are ready to learn when they understand how learning something will assist them in addressing their current life needs (Knowles, 1990). Higher education presents opportunities for learners to direct their learning choices as they select programs of study and consider future career paths.

Though Knowles (1990) suggested that the adult learner is best suited to identify their own readiness to learn (p. 195), his positioning of adult development as a scientific process that is unaffected by the context of one's life may oversimplify the experiences of nontraditional and multicultural learners (Pratt, 2002) and deny the agency of learners in general. For some, their readiness to learn may not be developing along the same timeline that Knowles assumed for all adults, especially when considering members of the neurodiverse community, whose life experiences diverge from the norm by nature of their identities. Readiness may not be determined by age range as rigidly as Knowles (1990) indicated but more due to a combination of the learner's self-concept and their mindset toward learning. But whatever its origin, readiness plays a key role in learners' levels of engagement.

Problem-Solving and Application Orientation to Learning

Andragogy also offers the assumption that adults prefer to learn topics that help them solve authentic problems and that they can apply to their daily lives. Knowles (1970) framed these problems as goals that benefit the individual. However, his interpretation of andragogy omitted the elements of social change that are more prevalent in European adult education theory (Loeng, 2018; Moll, 2024). Other scholars have introduced the notion that learners could benefit from considering common goals that unite individuals and reorient their learning to include a sense not of obligation to, but of mutual support within the communities to which they belong (Note et al., 2021). Rowland (2000) described the importance of group learning in Black American communities, for example, as demonstrating a communal orientation to learning that is underrepresented in andragogy. In any classroom, each student is likely to have a different orientation toward learning and a different way of expressing that orientation. These examples show that learners approach learning in complex ways, so educators need to better understand how learners express their learning preferences and develop strategies to support their diverse needs and styles. Higher education classrooms consist of a mix of students, some of whom may be more inclined to learning that solves problems, while others are more likely to respond to extended exploration of the subject matter.

Motivation

While both intrinsic and extrinsic motivators influence what and how learners engage in learning, Knowles (1990) suggested that adults are less constrained by extrinsic learning motivators and more intrinsically motivated in their learning than children. The assumption that extrinsic motivators become less important to adult learners implies that all adults have successful autonomy over their lives. This viewpoint, however, fails to consider the influence power and privilege have in the lives of most adults (Grace, 1996; Loeng, 2018) that requires learners to prioritize their motivations and learning actions.

Learners may be intrinsically motivated to fulfill personal learning interests while also satisfying less interesting learning requirements at work or in higher education with the extrinsic motivation to maintain their employment or achieve academic success. Lanford (2021) found that adult learners may deprioritize school as other external pressures become more prominent, yet they often seek out a new form of motivation to persist in their classes, such as new relationships they have established with their peers. By reprioritizing their motivations as needed, learners can refocus their learning on what is currently most relevant to them.

Need to Know

Knowles (1990) emphasized that adult learners must be able to find relevance in their learning to commit to it. He suggested educators proactively and transparently share learning objectives and course information (McGrath, 2009). McGrath further recommended the importance of convincing "adult learners to participate in a course by emphasizing the benefits of acquiring a qualification or learning new skills" (p. 99) determined through "participation of the learners in naming what is to be learned" (p. 4). Andragogical approaches to instruction can be enhanced by acknowledging the importance of involving learners in the process of identifying their needs and interests first and then identifying the expectations or needs of the discipline (context, community of practice, etc.), and subsequently using this information to design collaboratively a curriculum that ensures learners recognize learning for the value it offers them.

APPLYING THE ASSUMPTIONS OF ANDRAGOGY TO NEURODIVERGENT STUDENTS

While Neurodivergent learners share many characteristics with the stereotypical adult learner described by Knowles (1970), such as a desire for autonomy and a readiness to apply learning in real-world contexts, they often engage with these aspects in uniquely nuanced ways. Neurodivergent learners may also experience distinct challenges or approach learning with perspectives that enrich and broaden the traditional understanding of adult learner behaviors. This section aims to elucidate the relationship between theoretical assumptions and the observed behaviors exhibited by Neurodivergent students and to illustrate the ways in which these assumptions hold relevance to the lived experiences and learning behaviors of Neurodivergent students.

Autonomy and Learner Self-Concept

Neurodiversity's role as an umbrella term for myriad presentations, diagnoses, and identities (Clouder et al., 2020; Grummt, 2024; Miclea, 2024; Sidjaja, 2024) makes it impossible to synthesize them into a unified definition. Theorists of critical disability studies refer to this as the multidimensionality in the identities and experiences of people with disabilities (Hosking, 2008; Rocco; 2005). For that reason, making a single claim about the Neurodivergent learner's self-concept is impractical. Rather, each learner's self-concept is as distinctly and uniquely shaped by their identities as Neurodivergent people and the effort they invest in navigating neuromajority spaces throughout their lives (Grummt, 2024). Neurodivergent students clearly possess the ability to persist and achieve goals despite the challenges this presents for them, yet they are unfortunately often underestimated by those around them including educators (Clouder et al., 2020). Accepting that Neurodivergent students are capable of making decisions about what and how to learn, even if those decisions are not intuitive to others, empowers educators to meet students where they are and build upon their learning, leaning into the student's existing strengths. Making space for different ways of being and knowing among learners has the potential to positively shift classroom dynamics, increasing students' comfort level with sharing their ideas, and improving group cohesion through the camaraderie and collaboration that peer interaction generates.

The Value of Prior Experience

Andragogy highlights that experience is a source of learning for adults. Neurodivergent students rely on observation and experience to learn the invisible rules of neuromajority behavior and conform to them to avoid criticism or hostility, using a form of mimicking known as masking or camouflaging (Rasch, 2022; Spain et al., 2020). Drawing from prior experience in new situations is thus not an action specific to fully adult learners. And, just as andragogy encourages adult learners to leverage their prior experiences when learning new information, encouraging Neurodivergent students in HE to draw upon their prior experiences can be an effective way to help learners draw connections between new and known concepts, skills, and attitudes.

Choice and Readiness to Learn

Andragogy emphasizes that adults choose to learn about topics that are relevant to their current stage of life (Knowles, 1990). Similar to other learners of their age, HE Neurodivergent students' chosen areas of study represent one of the first major educational choices of their lives and can have lifelong consequences. Whereas the standardization of the United States K-12 curriculum tends to leave little room for individual student choice, HE provides a wealth of academic and extra-curricular options from which students can choose.

Up until this point in their lives, education for Neurodivergent students related to their life stages may have been focused on the rehabilitation or elimination of neurodiverse behaviors through therapy and/or prescription medications (Spaeth & Pearson, 2023). This can leave Neurodivergent students unprepared to demonstrate choice in their learning. A Neurodivergent learner may need to develop their skills with personal reflection and/or decision-making as an important first step toward recognizing and acting on their readiness to learn.

Problem-Centered Learning Orientation

Problem-centered learning addresses the practical needs of learners who approach learning with the goal of solving a problem or fulfilling a need that they have identified. This is markedly different from the subject-based instruction that students experience before HE. However, there are benefits to creating learning content and contexts that have clear, direct connections to the learner experience for neuromajority and Neurodivergent students that deserve further exploration.

Implementing problem-centered learning approaches that draw content from authentic real-world examples with which students have prior experience gives them opportunities to practice this type of learning, but Neurodivergent students may stand to benefit from it in additional ways. For example, a recent study by Morsanyi et al. (2022) showed that Neurodivergent students may have trouble processing metaphors and can require additional time to do so when compared to their neuromajority peers. Furthermore, Neurodivergent students with ADHD have been shown to succeed with problem-based learning in university classes (Nash-Luckenbach & Friedman, 2024). Grounding learning in realistic situations can lessen the burden of cognitive processing while also activating meaningful learning for students.

Sources of Motivation

Recognizing that motivation does not remain static throughout a person's life, andragogy indicates that a learner's motivations to learn become more intrinsic as they age (Knowles, 1990). Yet, Moll (2024) pointed out how intrinsically motivated learning tends to be nonformal in nature, and this insight could serve to inform the approach used by instructors of Neurodivergent students. Identifying and responding to the shift in Neurodivergent learners' motivation as their priorities change is key to improving student engagement (Wlodkowski & Ginsberg, 2017). Neurodivergent learners might demonstrate highs and lows in their engagement, but it would be a mistake to interpret this as a sign that students lack interest in what they are learning. Neuromajority instructors (and peers) may be unable to relate to the methods by which Neurodivergent learners process and express information, and this might lead them to view a change in engagement as the start of a permanent decline. It would be more beneficial to Neurodivergent students' long-term learning for instructors to understand more about neurodiverse learning behaviors and to allow for the fluctuations of engagement that occur over time.

Several neurodivergences including ADHD share the propensity to use hyper-focus or repetitive thinking to immerse oneself in a topic and become intimately familiar with its details (Ashinoff & Abu-Akel, 2021). Known as special interests, Neurodivergent learners employ hyperfixation in thinking processes in an effort to reduce anxiety, but the practice can also be leveraged to engage all learners more meaningfully with content that they can more easily relate to their existing interests (Boven, 2018; Cherewick, 2024). Recent research into the perceptions of autism among college students suggests that special interests are an expected and acceptable element of neurodiversity among individuals of that age range (Stockwell et al., 2021), which bodes well for the acceptance of Neurodivergent individuals who prefer to relate their learning to their nonacademic areas of interest.

Context and the Need to Know

Providing context and relevance for Neurodivergent learners related to the goals and intended outcomes of learning provides them with the time and space to prepare mentally and make informed decisions about their participation. A structured cognitive processing activity, often referred to as "mental rehearsal," involves mentally visualizing or "rehearsing" interactions, conversations, or scenarios before they happen. Many Autistic individuals use mental rehearsal to manage social interactions, reduce anxiety, and feel more prepared for various situations by anticipating outcomes (Spain et al., 2020). It can involve imagining potential outcomes, practicing appropriate responses, and identifying cues that can guide their reactions in the moment. This preparatory strategy can be especially useful for handling unfamiliar or challenging social situations and is common across several neurodivergences (Spain et al., 2020).

Scripting, the use of repeated scripted language, words, phrases, or sounds that provide a structured framework for communication "are presumed to be of vital importance for the development of shared meaning, communication, and social behaviour" within particular contexts (Trillingsgaard, 1999, p. 45), may be another avenue through which to support Neurodivergent students who are adjusting to the higher education environment. Scripting is especially common among Autistic individuals, but it is also a helpful coping strategy for other neurodiverse diagnoses, particularly for managing social or situational anxiety. Some individuals with ADHD use scripting to help with impulsivity and to organize their thoughts before engaging in situations where they may feel out of control or unfocused. People with social anxiety may also rehearse scenarios as a form of coping with anticipated stress in social interactions. For people with obsessive compulsive disorder (OCD) or generalized anxiety disorder (GAD), mental rehearsal may be useful to mitigate their anxiety by pre-planning how they will react (Spain et al., 2020). Working with policy experts and instructional designers, faculty can update the materials they share with learners to provide context for common university phrases and terms and socialize those terms across multiple channels, such as on department websites and within syllabi from different instructors. Phrases and terms like "office hours" or "counseling center" might be new to students, and they may need that extra context to feel comfortable taking advantage of such resources.

Also critical to this component of andragogy is to guide learners in finding the meaning in their learning – the need to know why – without responding with defensiveness. When students ask an instructor to explain the point of completing an assignment, it is not productive to consider it an accusation, or lack of respect, nor does it suggest that they expect the instructor to defend their choices. Recognition of the difference in communication styles between neuromajority and Neurodivergent individuals helps avoid such misunderstandings, which can undermine the quality of the instructor-student relationship and affect the student's motivation to continue with a specific class, area of study, or degree program.

PRACTICAL RECOMMENDATIONS

The following recommendations are intended for university faculty and staff to provide resources and enrichment activities on campus, design courses and align course objectives to student learning outcomes and facilitate and assess student learning in the classroom with an applied understanding how the assumptions of andragogy support the diverse needs and preferences of Neurodivergent students.

These recommendations consist of ways to develop inclusive university practices related to disability and neurodiversity, design learning content that is universally accessible to all students, build a cohesive classroom community, and foster self-directed learning in students.

Developing Inclusive University Practices

Authentic inclusion of Neurodivergent students must originate at the university level, with all departments and offices united under a shared mission of eliminating educational barriers for students with disabilities that is shared and supported by university leadership. Universities can do this by learning from their Neurodivergent student population directly and uniting all members of the campus community with a commitment to universal design for learning and a common understanding of neurodiversity.

Learn From Neurodivergent Students

The primary way that universities can improve their understanding of the issues facing Neurodivergent students and the solutions that would best meet their needs is by engaging directly with Neurodivergent students (Dwyer et al., 2023; Wilson & Dallman, 2024). Consulting with students to determine best practices for addressing their needs can improve the quality of support that students receive in the long term. Students' social and emotional skills also benefit from the chance to collaborate with others in the decision-making process, which are valuable experiences in shaping the self-concepts as independent, self-directed learners.

University faculty can collaborate in several ways to better understand the make-up and needs of their Neurodivergent students. Deans and professors can offer to speak at relevant student organization meetings, providing an opportunity to share their support for students and engage in direct conversations about their experiences. Professors can also arrange one-time private meetings with students who have disabilities, as identified through the Disability Office or accommodation letters, to establish their specific needs. Additionally, offices such as the Disability Office, Office of Research, and relevant colleges or departments can conduct targeted campus research, including student surveys focused on populations identified through the Disability Office or student groups, to gather valuable insights.

Strengthen Campus Bonds

Students, staff, and faculty cannot be forced to rely on informal, incidental learning about neurodiversity or relevant topics like Universal Design for Learning

(UDL). All members of the university need some level of formal training about these concepts (Accardo et al., 2024; Brandsen et al. 2024; Dwyer et al., 2023) with the goal of inspiring participants to become allies to Neurodivergent students and people with disabilities in general (Wolbring & Lillywhite, 2023). Other ways to dispel misconceptions about Neurodivergent students include publicly promoting aspects of neurodiversity or Neurodivergent people around campus and through digital channels like social media, creating positive messaging about Neurodivergent students that promotes their skills and abilities (Wilson & Dallman, 2024).

Campus events are an ideal environment to promote such attitudes. For example, incorporating neurodiversity as a theme in various academic lectures, panels, and cultural events for both faculty and students makes it a visible part of the campus culture. An academic panel could focus on the contributions of Neurodivergent individuals to various fields. It's also valuable to work with student groups across campus, especially those focused on disability advocacy, to organize campus-wide activities that celebrate Neurodivergent students. These events can promote Neurodivergent students' creative, intellectual, and leadership skills. A way for Neurodivergent students to further showcase their talents is to create platforms, such as art exhibitions, performance events, or hackathons. Publicize these events widely to highlight the diverse skills that Neurodivergent individuals bring to the campus community.

Consider creating and sharing positive narratives, such as student spotlights featuring stories of Neurodivergent students in newsletters, social media posts, or campus publications that showcase their achievements, talents, and experiences. These stories can be framed in a way that emphasizes their skills and contributions to campus life. Social media campaigns that highlight the diverse strengths of Neurodivergent students can include quotes, success stories, and testimonials that show how neurodiversity adds value to the university community. Working with Neurodivergent students to co-create content, such as blog posts, videos, or interviews, where they discuss their experiences, perspectives, and achievements, gives students a platform to speak for themselves and ensures their voices are heard. These actions demonstrate a clear commitment to inclusion to all members of the community and encourage them to participate in the effort.

Designing Universally Accessible Learning Content

The goal of universally accessible learning content is to create a learning environment that all students can access equally from the onset of instruction without needing individual adjustments. Creating learning that integrates supports for those needs can be accomplished by following established guidelines and recommendations for UDL and supplementing traditional in-person strategies with technology-based solutions in practical and innovative ways.

Leverage Universal Design for Learning Guidelines

Universal Design for Learning is a framework for designing and delivering instruction in a way that addresses multiple processing styles (CAST, 2024a). Guidelines for implementing UDL describe multiple means of engaging learning, representing learning content, and methods of learner action and expression (CAST, 2024b). Like the goals of andragogy, using these strategies leads to increased self-direction in learners (Cole et al., 2024) and improves Neurodivergent learners' engagement in learning (Cole et al., 2024; Wells, 2024).

Accessible learning content is content that is both relevant and meaningful to students while aligning with institutional standards and policies. One approach to enhancing accessibility is integrating real-world experiences into coursework. Taking a collaborative approach, faculty can incorporate student organization events, community volunteering opportunities, and other free local activities into assignments, providing students with hands-on, experiential learning. Encouraging students to explore issues within their own communities further reinforces the relevance of academic work to their lived experiences.

A particularly effective strategy is allowing students to design their own culminating projects for a course. This process involves three key steps: (1) selecting the subject matter and format of the project, ensuring that multiple pathways exist for achieving the same student learning outcomes (SLOs)—for example, in a writing course, students might submit a traditional written story, an audio recording, or a video with AI-generated narration, all meeting the objective of producing a compelling and well-structured narrative; (2) sharing their work with peers to receive constructive feedback; and (3) revising their project based on this feedback. This approach empowers students to take ownership of their learning, accommodates diverse learning styles, and fosters creativity, while also helping them develop essential social interaction skills through the collaborative process of giving and receiving feedback.

Additionally, offering enrichment options like further readings or videos that expand on a topic discussed in class can benefit students who show particular interest in a specific aspect of a course or who may require productive, self-directed engagement due to attention-related challenges. Faculty can also support students in developing research skills by guiding them in exploring special interests and hyperfixations through structured research opportunities across campus and within the community. These approaches not only foster deeper engagement with course material but also cultivate essential academic and professional skills in a way that respects diverse learning needs and preferences.

Although this may sound like it requires additional effort and planning for instructors, there are demonstrated benefits in HE spaces (Accardo et al., 2024; Sandland et al., 2023; Wells, 2024). Research demonstrates that implementing universally accessible teaching and learning practices is relatively simple (Clouder et al., 2020; Hamilton & Perry, 2024; Sarrett, 2018; Wells, 2024), reduces overall workload for instructors (Cole et al., 2024), and as an alternative to institutionally prescribed accommodations that are not tailored to learners and are therefore ineffective or inaccessible (Hamilton & Perry, 2024), has the potential to reduce demand on disability services offices (Cole et al., 2024). UDL may act as relief for the challenges that instructors face identifying student needs or next steps in the traditional academic accommodations process, while they work to truly accommodate all students in the way that benefits them while also protecting the confidentiality of a disability status (Fovet, 2024).

Learning about how to implement UDL practices can be another source of concern for faculty (Fovet, 2024). Additional opportunities to develop an understanding of UDL practices and how to enact them in academic spaces can reduce that concern. One way to foster understanding is by helping faculty to embrace the "universal" aspect of UDL and collaborating across colleges, departments, and roles to review the tenets of UDL and work together to create examples of how faculty can reach students by using multiple methods of fostering and maintaining student engagement, representing information, and encouraging interaction and communication among students. Student perspectives should be a part of this process as well, with faculty reaching out to students to listen to their opinions.

Use Technology to Enhance Learning

Although research has established that students' use and multitasking with technology can introduce distractions and affect their performance (Rourke et al., 2024), technology can also serve as a convenient tool to introduce practices consistent with UDL principles. Research shows that sharing presentation materials and/or recorded lectures from classes with Neurodivergent students supports them in processing and retaining the information (Clouder et al., 2020; Horlin et al., 2024; Sarrett, 2018). Faculty can accommodate students' diverse communication styles by offering online meetings as an alternative to in-person, holding multimodal office hours that students can join in person or using an online meeting tool, and using university-approved digital communication and collaboration tools such as their university's learning management system (LMS) to send announcements, set assignment due dates, and configure automatic reminders for students. Faculty can also take advantage of their LMS to collaborate in files, like using a shared document in which both the instructor and a student can share questions or comments they might not be able to share in person or verbally.

Building a Cohesive Academic Community

For those who are looking to help ameliorate the social challenges that Neurodivergent students encounter in HE, faculty, staff, and instructors need to acknowledge the influence of the group climate within student organizations, classrooms, and even in faculty-only settings. This can be done by setting ground rules that create explicit norms for the group and facilitating discussions that foster more balanced participation

Set Ground Rules

At the outset of any group formation, whether it is a class, student organization, committee, or other, begin by establishing discussion guidelines that emphasize the importance of equal participation and respectful listening. These guidelines should be co-created with the students to foster a sense of ownership. For example, the instructor can facilitate a group discussion in which students offer examples of classroom behaviors they consider conducive to learning, and those that are unproductive. Students should then review the agreements and provide additional feedback as an assignment for the next class meeting. This gives all students the opportunity to come to an agreement on the norms they want to uphold as a group, which can also serve as useful practice using their discussion and decision-making skills. It further provides multiple methods of adding to the discussion, which supports students who might need additional time to process the experience of the group discussion, who experience social anxiety, or are not as comfortable expressing themselves verbally or in group settings.

Facilitate Discussions

During group discussions, consider structuring group discussions to help maintain the flow of conversation. For example, use a round-robin format where each student has a set amount of time to share their thoughts, or call on students to participate based on random or demographic characteristics from the class, such as requesting a response from someone wearing red, or from a person whose last name begins with the letter R. This level of structure encourages participation from all students and prevents any one individual from dominating the conversation.

For a less prescribed discussion, establish routines that encourage students to use non-verbal cues, such as raising their hands or using a talking stick, to indicate they wish to contribute. It is also important for students to speak to each other, not the professor, to detect these cues. Note that the seating arrangement of a room can enhance students' ability to and comfort with speaking with each other; for example, a circular arrangement in which all students can face each other rather than the instructor helps students have discussions with their peers. This approach helps signal to students when it is appropriate to allow space for others to speak.

Nurturing Self-Directed Learning

Self-direction is both an attribute of learners and a process through which learners choose, plan, and implement learning tasks to meet a learning objective (Merriam & Bierema, 2014). The assumptions of andragogy hinge on the foundational assumption that adult learners are more likely to want to be self-directed and are more capable of successfully implementing self-directed learning than children (Knowles, 1980). Postsecondary instructors play an important role in guiding students through the transition from dependent to independent and self-directed learners through coaching, goal setting, reflection, and self-evaluation of learning (Grow, 1991). They can support Neurodivergent students in particular by providing opportunities for students to hone their confidence and skills at self-directed learning.

In the classroom, encouraging the use of self-reflection and assessment tools like journals, checklists, or portfolios can help students develop self-awareness and identify areas for improvement. Collaborative learning through group projects, peer coaching, and mentorship can provide Neurodivergent students with opportunities to learn from others and engage in self-directed learning in a social context. Student involvement in academic clubs, conferences, or internships helps students pursue learning beyond the classroom and make connections with other students with similar backgrounds or interests, and faculty can promote these types of events to raise awareness across the university. Peer coaching and mentoring programs that pair more senior Neurodivergent students with newer students may provide another way for students to develop social relationships and receive practical advice from a peer they can relate to.

Another way to address Neurodivergent students' skill development is to consider a holistic approach that considers the learner's mental, physical, and academic wellbeing. University disability services offices can proactively collaborate with student affairs as well as the university's recreation, writing, counseling, and/or tutoring centers to identify existing events and resources for Neurodivergent students that provide this type of support. Better yet, these groups can work together to identify new events and resources to satisfy unmet needs, such as organizing a mixer for Neurodivergent students on campus so that students in different colleges can meet and interact.

Scaffold Support

All learners demonstrate differing levels of self-direction in their learning (Grow, 1991). Using a staged model that identifies four broad levels of self-direction that learners exhibit, from learners who are completely unable or unwilling to self-direct their learning to learners who are experts at doing so, Grow (1991) offered strategies that educators can use to encourage learners to successfully develop the skills of self-directed learning beyond their current level. These strategies begin with providing coaching and objective feedback to dependent learners, followed by increased personal interaction and goal setting, instructor facilitation of learning, and finally cultivation and support for independent learners (Grow, 1991). For example, a first-year public speaking student begins as a dependent learner, receiving structured coaching and objective feedback on speech organization and delivery. As their confidence grows, personal interaction and goal setting encourage self-reflection and peer collaboration. In the involved stage, the instructor shifts to a facilitative role, prompting critical thinking as the student develops original presentations. Finally, as a self-directed learner, the student takes full ownership of their learning—researching topics, delivering compelling speeches, and mentoring peers—with the instructor serving as a mentor. This process fosters increasing autonomy, transforming a novice into a confident, self-sufficient speaker. Similarly, Neurodivergent students may express varying levels of comfort with self-direction that instructors can identify and target with coaching, motivation, consultation, or mentoring, based on their needs.

Active Learning

Create opportunities for students to practice self-directed learning through active learning activities with their peers. This can occur through formal group work or by employing interactive lecturing teaching strategies that insert student-centered activities at strategic points within a traditional lecture (Coryell, 2024). During these activities, instructors can guide students as they become more active participants in their learning and engage with their peers to ask questions, discuss new concepts in their own words, engage in problem-solving activities, participate in group debate, role-playing, or simulations, research real-world examples connected with the content, and evaluate ideas. Choose activities that are appropriate for the size of your groups and what they are learning, such as by asking pairs of students to discuss two opposing theories or asking larger groups to develop a case study. This also gives instructors the chance to observe their students as they work together and become better acquainted with the social dynamics among students and help maintain productive relationships among them.

Addressing Challenges

We acknowledge the potential challenges inherent in implementing a more neurodiverse instructional style. For that reason, we offer some advice for how HE educators can navigate common issues that present themselves including matters of disability disclosure and classroom size.

Disclosure

Disclosing a disability is at the prerogative of the HE student. To disclose a disability, one must provide documents that explain the disability, potentially requiring a diagnosis, and accommodations the student may desire. Students should be encouraged to consider official disclosure and talk with instructors about how their disability or disabilities affect their learning. If the disability is disclosed, the institution must provide accommodations, but they may not be required to provide the student with the same supports they had in previous educational settings.

It is likely faculty will have many diverse students in their classrooms including neuromajority learners as well as Neurodivergent learners who may or may not disclose their disabilities or in some cases, even know they have a disability (Learning Disabilities Association of America, n.d.). Importantly, the recommendations and strategies offered in this chapter are supportive for all learners in HE, regardless of ability. Based on the tenets of andragogy, incorporating these strategies in diverse classrooms, with continual focus on getting to know the students and meeting learners where they are, will provide a strong foundation for success for all.

Scaling Recommendations for Larger Classes

Designing for and teaching large groups of students can be challenging. However, designing instruction and incorporating teaching strategies linked with this chapter's discussion on andragogy can promote learning with classes of any size. Instructors, in supporting the andragogical tenets of prior experience, motivation, and self-concept can begin the course by surveying students prior to the beginning of the semester asking them to reflect on what they already know or have experienced with the subject of the course; their personal interests, motivations, and learning goals; and their learning strengths, weaknesses, resources, and challenges they would like the instructor to know about them to support them in their learning. This information can then be used to provide information about available learning resources and supports offered at the institution; referred to in-class when introducing a new concept; discussed when articulating learning goals and applications in future occupations; and incorporated into case studies and real-world problems throughout the course.

Offering opportunities for all learners to be active in their learning is supported by learning principles of experience, readiness to learn, problem-solving and application learning orientations, and need to know. Recommendations include designing interactive lectures with periodic pauses that ask students to work together in pairs or small groups to engage in active learning techniques including discussion, comparison, problem-solving, analysis of real-world issues, peer feedback, etc.

Finally, promoting self-directed learning and offering learners choices in how they provide evidence of their learning provides support for diverse ways of thinking and knowing. Including at least one assignment that allows students to conduct their own research, individually or in small groups, about a real-world problem that is linked with course content progresses with andragogical suppositions of self-directedness, problem-solving, and learning application.

CONCLUSION

Andragogy assumes that learners prefer to learn in a way that deviates from the norm of instructional practices in the formal education students experience in primary and secondary schooling. For Neurodivergent students, andragogy is a drastic change from the educational system of their childhood that rewards obedience and sameness and discourages critical thinking.

As we have asserted in this chapter, Neurodivergent learners can flourish when they can devote their time and attention to learning and developing their skills, rather than constantly striving to hide or minimize the neurodiverse aspects of their personalities around others. Andragogy highlights strategies from nonformal learning (Moll, 2024) that, when applied to formal settings such as HE, can engage Neurodivergent learners more meaningfully than traditional methods. Instructional strategies based on the assumptions of andragogy are well-suited for use with Neurodivergent students, but andragogy also serves as a foundation upon which instructors can build their own understandings of relating to Neurodivergent and neuromajority students in ways that respond to the needs of young adulthood.

Adapting andragogy's principles for Neurodivergent learners has many implications for how educators and administrative decision-makers design, implement, and assess the results of instruction. To reach the diverse learners whose needs and perspectives have heretofore been un- or under supported by andragogy, it could be helpful for educators to dedicate more time to evaluating their personal assumptions about education and the adult learner and identifying any biases or blind spots that might inhibit their students' learning (Pratt, 2024). Related to this is the concept of action with reflection known as praxis (Vella, 2002), which gives learners the opportunity to practice critically, reviewing new experiences in order to learn from them. Praxis reorients learners to learn from their experience instead of using their experience as proof of prior learning. Adult educators can also use praxis to explore their teaching styles directly with learners and develop a more comprehensive understanding of their students (Lanford, 2021).

Collaboration is fundamental to both education and professional growth, as it involves communication, resource-sharing, and collective problem-solving. In higher education, faculty and staff must work together to create inclusive learning environments, particularly for Neurodivergent students. To achieve this, institutions need policies that support expanded professional development (PD) opportunities for faculty, along with structured, collaborative learning experiences that equip educators with the knowledge and skills to support Neurodivergent students effectively.

A well-designed professional development framework should help faculty:

- **Develop expertise in neurodivergence** by learning from student speakers, experts, and disability services staff, fostering allyship and informed teaching practices.
- **Understand and accommodate neurodiverse learning behaviors** with sessions led by Neurodivergent students, disability office staff, and external experts, which can provide valuable insights.
- **Facilitate and lead groups of Neurodivergent students** by collaborating with departments, student affairs professionals, and the Disability Resource Office (DRO) to implement inclusive leadership strategies tailored to neurodiverse needs.
- **Implement problem-centered learning approaches** that connect academic content to real-world experiences. This requires learning about students' special interests, skills, and backgrounds and collaborating with instructional designers and accessibility specialists to develop both in-person and online learning activities.
- **Build partnerships with community and industry professionals** to create experiential learning opportunities. Faculty can work with university business experts to identify potential collaborators or coordinate with career services and disability offices to establish volunteer and internship opportunities for Neurodivergent students.

Beyond faculty training, institutional support is essential for sustaining inclusive practices. Universities should invest in cross-college and interdepartmental initiatives that foster collaboration among faculty, staff, and students. Additionally, encouraging faculty participation in research on neurodivergence can contribute to a broader understanding of effective teaching strategies and institutional policies and neurodivergence in higher education spaces. By embracing the neurodiversity of the current HE classroom and developing their own understanding of neurodivergence and andragogy, administrators and instructors can help Neurodivergent HE learners achieve new heights of success.

CASE STUDIES AND DISCUSSION QUESTIONS

Case Study 1: Navigating Group Dynamics in a Neurodiverse Classroom

In a university course on psychology, Professor Johnson leads a diverse group of students, including Sophia, a Neurodivergent student with a keen interest in the subject matter. Sophia often dominates group discussions, speaking at length about her opinions and insights. While her contributions are insightful and show a deep understanding of the material, they tend to overshadow other students, resulting in a lack of equitable participation. Professor Johnson recognizes the need to address this dynamic to foster a more inclusive learning environment. Some of the specific challenges he notes are Sophia's skills in discussion and active listening, and his ability to manage the needs of both Sophia and the other students in the class. Sophia frequently speaks for extended periods, often neglecting to pause for input from her peers. This leads to other students feeling sidelined and less willing to contribute. Sophia 's approach to discussions does not reflect active listening; she often fails to acknowledge or respond to her classmates' ideas. This creates a sense of frustration and disengagement among other group members. At times, other students use nonverbal cues and facial expressions that indicate their disinterest in what Sophia is saying, but Sophia has not reacted to them. Professor Johnson overheard a student in the class mention a group text from which Sophia is evidently excluded and in which they vent about, among other complaints common among university students, Sophia's dominance in conversations. Professor Johnson values Sophia's contributions but also wants to ensure that all students feel comfortable sharing their thoughts and opinions.

Questions

1. What actions should Professor Johnson take to learn more about the conflict he sees?
2. How can instructors use principles of adult learning to create more inclusive, balanced discussions that respect the varied communication styles of both neuromajority and Neurodivergent students?
3. What measures can the university take to assist instructors in promoting classroom strategies that foster fair participation and respect for diverse communication needs?

Case Study 2: Creating Inclusive Orientation Experiences for Neurodivergent Students

A university administrator in the Office of Student Affairs was approached by Hector, a first-year student with social anxiety disorder who had recently attended an orientation for incoming freshmen. Hector voiced a desire for more inclusive orientation activities tailored to Neurodivergent students. Hector expressed challenges he faced with traditional large-group events, which tend to be loud, overwhelming, and filled with unstructured social interactions.

Despite his disorder, Hector was hopeful that he would make new friends at school that understood, if not shared, his experiences with anxiety. The administrator listened attentively as Hector outlined how such settings heightened his anxiety and posed barriers to meeting other students and navigating the campus comfortably. Hector further explained that they felt the lack of specific resources for Neurodivergent students, including those with conditions such as autism, ADHD, and anxiety disorders, resulted in many students missing out on vital social integration and support opportunities. He also expressed a desire for orientation content that better supports the unique ways Neurodivergent students process information and engage with new material. He shared that traditional formats, which often rely on rapid verbal presentations and large amounts of unstructured social interaction, can be difficult to absorb or retain. Hector described feeling overwhelmed and "drained" after attending orientation, less confident about his ability to thrive as a student.

Questions

1. In what ways can the orientation program be modified to better support Neurodivergent students, such as those with social anxiety disorder, autism, or ADHD, in navigating and engaging with the campus environment?

2. How might structured, smaller-scale social activities or quiet spaces be integrated into the orientation schedule to accommodate students who may find large-group events overwhelming?
3. What specific resources or ongoing support mechanisms could be developed to help Neurodivergent students like Hector build confidence and establish connections with peers throughout their first year?

Case Study 3: Designing Real-World Learning Experiences in Engineering Education

Dr. Patel, an associate professor of mechanical engineering at a large university, is in the process of redesigning a key assignment for the junior-level Thermal Systems Design course. The course focuses on applying thermodynamics and heat transfer principles to real-world engineering challenges, and Dr. Patel wants to ensure that students not only understand the theoretical concepts but also gain experience with problem-solving in professional contexts.

One of Dr. Patel's main concerns is ensuring that the assignment provides practical experience that mirrors the types of work students will encounter after graduation. They envision an assignment where students analyze and propose energy-efficient solutions for real-world heating and cooling systems, possibly in collaboration with local companies or campus facilities. However, they are unsure how to structure the project so that all students, including those who are Neurodivergent, can effectively engage with and benefit from the experience.

During a faculty meeting, Dr. Patel discusses ideas with colleagues in both engineering and instructional design. A colleague suggests incorporating elements of industry-style project management, while another raises the importance of ensuring accessibility and flexibility in how students engage with the assignment. Dr. Patel begins to consider different ways to balance structure with autonomy, provide multiple modes of engagement, and ensure that all students can develop the professional skills necessary for engineering careers.

Questions

1. How can the project be designed to provide meaningful, real-world experience without overwhelming students?
2. What strategies can ensure that Neurodivergent students receive the support they need while still developing independence?
3. How can faculty help all students gain confidence in their ability to transition from academic learning to professional engineering practice?

REFERENCES

Accardo, A. L., Bomgardner, E. M., Rubinstein, M. B., & Woodruff, J. (2024). Valuing neurodiversity on campus: Perspectives and priorities of neurodivergent students, faculty, and professional staff. *Journal of Diversity in Higher Education.* Advance online publication. https://doi-org.DOI: 10.1037/dhe0000571

Ashinoff, B. K., & Abu-Akel, A. (2021). Hyperfocus: The forgotten frontier of attention. *Psychological Research, 85*(1), 1–19. DOI: 10.1007/s00426-019-01245-8 PMID: 31541305

Boven, F. (2018). Special interests and inclusive academic learning: An autistic perspective. *Advances in Autism, 4*(4), 155–164. https://doi-org.DOI: 10.1108/AIA-05-2018-0020

Brandsen, S., Blackshear, K., Coleman, R., Hallur, S., & Chandrasekhar, T. (2024). Developing an inclusive campus for autistic students. *Journal of Diversity in Higher Education.* Advance online publication. https://doi-org.DOI: 10.1037/dhe0000551

Butcher, L., & Lane, S. (2024). Neurodivergent (Autism and ADHD) student experiences of access and inclusion in higher education: An ecological systems theory perspective. *Higher Education: The International Journal of Higher Education Research,* 1–21. https://doi-org.DOI: 10.1007/s10734-024-01319-6

CAST. (2024a). About CAST. https://www.cast.org/about/about-cast

CAST. (2024b). Universal Design for Learning Guidelines version 3.0. https://udlguidelines.cast.org/

Cheang, R. T. S., Skjevling, M., Blakemore, A. I. F., Kumari, V., & Puzzo, I. (2024). Do you feel me? Autism, empathic accuracy and the double empathy problem. *AUTISM.* Advance online publication. https://doi-org.DOI: 10.1177/13623613241252320

Cherewick, M. (2024). Future directions for neurodiversity affirming autism interventions: Adolescence is a second sensitive period to support positive developmental trajectories. *Current Psychology: A Journal for Diverse Perspectives on Diverse Psychological Issues, 43*(10), 9191–9198. https://doi-org.DOI: 10.1007/s12144-023-05053-7

Clouder, L., Karakus, M., Cinotti, A., Ferreyra, M. V., Fierros, G. A., & Rojo, P. (2020). Neurodiversity in higher education: A narrative synthesis. *Higher Education, 80*(4), 757–778. DOI: 10.1007/s10734-020-00513-6

Cole, J. Y., Graham, J., Norvell, S., & Schaber, P. (2024). Universal design for learning principles impact on students with neurodiverse learning styles. *Journal of Occupational Therapy Education, 8*(2), 1–21. DOI: 10.26681/jote.2024.080204

Cook, A. (2024). Conceptualisations of neurodiversity and barriers to inclusive pedagogy in schools: A perspective article. *Journal of Research in Special Educational Needs, 24*(3), 627–636. https://doi-org.DOI: 10.1111/1471-3802.12656

Coryell, J. E. (2024). Interactive lecture: Engaging active learning/interactive teaching and learning with lecture. In Coryell, J. E., Baumgartner, L. M., & Bohonos, J. W. (Eds.), *Methods for facilitating adult learning: Strategies for enhancing instruction and instructor effectiveness* (pp. 27–37). Routledge. DOI: 10.4324/9781003446019-3

Drader-Mazza, N., Lopez-Kidwell, V., Kanwal, F., Reger, R. K., & Vogus, T. J. (2024). The double empathy problem and person-environment fit: Mutual understanding and bidirectional adjustment in autistic talent acquisition. *Human Resource Management.* Advance online publication. https://doi-org.DOI: 10.1002/hrm.22258

Dwyer, P., Mineo, E., Mifsud, K., Lindholm, C., Gurba, A., & Waisman, T. C. (2023). Building neurodiversity-inclusive postsecondary campuses: Recommendations for leaders in higher education. *Autism in Adulthood: Challenges and Management, 5*(1), 1–14. DOI: 10.1089/aut.2021.0042 PMID: 36941859

Evans, D., Granson, M., Langford, D., & Hirsch, S. (2023). Autism spectrum disorder: Reconceptualising support for neurodiverse students in higher education. *Journal of Higher Education Policy and Management, 45*(2), 243–257. https://doi-org.DOI: 10.1080/1360080X.2023.2180168

Feuer, D., & Geber, B. (1988). Uh-oh… Second thoughts about adult learning theory. *Training (New York, N.Y.), 25*(12), 31–39.

Foote, L. S. (2015). Re-storying life as a means of critical reflection: The power of narrative learning. *Christian Higher Education, 14*(3), 116–126. DOI: 10.1080/15363759.2015.1028580

Fovet, F. (2024) Accommodations 2.0: Reflecting on the future of post-secondary accommodations in a UDL landscape. *AHEAD Journal*, 17.

Franz, D. J., Lenhard, W., Marx, P., & Richter, T. (2023). Here I sit, making men in my own image: How learning disorder labels affect teacher student's expectancies. *Current Psychology: A Journal for Diverse Perspectives on Diverse Psychological Issues, 42*(12), 9795–9809. https://doi-org./DOI: 10.1007/s12144-021-02250-0

Friedman, Z. L., & Nash-Luckenbach, D. (2024). Has the time come for heutagogy? Supporting neurodivergent learners in higher education. *Higher Education, 87*(6), 1905–1920. https://doi-org.DOI: 10.1007/s10734-023-01097-7

Galbraith, M. W., & Jones, M. S. (2008). First things first in becoming a teacher of adults. *Journal of Adult Education, 37*(1), 1–12. https://eric.ed.gov/?id=EJ891070

Gavín-Chocano, Ó., García-Martínez, I., & de la Rosa, A. L. (2024). Self-regulated learning as an inherent factor of academic self-concept in university students. *Current Psychology (New Brunswick, N.J.), 43*(34), 27469–27480. DOI: 10.1007/s12144-024-06352-3

Grace, A. P. (1996). Taking a critical pose: Andragogy—missing links, missing values. *International Journal of Lifelong Education, 15*(5), 382–392. DOI: 10.1080/0260137960150506

Grow, G. (1991). Teaching learners to be self-directed. *Adult Education Quarterly, 41*(3), 125–149. DOI: 10.1177/0001848191041003001

Grummt, M. (2024). Sociocultural perspectives on neurodiversity-An analysis, interpretation and synthesis of the basic terms, discourses and theoretical positions. *Sociology Compass, 18*(8), 1–17. DOI: 10.1111/soc4.13249

Hamilton, L. G., & Petty, S. (2024). Corrigendum: Compassionate pedagogy for neurodiversity in higher education: A conceptual analysis. *Frontiers in Psychology, 14*, 1–2. DOI: 10.3389/fpsyg.2023.1345256 PMID: 38444880

Henning, C., Summerfeldt, L. J., & Parker, J. D. (2022). ADHD and academic success in university students: The important role of impaired attention. *Journal of Attention Disorders, 26*(6), 893–901. DOI: 10.1177/10870547211036758 PMID: 34384265

Horlin, C., Hronska, B., & Nordmann, E. (2024). I can be a "normal" student: The role of lecture capture in supporting disabled and neurodivergent students' participation in higher education. *Higher Education: The International Journal of Higher Education Research,* 1–18. https://doi-org.DOI: 10.1007/s10734-024-01201-5

Hosking, D. L. (2008). *Critical disability theory*. [Paper presentation]. 4th Biennial Disability Studies Conference, Lancaster University. https://www.lancaster.ac.uk/fass/events/disabilityconference_archive/2008/papers/hosking2008.pdf

Hotez, E., Rava, J., & Kuo, A. A. (2023). Brief research report: Investigating neurodiversity acceptance in the college classroom: An exploratory study. *Frontiers in Education, 8*, 1223175. Advance online publication. DOI: 10.3389/feduc.2023.1223175

Jones, D. R., Botha, M., Ackerman, R. A., King, K., & Sasson, N. J. (2024). Non-autistic observers both detect and demonstrate the double empathy problem when evaluating interactions between autistic and non-autistic adults. *Autism: The International Journal of Research and Practice, 28*(8), 2053–2065. https://doi-org.DOI: 10.1177/13623613231219743

Knowles, M. (1980). *Andragogy*, not pedagogy. *Adult Leadership, 17*(1), 350–352.

Knowles, M. S. (1970). *The modern practice of adult education: Andragogy versus pedagogy*. The Association Press.

Knowles, M. S. (1990). *The adult learner: A neglected species* (4th ed.). Gulf.

Lanford, M. (2021). In pursuit of respect: The adult learner attending community college in the "new economy.". *The Educational Forum, 85*(1), 34–48. DOI: 10.1080/00131725.2020.1775329

Learning Disabilities Association of America. (n.d.). The adult learning disability assessment process. https://ldaamerica.org/info/adult-learning-disability-assessment-process/

Lindeman, E. C. (1926). *The meaning of adult education*. New Republic, Inc.

Loeng, S. (2018). Various ways of understanding the concept of andragogy. *Cogent Education, 5*(1), 1496643. Advance online publication. DOI: 10.1080/2331186X.2018.1496643

McGrath, V. (2009). Reviewing the evidence on how adult students learn: An examination of Knowles' model of andragogy. *Adult Learner: The Irish Journal of Adult and Community Education,* 99–110.

Merriam, S. B., & Bierema, L. L. (2014). *Adult learning: Linking theory and practice* (1st ed.). Jossey-Bass.

Miclea, B. (2024). Neurodiversity and mental disorders. *BRAIN: Broad Research in Artificial Intelligence & Neuroscience, 15*(2), 225–233. https://doi-org.DOI: 10.18662/brain/15.2/574

Milligan, F. (1995). In defence of andragogy. *Nurse Education Today, 15*(1), 22–27. DOI: 10.1016/S0260-6917(95)80074-3 PMID: 7708024

Milton, D. E. M. (2012). On the ontological status of autism: The 'double empathy problem.'. *Disability & Society, 27*(6), 883–887. DOI: 10.1080/09687599.2012.710008

Moll, I. (2024). A psychological critique of Knowles' andragogy as a theory of learning. *Andragoška spoznanja/Studies in Adult Education and Learning, 30*(1), 151–170. DOI: 10.4312/as/16396

Morsanyi, K., Hamilton, J., Stamenković, D., & Holyoak, K. J. (2022). Linking metaphor comprehension with analogical reasoning: Evidence from typical development and autism spectrum disorder. *British Journal of Psychology (London, England: 1953), 113*(2), 479–495. https://doi-org.libproxy.txstate.edu/10.1111/bjop.12542

Nafukho, F., Amutabi, M., & Otunga, R. (2005). *Foundations of adult education in Africa*. Pearson; UNESCO Institute for Education.

Nash-Luckenbach, D. M., & Friedman, Z. L. (2024). The neurodivergent college learner: Faculty Perceptions of supporting individuals with ADHD in higher education. *Quality Assurance in Education: An International Perspective, 32*(4), 597–610. https://doi-org.DOI: 10.1108/QAE-01-2024-0014

Note, N., De Backer, F., & Donder, L. D. (2021). A novel viewpoint on andragogy: Enabling moments of community. *Adult Education Quarterly, 71*(1), 3-19. https://doi-org.DOI: 10.1177/0741713620921361

Pratt, D. D. (1993). Andragogy after twenty-five years. *New Directions for Adult and Continuing Education*, *57*(57), 15–23. DOI: 10.1002/ace.36719935704

Pratt, D. D. (2002). Good teaching: One size fits all? *New Directions for Adult and Continuing Education, 2002*(93), 5-16. https://doi-org.DOI: 10.1002/ace.45

Pratt, D. D. (2024). Teaching perspectives: A philosophical foundation for methods. In Coryell, J. E., Baumgartner, L. M., & Bohonos, J. W. (Eds.), *Methods for facilitating adult learning: Strategies for enhancing instruction and instructor effectiveness* (pp. 69–86). Routledge. DOI: 10.4324/9781003446019-6

Rachal, J. R. (2014). Book review: Malcolm Shepherd Knowles: A history of his thought. *Adult Education Quarterly, 64*(1), 80-84. https://doi-org.DOI: 10.1177/0741713613496616

Rasch, E. V. (2022). The lights are too loud: Neurodivergence in the student affairs profession. *Vermont Connection, 43*(1), 189–203.

Rocco, T. S. (2005). From disability studies to critical race theory: Working towards critical disability theory. *Proceedings of the 46th Annual Adult Education Research Conference*. https://newprairiepress.org/aerc/2005/papers/17

Röhm, A., Grengel, M., Möhring, M., Zensen-Möhring, J., Nellen, C., & Hastall, M. R. (2022). Applying the mixed-blessings model and labeling theory to stigma in inclusive education: An experimental study of student and trainee teachers' perceptions of pupils with ADHD, DLD, and intellectual disability. *Frontiers in Psychology, 13*, 1-14. https://doi-org.DOI: 10.3389/fpsyg.2022.910702

Ross-Gordon, J., Rose, A. D., & Kasworm, C. E. (2017). *Foundations of adult and continuing education*. Jossey-Bass.

Rourke, B., Bellur, S., & Nowak, K. (2024). All distractions are not equal: The moderating role of autistic traits and technology multitasking on academic performance among college students. *Atlantic Journal of Communication*, *32*(3), 325–347. DOI: 10.1080/15456870.2023.2177292

Rowland, M. L., & ERIC Clearinghouse on Adult, Career, and Vocational Education, Columbus, OH (2000). African Americans and self-help education: The missing link in adult education. *ERIC Digest No. 222*.

Sandland, B., MacLeod, A., & Hall, N. (2023). Neurodiverse students within higher education: Initial thoughts from a collaborative project. *Good Autism Practice, 24(*2), 13–22. https://www.ingentaconnect.com/content/bild/gap/2023/00000024/00000002/art00004# Sandlin, J. A. (2005). Andragogy and its discontents: An analysis of andragogy from three critical perspectives. *PAACE Journal of Lifelong Learning, 14,* 25–42.

Sarrett, J. C. (2018). Autism and accommodations in higher education: Insights from the autism community. *Journal of Autism and Developmental Disorders, 48*(3), 679–693. https://doi-org.DOI: 10.1007/s10803-017-3353-4

Seelmeyer, L. (2024). Disability and neurodiversity in the academic library: Fostering new and continuing engagement. *Public Services Quarterly, 20*(3), 217–224. https://doi-org.DOI: 10.1080/15228959.2024.2367530

Shepherd, J., Sutton, B., Smith, S., & Szlenkier, M. (2024). 'Sea-glass survivors': Autistic testimonies about education experiences. *British Journal of Special Education, 51*(2), 142–155. https://doi-org.DOI: 10.1111/1467-8578.12506

Sidjaja, F. F. (2024). The growing definition of autism. *International Journal of Disability Development and Education,* •••, 1–7. https://doi-org.libproxy.txstate.edu/10.1080/1034912X.2024.2393382. DOI: 10.1080/1034912X.2024.2393382

Spaeth, E., & Pearson, A. (2023). A reflective analysis on how to promote a positive learning experience for neurodivergent students. *Journal of Perspectives in Applied Academic Practice, 11*(2), 109–120. https://doi-org.DOI: 10.56433/jpaap.v11i2.517

Spain, D., Zıvralı Yarar, E., & Happé, F. (2020). Social anxiety in adults with autism: A qualitative study. *International Journal of Qualitative Studies on Health and Well-being, 15*(1), 1–15. DOI: 10.1080/17482631.2020.1803669 PMID: 32815779

Stockwell, K. M., Bottini, S., Jaswal, V. K., & Gillis, J. M. (2021). Brief report: Social behavior and special interests in the stigmatization of autistic college students. *Journal of Autism & Developmental Disorders, 51*(9), 3356–3364. https://doi-org .DOI: 10.1007/s10803-020-04769-w

Sullivan, J. (2024). Organisational neurotypicalness: Fighting unintentional ableism in working spaces. *Disability & Society, 1–4*. Advance online publication. DOI: 10.1080/09687599.2024.2373769

Taylor, B., & Kroth, M. (2009). Andragogy's transition into the future: Meta-analysis of andragogy and its search for a measurable instrument. *Journal of Adult Education, 38*(1), 1–11. https://eric.ed.gov/?id=EJ891073

Tipton, W., & Wideman, S. (2021). Toward an invitational andragogy: Articulating a teaching philosophy for the andragogic classroom. *Journal of Communication Pedagogy, 5*, 156–163. DOI: 10.31446/JCP.2021.2.16

Trillingsgaard, A. (1999). The script model in relation to autism. *European Child & Adolescent Psychiatry, 8*(1), 45–49. DOI: 10.1007/s007870050082 PMID: 10367740

Vella, J. (2002). *Learning to listen. Learning to teach. The power of dialogue in educating adults* (Revised ed.). Jossey-Bass.

Wells, M. B. (2024). Supporting higher education students with attention deficit hyperactivity disorder through universal design for learning. *College Teaching, 72*(3), 227–230. https://doi-org.DOI: 10.1080/87567555.2022.2160959

Wilson, K., & Dallman, A. (2024). Strategies for promoting neurodiversity and autism acceptance in higher education. *Journal of Diversity in Higher Education*. Advance online publication. DOI: 10.1037/dhe0000550

Wlodkowski, R. J., & Ginsberg, M. B. (2017). *Enhancing adult motivation to learn: A comprehensive guide for teaching all adults* (4th ed.). Jossey-Bass.

Wolbring, G., & Lillywhite, A. (2023). Coverage of allies, allyship and disabled people: A scoping review. *Societies (Basel, Switzerland), 13*(11), 241. DOI: 10.3390/soc13110241

ADDITIONAL READING

CAST. (2024). Universal Design for Learning Guidelines version 3.0. https://udlguidelines.cast.org/

Coryell, J. E., Baumgartner, L., & Bohonos, J. (2024). *Methods for facilitating adult learning: Strategies for enhancing instruction and instructor effectiveness*. Routledge. DOI: 10.4324/9781003446019

Dwyer, P., Mineo, E., Mifsud, K., Lindholm, C., Gurba, A., & Waisman, T. C. (2023). Building neurodiversity-inclusive postsecondary campuses: Recommendations for leaders in higher education. *Autism in Adulthood: Challenges and Management*, *5*(1), 1–14. DOI: 10.1089/aut.2021.0042 PMID: 36941859

Knowles, M. S. (1990). *The adult learner: A neglected species* (4th ed.). Gulf.

Shepherd, J., Sutton, B., Smith, S., & Szlenkier, M. (2024). 'Sea-glass survivors': Autistic testimonies about education experiences. *British Journal of Special Education, 51*(2), 142–155. https://doi-org.DOI: 10.1111/1467-8578.12506

Wlodkowski, R. J., & Ginsberg, M. B. (2017). *Enhancing adult motivation to learn: A comprehensive guide for teaching all adults* (4th ed.). Jossey-Bass.

Chapter 3
Context and Coping Skills:
A (New) Theoretical Approach to Program Development

Simone R. Dufresne
https://orcid.org/0000-0003-2880-7917
Tufts University, USA

Eileen T. Crehan
https://orcid.org/0000-0002-1744-7621
UMass Chan Medical School, USA & Tufts University, USA

ABSTRACT

With the rise in neurodiversity in higher education, it is increasingly important to understand how students are coping within this context. This chapter explores the experiences and support of Neurodivergent students in mainstream higher education through a new application of the theoretical framework Phenomenological Variant of Ecological Systems Theory (PVEST) (Spencer, 2006). College personnel can use PVEST as a framework for examining the impact of students' context and supporting students' development of adaptive coping mechanisms to improve negative outcomes. A successful pilot called "Navigating Tufts for Neurodivergent Students," developed with PVEST in mind, is presented as an example of a collaborative campus support program with recommendations for adaptation. This chapter provides readers with an understanding of how the PVEST model has been and could be applied to shape programs. Lessons learned from the example program will empower readers to utilize similar participatory approaches to design collaborative, affirming, and practical programming in other academic settings.

DOI: 10.4018/979-8-3693-8920-1.ch003

INTRODUCTION

As discussed throughout this book, Neurodivergent students are increasingly enrolling in mainstream colleges and universities (Bakker et al., 2019; Cox et al., 2017; Dwyer et al., 2023) but report that they are not receiving adequate support on campus (Dexter et al., 2024; Newman et al., 2019). In this chapter, the terms "higher education," "college," and "university," are used interchangeably. This practice reflects colloquial understanding in the United States that all terms are describing a setting/ time period in which young people, most often ages 18-22, elect to continue their education to earn an advanced degree such as a Bachelor of Arts or Science. Despite an increased presence, approximately 20% fewer Neurodivergent students complete their college degree than neuromajority students (DuPaul et al., 2018; Dwyer et al., 2023; National Center for Education Statistics [NCES], 2017; Newman et al., 2019; UC Academic Senate, 2021). Students must navigate through many complex systems to get the support they need, but often these processes are arranged in a way that is not conducive to Neurodivergent students' success (Clouder et al., 2020; Coghill & Coghill, 2020). This is particularly true at high-ranking "elite" institutions where supports are sparse (Nachman, 2020). More neurodiversity-friendly systems, such as access to information curated specifically for Neurodivergent students, would likely improve the navigability of four-year college campuses and could improve the feeling of connection to campus for Neurodivergent students (Butcher & Lane, 2024).

One promising framework that could serve as a foundation for services that improve the college experience is the Phenomenological Variant of Ecological Systems Theory (PVEST; Spencer, 2006). PVEST examines how individuals, based on their context and experience of this context, develop short-term and long-term coping mechanisms that lead to stage-specific outcomes. Centering the experience of Neurodivergent students is at the core of this approach. PVEST also accounts for the effects of others' involvement on the individual, highlighting the responsibility of faculty and staff in higher education to support the needs of students in ways that are conducive to their optimal functioning.

In this chapter, we will discuss how college personnel can use PVEST as a framework for examining the impact of students' context (i.e., risk and protective factors) and supporting students' development of adaptive coping mechanisms to improve negative outcomes. A successful pilot program called "Navigating Tufts for Neurodivergent Students," developed with PVEST in mind, will be presented as an example with recommendations for adaptation. This chapter will provide readers with an understanding of how the PVEST model has been and could be applied to shape programs. Lessons learned from the example program will empower readers to utilize similar participatory approaches to design collaborative, affirming, and practical programming in other academic settings. This chapter is based largely on the PhD dissertation of our first author, Dr. Simone Dufresne (Dufresne, 2024). Some content is replicated exactly from the previous work; this work has not been published elsewhere but is available in its entirety via ProQuest Dissertations & Theses Global (Dissertation number: 31239840) and the Tufts University Digital Library (ID: n583z8516).

PVEST APPLICATIONS FOR NEURODIVERSITY IN HIGHER EDUCATION

With the rise in neurodiversity on college campuses, it has become increasingly important to understand how Neurodivergent students are experiencing and coping within this developmental context, particularly in areas such as academics, social life, and independence (Flegenheimer & Scherf, 2022; Lei et al., 2020). To frame these experiences, we propose a new application of the Phenomenological Variant of Ecological Systems Theory (PVEST) (See Figure 1), developed by Margaret Beale Spencer (2006) as a model for the development of marginalized youth who have been historically overlooked in developmental theories. PVEST examines an individual's development through their objective context (*net vulnerability*), experience of this context (*net stress*), acute coping mechanisms and problem-solving strategies (*reactive coping processes*), long term coping strategies (*stable coping responses and emergent identities*), and *stage-specific coping outcomes* (Spencer, 2006).

Figure 1. Phenomenological Variant of Ecological Systems Theory

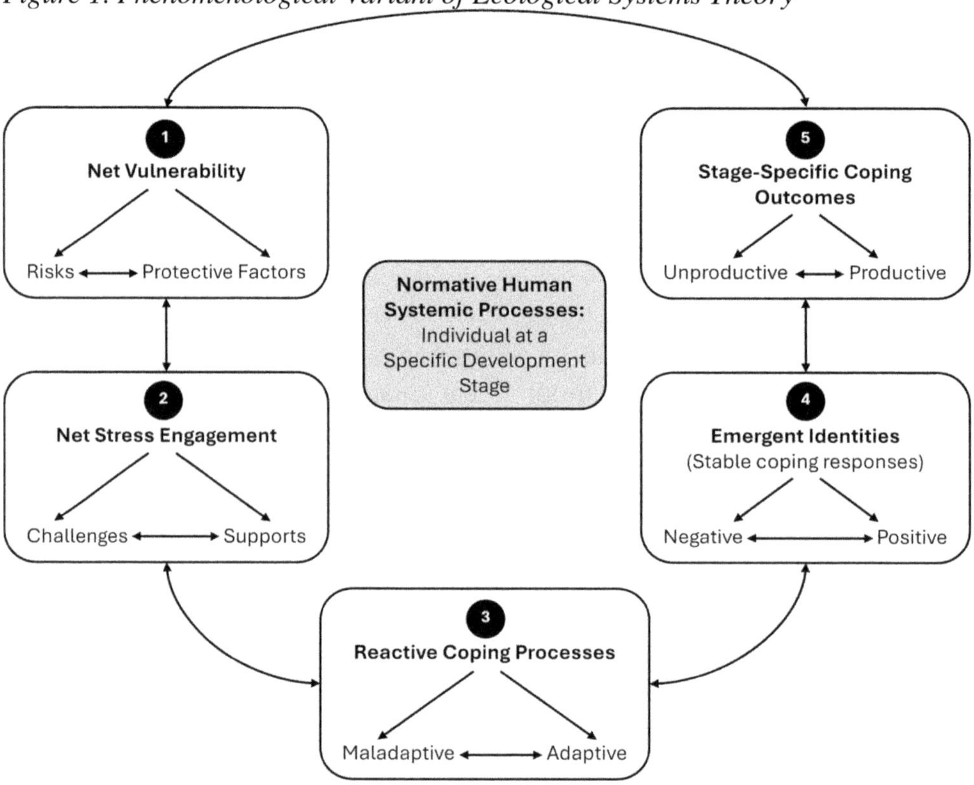

Note. This figure was adapted from Spencer's work on the development of diverse groups (Spencer, 2006, p. 708).

Developmental frameworks can provide a rich context within which to understand systems. Systems theorists such as Bronfenbrenner (1977) have historically brought important insights into how individuals and environments affect each other. Also, as a systems theory, PVEST was originally developed to explore the development of marginalized children of color. Prior developmental theories took a deficit perspective on youth of color and did not take into consideration the effects of specific systemic factors like racism; studies of Neurodivergent students reflect similar shortfalls in the literature (e.g., emphasis on atypical behavior and symptomatology, comparisons to neuromajority "controls," and discounting the impact of ableism on development) (Youngblood II & Spencer, 2002). The application of PVEST offers a strengths-based way to conceptualize how to best support coping for marginalized youth.

PVEST can be a useful framework in research studies to understand specific developmental phenomena (Hope & Spencer, 2017; Morton & Parsons, 2018; Ozaki et al., 2020). In addition to looking at development cyclically, it is also possible to begin examination of a developmental component at any point in the cycle. For example, one could identify a reactive coping process and then look both backward to net stress and forward to stable coping responses to understand why the reactive coping process is happening and whether it is adaptive or maladaptive (Spencer, 2006).

While PVEST has not been systematically used to examine the experiences of Neurodivergent youth in higher education, its components can be applied to existing literature in order to identify knowledge gaps and opportunities for intervention. There is a growing knowledge base of the contextual factors (net vulnerability) and outcomes (stage-specific outcomes) for students generally, and scholars are beginning to explore students' subjective experiences of their context in higher education (net stress). However, there is a gap in knowledge about the resulting coping mechanisms and problem-solving strategies that students use to mitigate stress and improve their outcomes (reactive coping processes and stable coping responses), as well as how they learn about and/or develop these strategies, which this chapter attempts to address.

Higher Education Context

Net vulnerability is determined by assessing the balance of risk and protective factors that an individual experiences in their daily life (Dupree et al., 2015; Spencer, 2006). Risk and protective factors are objective measures of a young person's context based on the environment they are in, with risk factors having a negative influence on an individual and protective factors having a positive influence. Youth with more protective factors than risk factors have lower net vulnerability. Protective factors act as buffers against vulnerability, but often these factors are neither assumed nor explored for marginalized youth when viewing them through a deficit lens (Spencer, 2006).

Like neuromajority students, Neurodivergent students come into higher education with a wide range of backgrounds, experiences, and levels of preparedness (Caldora II & Coghill, 2020). However, because their neurocognitive functioning differs from that of neuromajority students (for whom college learning environments were primarily designed) aspects of their higher education experience can be uniquely challenging (Lawson, 2010). Thus, Neurodivergent students may require adjustments to the college environment to address aspects of their neurodivergence, such as sensory sensitivities, executive functioning challenges, and social difficulties. These difficulties are described further in the section below, "Neurodivergent Students' Personal Experiences of Higher Education."

Areas of accommodation for neurodivergence in higher education can include academic (e.g., extended time on exams, note-taking support), housing (e.g., single rooms or sensory friendly accommodations), nutrition (e.g., specialized diets), and transportation (e.g., door-to-door transportation for co-occurring mobility needs)

(DuPaul et al., 2009; Newman et al., 2019; Sarrett, 2018). Accommodations are highly individualized to the person, and the process of requesting accommodations varies between institutions, but plans are typically determined by disability services offices. Currently, in the U.S., being considered for formal accommodations in a higher education setting requires comprehensive adult psychological testing and documentation from clinical professionals (NCLD, 2023). Although there are some initiatives aimed at making higher education more accessible for students with disabilities (NCLD, 2023), there are no clear timetables for the passage of pending legislation aimed at expanding access.

Outside of disability services offices, institutions' approaches to neurodiversity and disability inclusion vary considerably (Dwyer et al., 2023). Neurodiversity-focused awareness training for higher education professionals, particularly faculty, is limited, not standardized (Clouder et al., 2020; Dwyer et al., 2023), and relies on the institution to see the importance of providing this training. Inclusivity efforts in higher education often do not include disability or accessibility, instead focusing on elements such as race, ethnicity, gender, and sexuality (Scheef et al., 2020). Additionally, supports for Neurodivergent students are often provided in silos and are not centralized or consistent between different campus departments or offices (Clouder et al., 2020). Self-help books, how-to guides, and first-person accounts of navigating higher education as Neurodivergent students are available (e.g., ASAN, 2013; Nadeau, 2006). However, there are few pre-existing curricula designed to support Neurodivergent students before and during their time in higher education that are widely available for U.S. students (see "Attempts to Improve Neurodivergent Student Experience and Outcomes" section below for more information on curriculums).

A lack of centralized recommendations for campuses, hugely variable accommodation offerings for students, and a general misfit of the design of academic and social college environments for neurodivergent profiles constitute vulnerabilities for students. In the absence of critical policy changes, programming developed using the PVEST model will need to account for these vulnerabilities which contribute to challenges navigating college for Neurodivergent students.

Higher Education Outcomes

Life-stage specific coping outcomes are larger-scale productive or unproductive outcomes that shape a young person's future. These outcomes can include things like school performance, employment status, and relationships with others (Spencer, 2006). While Neurodivergent students certainly can be and are successful in a college setting, higher-education outcomes for Neurodivergent students overall are worse than for their neuromajority counterparts. Students with autism and/or ADHD are significantly less likely to both enroll in college and graduate than their neuromajority peers (DuPaul et al., 2018; Shattuck et al., 2012); while precise disparities are difficult to calculate because not all Neurodivergent students are identified by their institutions, studies estimate that graduation rates for Neurodivergent students are approximately 20% lower than those for neuromajority students (National Center for Education Statistics, 2017; Newman et al., 2019; UC Academic Senate, 2021). Neurodivergent students also tend to have more academic challenges such as failed classes and lower grade point averages (DuPaul et al., 2021; McLeod et al., 2019). Although postsecondary enrollment rates of students with learning disabilities have been increasing over the past few decades, completion rates have remained relatively stagnant (Newman et al., 2010, 2019).

Additionally, individual challenges that Neurodivergent students may experience in higher education (e.g., executive dysfunction, social challenges) can lead to burnout, reduced capacity for engagement in courses and social life, higher interpersonal conflict, lower academic achievement, and higher drop-out rates than for neuromajority peers (DuPaul et al., 2018; Hamilton & Petty, 2023; Irvine & MacLeod, 2022; Newman et al., 2019). Importantly, these negative outcomes can further exacerbate negative physical and mental health conditions, including increased risk of anxiety, depression, and suicide (Aguilar & Lipson, 2021; McLeod et al., 2019; Rosenau et al., 2023). As students learn more or less productive strategies to navigate the developmental process of "being in college," programming that at least offers opportunities relating to mental health and skill building can help move Neurodivergent students through to the next stage and into independent adulthood.

Neurodivergent Students' Personal Experiences of Higher Education

Net stress engagement is a young person's own assessment of support and challenge in their life, or how they perceive and experience their context (Dupree et al., 2015). This component is where phenomenology, or the examination of an individual's experience, such as of an event, or context, is incorporated, as net stress is determined based on how the youth feels about their circumstances. What one young person feels is a large challenge in their life could feel like less of a challenge for someone else who either experiences that challenge less acutely or feels more supported in meeting that challenge. Experiences of challenge and support can also be influenced by society, in that how an individual's surrounding community perceives the person's circumstances can impact the individual's own perception (Spencer, 2006).

Despite being at higher risk for negative outcomes, many Neurodivergent students find higher education to be a positive setting where they can find other people with similar interests, focus on academic subjects and coursework that they find interesting, and learn valuable skills for future employment and personal success (Anderson et al., 2017; Armstrong, 2010; Irvine & MacLeod, 2022). In order to feel successful, however, Neurodivergent students have needs that may or may not be different (or accessed differently) from their neuromajority peers.

In their qualitative study with 48 Autistic college students across four US universities, Accardo and colleagues (2019) found that students discussed three factors that they felt helped them to achieve success in higher education: developing a social network, using self-determination and executive functioning skills, and engaging in self-advocacy for the accommodations and support services that they needed. While many of these elements are similar for neuromajority students, Neurodivergent students often have added barriers to success. For example, students must initiate the accommodations process for themselves, which requires self-awareness and advocacy, as well as the executive functioning to sequence and follow through on complex processes (Dexter et al., 2024; Hamilton & Petty, 2023; Newman et al., 2019). Additionally, Neurodivergent students often report higher levels of loneliness and isolation than their neuromajority peers (Gelbar et al., 2015; Jobe & Williams White, 2007; Stice & Lavner, 2019). Connecting with others with diverse neurotypes can be difficult due to concerns about social rejection and stigma, a lack of support in building relationships, and sensory sensitivities that can make it difficult to be in busy public spaces where students gather (e.g., dining halls, open student centers, and parties) (Anderson et al., 2017; Flegenheimer & Scherf, 2022; Gelbar et al., 2015).

Many processes and protocols for how to be successful in college are part of the "hidden curriculum," which refers to the unspoken, often implicit rules or practices that individuals are expected to intuit or learn from their context (Jackson, 1968). Information about the administrative processes of higher education and available services is not always communicated in ways that are accessible to Neurodivergent students (Anderson et al., 2017; Berg et al., 2017; Sarrett, 2018). As such, Neurodivergent students may or may not know about these resources, if they exist at all (Clouder et al., 2020; Coghill & Coghill, 2020). Additionally, students are required to self-disclose their neurodivergence to access many services in college. Disclosure can be met with stigma and a lack of acceptance, which may lead students to conceal their identities and forgo support altogether (Dwyer et al., 2023; Gillespie-Lynch et al., 2021; Newman et al., 2019; Thompson & Lefler, 2016). This process of gathering information piecemeal is seemingly at odds with some core experiences of neurodivergence (Clouder et al., 2020; Hamilton & Petty, 2023). There is a significant need for supports to navigate a murky accessibility services system, but this is a not a resource that receives enough financial support on most campuses (Chiwandire & Vincent, 2019). Peer learning holds tremendous potential as a way for more senior students who know the particulars of their own college campus and have paved their own successful path with or without institutional support to pass that information along to students earlier in their college careers (Hillier et al., 2019).

Attempts to Improve Neurodivergent Student Experience and Outcomes

Reactive coping processes describes the specific self-regulation coping mechanisms that youth use in the moment to respond to challenges (Dupree et al., 2015), which can be adaptive or maladaptive depending on their impact on the youth's circumstances. Coping processes are used in response to acute stressors, such as isolation or withdrawal (maladaptive) or seeking out support (adaptive) (Steinberg, 2022). These coping strategies work reciprocally with *net stress*, as "adaptive coping strategies can mitigate stress experienced and maladaptive coping strategies can exacerbate stress experienced" (Dupree et al., 2015).

Reactive coping mechanisms lead to *stable coping responses*, which are "general and redundant coping processes, [that develop as a] response to pervasive and consistent exposure" (Dupree et al., 2015), and the subsequent sense of self that youth develop after adopting these long-term coping strategies. As youth test out their reactive coping strategies, they see which strategies produce an outcome that mitigates stress. Stable coping strategies can be negative or positive, again depending on how they impact the youth's circumstances. Identity formation begins as a result of these stable coping strategies; young people begin to internalize how they consistently respond to their context and stressors, which then further influences how they think about and respond to their circumstances based on whether these responses fit within their developing concept of their identity, and their responses become more automatic (Dupree et al., 2015).

Despite significant room for more support, there are some programs that reflect the needs of Neurodivergent students specifically in developing and using reactive and stable coping mechanisms. To address both individual and systemic challenges, there is a growing movement to implement more comprehensive support for Neurodivergent students in many educational settings. In the United Kingdom, students may receive Specialist Mentoring services through their government-funded Disabled Students Allowance; these services support Autistic and otherwise Neurodivergent students and students with other mental health needs (Lucas & James, 2018). The Autism and Uni Project, which has been adopted by at least 15 universities in the UK, Ireland, Poland, and Switzerland, provides a free toolkit that universities can populate with information about their own resources and supports for Autistic students to access (Fabri et al., 2016).

In the United States, many individual institutions are implementing programs, such as the Peer to Peer (Hillier et al., 2019) and Horizons Plus mentoring programs at the University of Massachusetts Lowell and the Mentoring, Organization, and Social Support for Autism/All Inclusion on Campus (MOSSAIC) program (Locke et al., 2023) at the University of Montana. Unfortunately, as Nachman and colleagues (2022) found in their search for autism-specific college support programs at U.S. colleges and universities, only 74 of these programs exist, representing 2.2% of higher education institutions. Additionally, only about a quarter of these programs exist at private institutions and very few at competitive "elite" institutions (e.g., colleges and universities highly ranked by entities such as *US News and World Report* and *Forbes*) (Nachman et al., 2022). Colleges and universities in the Northeast in particular, of which there are many, are overall lacking in specific programming for Neurodivergent students (College Autism Network, n.d.; Crehan et al., in preparation). Thus, there is a sizable gap in support and ample opportunity for program development.

THE "NAVIGATING TUFTS FOR NEURODIVERGENT STUDENTS" WORKSHOP SERIES

In light of the growing body of evidence on Neurodivergent student needs in higher education, particularly in high-ranking private institutions, we developed and piloted a program informed by PVEST and Neurodivergent students on our own private college campus during the 2023-24 academic year. It is important to note that this program was conceived of and carried out primarily by the first author in service of her doctoral dissertation (Dufresne, 2024), with the second author serving as faculty mentor. Creating this program as part of a dissertation allowed for many unique opportunities (e.g., collaborative design, more flexible inclusion criteria for participants, mixed methods evaluation, low cost to the university) while resulting in some challenges (e.g., that the program was dependent on an individual facilitator instead of embedded in a university system and thus was not guaranteed longevity).

These workshops were designed to foster students' coping and problem-solving skills (both reactive and stable, per the PVEST model) by providing specific, targeted, and accessible information that students may want or need to be successful in college. While there is much work to be done on a systemic level to make higher education institutions more accessible to Neurodivergent students, current students are looking for support and resources now in order to engage optimally with their college experience. We developed and piloted this program at Tufts University, with the idea that the framework could be adapted for other colleges and universities where programming is limited. Collaborative and consultative models of participation were used during the process of designing and implementing the program. Throughout the process, we sought to understand whether the workshops had any perceived impact on how the participants approach their time in higher education

– in particular, whether the workshops taught or reinforced any potential coping strategies for students, from their perspectives. We present our findings here to help readers learn from our experience and encourage them to build similar programming in their own institutions.

Program Setting

Tufts University ("Tufts") is a private research university in the northeast United States. In 2025, *US News & World Report* ranked Tufts at #37 on their lists of undergraduate universities in the country (*US News & World Report*, 2025), and the acceptance rate for the class of 2029 was 10.5% (Eng & Onysko, 2025). In 2023, 11.5% of first-year and 9.6% of sophomore students identified as Neurodivergent according to large-scale surveys conducted by the University's Office of Institutional Research (Tufts OIR, 2023a, 2023b). For context, the response rate for the first-year survey was 607, 36.43% of the first-year student body, and the response rate for the sophomore survey was 551, 31.31% of the sophomore student body.

At Tufts, Neurodivergent students can receive disability-related support from two main entities: the accessibility center and student organizations (one group specifically for Neurodivergent students, a general disability organization, and an LGBTQ+ disability group). These organizations provide spaces for students with disabilities to connect with each other, form community, and engage in activism on campus. Tufts also offers a Neurodiverse House, which is special-interest housing for Neurodivergent students. Additionally, there are numerous identity-specific centers across campus where students seek support; however, there is currently no disability-specific identity or cultural center where programming and resources are centralized. Moreover, some Neurodivergent students choose not to engage in any disability-specific services or identity spaces. Although we do not have any specific data on why some Tufts students do not engage in services, a systematic review by Anderson and colleagues (2017) found that ineligibility (e.g., because of a lack of a clinical diagnosis), being unaware of available services and supports, and concerns about stigma are common factors.

Pre-Program Planning

Approximately one and a half years before beginning the workshop development process, our research lab, accessibility center, and Neurodivergent student group held a campus-wide informal needs assessment with students and faculty/staff on neurodiversity issues on campus. At this event, participants described their experience with neurodiversity at Tufts and made recommendations for future programming and support (Aladin et al., 2022). Identified priorities included: 1. improving accessibility of the housing process (e.g., better guidance on accessing housing accommodations and navigating independent living both on and off campus); 2. more streamlined sources of information (e.g., a directory) that would point students toward the most relevant neurodiversity-related information; 3. point-people (e.g., advocates or mentors) who could support students across multiple areas of student life; 4. increased support and resources for students dealing with substance use; 5. more comprehensive orientation programming; and 6. workshops for students on topics like self-advocacy (Aladin et al., 2022). These findings informed the beginnings of the workshop design.

Workshop Development

The first step in developing the workshop series was the creation of a project advisory board of current Neurodivergent Tufts students. Because the workshop series was for the Tufts Neurodivergent community, it was essential that members of this community were involved in the creation and evaluation of the workshops (Fletcher-Watson et al., 2019; Wright et al., 2021). An advisory board was incorporated at the start of the project to ensure that the workshops themselves were addressing topics that were of genuine interest to the Tufts Neurodivergent community and that the workshops were formatted and facilitated in a way that was appropriate and accessible. The advisory board consisted of four Tufts undergraduate students who identify as Neurodivergent (e.g., having a diagnosis of autism, ADHD, learning disabilities, and/or Tourette Syndrome). Advisory board members were recruited through Tufts neurodiversity and disability-focused student groups and were a mix of clinically diagnosed and self-identifying. We felt that this representation was necessary to ensure that the program was relevant for the widest array of students.

Advisory board members participated in four virtual advising activities during the summer before the workshop series, each lasting one hour (Table 1). According to the principles outlined by Wallerstein and colleagues (2018), we took a community-engaged approach at the consultation level. As the PI and faculty advisor, we brought the idea of the workshop series and topic ideas from the Tufts-specific informal needs assessment and review of the broader literature to the advisory board initially. We also largely wrote or adapted the activities (e.g., self-advocacy scenarios for group discussion) based on the ideas and feedback from advisory board members, as well as developed the evaluation plan and measures (survey and interview questions) following guidelines from PVEST (Spencer, 2006) and the British Medical Research Council (Skivington et al., 2021). Advisory board members independently reviewed the activities and evaluation plan between meetings.

Table 1. Advising activities

Activity	Topic/Purpose
Meeting 1	Development of workshop topics and structure, identification of campus partners
Meeting 2	Group review of draft of workshop curriculum
Meeting 3	Group review of draft of workshop curriculum
Independent Work	Review/feedback of final workshop materials and evaluation tools (surveys and interview questions)
Meeting 4	Post-workshop debrief and review of participant feedback/interview results

Note. The structure and overall content of the workshops were co-developed with the board during advisory board meetings, including the order of topics, which campus partners to invite in based on these topics (e.g., the accessibility and counseling centers, student life, and residential life), and the types of activities.

After the workshop series and evaluation were completed, a final meeting was held for both advisory board members and workshop participants. The purpose of this meeting was to share the results of the evaluation for data-checking and community interpretation, discuss questions that came up during the course of the project, and gather any additional feedback about the process of participating in the program.

Running the Workshop

Participants

Students were eligible to participate if they identified as Neurodivergent, were a Tufts student, and were able to attend the sessions in-person. The definition of "neurodivergent" was kept intentionally vague (i.e., no specific definition or diagnoses were included in the recruitment materials) to be inclusive of different interpretations of neurodivergence, and participants could be clinically diagnosed or self-identify as neurodivergent. We recommend this approach, as about half of our participants did not have a formal diagnosis or were in the process of being assessed. These students described challenges consistent with the clinically diagnosed students but were not able to access formal accommodations at our institution, so having access to this workshop series helped to bridge that gap in support. Research has shown support for the utility of self-identification for neurodivergence (particularly autism) in contexts like ours (Ardeleanu et al., 2024; Lewis, 2016b, 2016a; Overton et al., 2024; Sturm et al., 2024), and we feel confident that the effects of the workshop were largely consistent between self-identified and clinically diagnosed participants. Although the workshop series was primarily aimed at undergraduate students, graduate students were welcome. Advisory board members were also able to participate in the workshops if they chose but were not required to do so. A multi-faceted recruitment approach was used, including lab social media, flyers, campus groups, and information to large introductory classes on campus. In our pilot, fifteen students registered in advance for the series, nine individual students participated across all sessions, and sessions had an average of four participants in attendance.

Workshop Structure and Curriculum

Five weekly workshop sessions were conducted in person during the fall semester. Each session lasted two hours and took place in the afternoon, in the same location each time. Varied times were offered to accommodate varying student schedules. Participants were asked to register in advance (though drop-ins were welcomed), sign an online consent form for their participation in the research project, and complete pre-surveys on demographics and goals for the workshops. Participants were encouraged to attend all sessions, but they did not need to attend all sessions to participate in the series. This decision was made to maximize attendance at individual sessions to ensure that as many people were able to receive the information as possible, and so that students were not discouraged from attending if they had to miss a session.

Components of each session were meant to fit within the PVEST framework. For instance, to minimize risk factors and increase protective factors (net vulnerability), tailored, neurodiversity-informed information directly from institutional representatives and campus partners was incorporated in the form of speakers or visual summaries of processes. Direct skills practice using evidence-based methods was used in relation to stage-specific outcomes, and integrating student groups and perspectives was meant to improve access to reactive coping processes. Specific details about workshop components can be found in Table 2.

Table 2. Overview of workshop series curriculum

Workshop 1: Self-advocacy & disclosure	
Guest Speaker	Master's student & Autistic self-advocate
Activity	Self-advocacy scenarios (group discussion)
Self-Reflection	Disclosure worksheet
Workshop 2: Accessing formal accommodations	
Campus Partner	Associate Dean of Student Accessibility and Academic Resources
Self-Reflection	Accommodations worksheet
Workshop 3: Social life & campus community	

continued on following page

Table 2. Continued

Campus Partners	Representatives from Tufts student organizations: Diverse Minds, Disability Student Coalition, Disability Queers, Tufts Sex Health Reps, Trans and Nonbinary Group (TANG), Tufts Tabletop Club (tabletop gaming), Tufts Anime Brigade, Torn Ticket II & 3Ps (student theater groups), LCS Tutoring, and Laidlaw Scholars (student research and leadership program)
Activity	Neurodiversity on campus (group discussion)
Workshop 4: Executive functioning & self-care	
Campus Partner	Senior Associate Director of Academic Support
Campus Partner	Staff Clinician, Counseling and Mental Health Services
Self-Reflection	Situational stress test worksheet
Workshop 5: Housing & living on your own	
Self-Reflection	Housing survey
Activity	Housing scenarios (group discussion)

Note. Participants rated their satisfaction with and the usefulness of each session both quantitatively and qualitatively. Full results can be found in Dufresne (2024).

Key Themes

Self-Help and Skill-Building

One of the key components of our program, identified by participants as highly impactful, was introducing information and resources that could be used as reactive and stable coping mechanisms, addressing key components of PVEST. Session 3 involved presentations from a number of student organizations, both disability/neurodiversity-focused and hobby/academic clubs. Many colleges and universities (including Tufts) hold a student organization or club fair in the fall semester, which can be helpful for many students in that it provides an opportunity to see all of the options available and talk directly with students in those clubs. However, for Neurodivergent students, these large events can be loud and crowded, leading to social and/or sensory overwhelm. Introducing students to available groups and helping them connect with the relevant student leaders in a relaxed and comfortable setting can be more effective. In our case, one student ended up joining a new student organization because this group had presented during the workshop.

Session 4 on Executive Functioning & Self Care was overall the most popular workshop in the series, in terms of attendance, satisfaction ratings, and perceived impact. To plan the session, we collaborated with staff in the academic resource and counseling centers who focus on neurodiversity-specific strategies and support in their work with students. These campus partners engaged participants in discussions about the session's topics and provided examples of concrete resources, strategies, and tools that they could use in their daily lives. Executive functioning is a common area of challenge for students across the Neurodivergent spectrum (Dijkhuis et al., 2020; Southon, 2022), and because Neurodivergent students experience higher levels of stress, anxiety, and burnout (DuPaul et al., 2018; Irvine & MacLeod, 2022; Newman et al., 2019), it follows that learning self-care strategies would be seen as highly impactful to students' wellbeing.

What these sessions did was introduce resources at Tufts (student groups, academic coaching, counseling services) that participants may not have known about or not known how to access before attending. Learning about available resources and navigating complex or confusing university systems to access them is often challenging for Neurodivergent students (Butcher & Lane, 2024; Cox et al., 2021; Dwyer et al., 2023; Newman et al., 2019). By bringing student leaders and campus professionals into a neutral space, however, the tools and information presented can feel more approachable, and students may be more likely to utilize these resources in the future. This more personalized navigation-type support at other institutions has been shown to be effective at increasing students' confidence and capacity through mechanisms like mentoring programs and coaching (Hillier et al., 2019; Locke et al., 2023; Lucas & James, 2018; Rando et al., 2016). Ideally, knowing more about where to look for support will help students make better use of available resources more consistently, feel more supported in their own context, and develop stronger coping mechanisms that can help them be more successful in the long run.

However, the goal of introducing information and resources that could be used as coping processes was not easily achieved in all sessions, which leaves room for future improvement. Specifically, our session on Self-Advocacy & Disclosure was seen by students as less successful, largely due to the lack of concrete strategies and resources. These topics are crucial for Neurodivergent students' success (Caldora II & Coghill, 2020; Cox et al., 2017), and as such are often part of support programs (Gillespie-Lynch et al., 2021; Hotez et al., 2018; Locke et al., 2023), but it is important to consider how these conversations are happening and with whom. Every individual's comfort with decisions around disclosure and self-advocacy are personal; looking at this topic through a PVEST lens, participants' phenomenological experiences of their context (i.e., their different experiences with disclosing in the past) would impact their responses (whether and how to disclose) moving forward. Neurodifferences are still met with stigma and prejudice on college campuses (Clouder et al., 2020; Evans et al., 2023; Gillespie-Lynch et al., 2021; Thompson & Lefler, 2016), and as such, students are not always willing to disclose or to engage in self-advocacy.

To avoid seeming like we were pressuring students into doing something they were not ready to do, our session did not contain much "advice," but instead provided opportunities for participants to share experiences and ideas with each other. Participants reported enjoying the discussions and hearing from the guest speaker, a Neurodivergent graduate student who spoke about her own experiences with the topics and answered questions; however, they specifically mentioned wanting more concrete strategies for approaching self-advocacy and disclosure, particularly ways to respond to others' negative reactions to disclosure.

For future iterations or adaptations, it would be important to prioritize sharing more strategies that are neurodiversity-affirming and reasonable to expect of students. This could be accomplished in a few different ways. One would be to adopt a tool like Han and colleagues' (2024) disclosure intervention which was designed to reduce participants' feelings of stigmatization by empowering them to make disclosure-related decisions. Another could be to expand the guest speaker component to be more of a panel; collaborating with more Neurodivergent students (e.g., previous workshop participants) and Neurodivergent faculty and/or staff at the institution who could offer a more diverse array of perspectives and advice from personal experience. Additionally, while our office of equal opportunity elected to send written resources for students and remain available for individual consultations, collaborations with representatives from this or other similar offices (e.g., human resources) at other institutions may be good options for developing workshop content.

A Space for Neurodivergent Students and Connecting with Others

Something that was achieved more equally across all sessions was providing the participants a space specifically for Neurodivergent students to connect with each other, learn together, and share information and advice, which presented another opportunity for coping skill development. One intentional choice we made in developing the series was advertising it as a support for "Neurodivergent students" without including a specific definition of the term. We recommend using the term "Neurodivergent" as opposed to any specific diagnoses because some people find it easier to publicly identify as Neurodivergent than a particular diagnostic label, as "Neurodivergent" can feel like more of an identity than a clinical term (Beck, 2023). This way, students do not have to disclose their specific Neurodivergent presentation to others in the group in order to attend the workshop series, as neurodivergence, while part of someone's identity, is often based on a private medical diagnosis. It is important to protect the participants' privacy and comfort in the group, as concerns about stigma have been shown to contribute to less disclosure and engagement with support (Clouder et al., 2020; Evans et al., 2023; Van Hees et al., 2015). This practice can help to honor and mitigate students' net stress, as it is sensitive to different students' experiences and perspectives. Additionally, because services in higher education are often limited to those who have a clinical diagnosis

(NCLD, 2023), opening up programming to anyone who identifies as Neurodivergent allows universities to serve students who may not be able to access other supports; in our program, almost half of the participants were not clinically diagnosed but still discussed positive impacts.

We found that the use of "Neurodivergent" specifically was a motivating factor for some attendees. During the post-series debrief, participants shared that they appreciated the use of this particular term because the target audience of the workshop series was clear. Using a current, affirming term can increase participants' confidence that a workshop series designed for Neurodivergent students might have tips and strategies that are designed for their Neurodivergent brains, as opposed to workshops and information sessions that try to appeal to a more general (and often neuromajority) audience. For example, neurodiversity-informed support should include providing different methods of information delivery and focusing on the root causes of neurodivergence-related challenges instead of only surface level behaviors (Hamilton & Petty, 2023; Stowers, 2022). The use of "Neurodivergent" can also indicate that the person running this series is aware of and oriented toward neurodiversity frameworks and is more likely to be strengths-based than deficit-focused (den Houting, 2019; Naylor, 2023), as long as practitioners do the work to actually incorporate these frameworks.

In their motivations for participating in the workshop series, many participants also mentioned wanting to connect with other Neurodivergent students. Considering that Neurodivergent students often find socializing and creating community more difficult than neuromajority students (Flegenheimer & Scherf, 2022; Reeble et al., 2023) despite wanting to do so, creating opportunities for students to connect with each other through programming is an important factor. Spending time with other Neurodivergent people can provide a sense of understanding and comfort unique from spending time with neuromajority people (Crompton et al., 2020; McKee, 2017), as these spaces can reduce the need to mask Neurodivergent traits and allow people to engage as their more authentic selves.

Research with other minoritized groups has shown that affinity spaces can provide buffering effects against negative societal reactions (Salusky et al., 2022; Woo et al., 2019). In the higher education space, spending time in cultural or identity centers can increase students' sense of belonging and success on campus (Patton, 2023). In the absence of centralized communities like disability cultural centers, which have been shown to be effective at other institutions (Elmore et al., 2018), programming like this workshop series can help to fill in gaps by providing a space for Neurodivergent students to gather, introducing them to other opportunities for connection, and offering supportive contexts. These outcomes have also been observed in other similar programs (Brownlow et al., 2023; Gillespie-Lynch et al., 2017; Hotez et al., 2018).

PILOT PROGRAM LESSONS LEARNED & CONSIDERATIONS FOR FUTURE PROGRAMMING

While there were many positive results from the workshop series, running this pilot program was not without its challenges, which we want to be transparent about in the hopes that others may be able to address these challenges.

Workshop Format, Recruitment, and Retention

Retention was difficult for both the advisory board and workshop sessions. While many students were initially interested in being involved in the project, the actual participation rates did not match this initial enthusiasm. We found that despite publishing the workshop dates and times in advance, offering incentives, and seeking out advisory board members' availability before meetings, on average only about 50% of students who registered actually attended the program, and two advisory board members were lost to follow-up after the second meeting. While it is unclear from the literature whether retention is a universal challenge in programming for Neurodivergent students, students in settings like Tufts are extremely busy, have many options for how to spend their non-academic time, and are often overcommitted (Adam, 2021; Hilton, 2023). Thus, considering ways to make programming optimally accessible is key to success.

There are a few pieces to consider when attempting to maximize accessibility for busy students: location, modality, and format. As we discovered, the location of the workshops was an important design component that had a large impact on student satisfaction with the program. For us, the building where the workshop was held was somewhat on the outskirts of campus, and students consistently described this as less than satisfactory. Our students shared that they were looking for something more convenient, and the location may have impacted other students' willingness to attend the program. Others seeking to implement this type of programming should consider areas where students tend to gather and opportunities for collaboration with staff at those locations; running programs in student centers, libraries, popular academic buildings, and even dorms that are central and easily accessible may help to increase attendance.

Additionally, while the students who attended our program enjoyed the in-person format, future iterations of this workshop series could also experiment with an online or asynchronous modality to increase accessibility. Delivering online or asynchronous interventions have had mixed results; some participants prefer to work independently at their own pace (Han et al., 2024) and online delivery reduces access burdens of scheduling and travel to an in-person location (Crane et al., 2023), but engagement and satisfaction can be lower (Brownlow et al., 2023;

White et al., 2016). However, this may prove to be a more feasible option for busy college students. Working with partners in education or information technology to incorporate best practices for online and hybrid learning could make these formats maximally accessible and engaging for learners.

It also may be beneficial to explore other formats for the workshop series to find the optimal form of service delivery; some alternatives could include orientation programs or a for-credit course, both of which would establish a cohort model that could help to build relationships, foster accountability, and improve retention. Orientation program staff would likely have valuable input on establishing strong inter-group connections, and faculty who teach required skill-building courses (e.g., department-specific professional seminars) could advise on maximizing engagement in required courses. While our board liked those format ideas, they thought that other programming should not replace but augment the current model of drop-in sessions on specific topics for students to pick-and-choose what would be most relevant to them. Valuing topic choice has been shared in other literature on support programs for Neurodivergent higher education students (Brownlow et al., 2023), which speaks to the importance of recognizing and considering phenomenology in the development and provision of programming. Because every student will approach and engage with supports differently based on their own context and experience, including as much choice as possible is key for continued feasibility and acceptability of programming. This experience reflects students' stage-specific coping outcomes and allows room for students at different stages of their developmental journey through college to engage when they might want to. Given our low attendance rates and small group numbers, diversifying the instructional methods and intervention construction may prove fruitful and could be studied with a comparative design, similar to work by Brownlow and colleagues (2023) and Crane and colleagues (2023). Consulting with faculty and staff from college/university centers for teaching and learning could help to adapt programming optimally for the home university, whereas collaborating with national groups such as the Neurodiversity Network or College Autism Network could allow for the sharing of best practices across institutions.

The Importance and Challenges of Student Engagement in Program Development

In general, Neurodivergent individuals are part of a marginalized group who have received many interventions not co-created with members of the community, leading to questions about relevance and social validity of the interventions (Fletcher-Watson et al., 2019; Raymaker & Nicolaidis, 2013; Wright et al., 2021). While there is a growing body of participatory intervention research being done with the Neurodivergent community (Brown et al., 2016; Brownlow et al., 2023; Crane et al., 2021; Han et al., 2024; Hotez et al., 2018), doing this work with college students requires a particular sensitivity to students' capacity, especially given the previous discussion of student overcommitment. Additionally, Neurodivergent students are already having to fight for services and support on campus (Dwyer et al., 2023; Kuder et al., 2021), when they should be able to spend their time accessing the full college experience. As one of our participants put it:

> *One thing that a lot of universities, schools focus on is, like, self-advocacy, and it's putting the work on the person, and that's very exhausting. And I feel like I've had to do that my whole life, and it's frustrating, it's challenging, and it takes a lot of effort and extra work, and I already have to do more work than other people just to be at the same level... I think one thing would be shifting the focus from advocating for yourself to, 'How can we support you? What can we do for you?' I feel like that's not really done enough, really anywhere...*

As such, asking or expecting students to take on the heavy lifting of creating and running programming for themselves and others is unfair, particularly when they are asking for more from their institutions. At the same time, being prescriptive in telling students what we think they need without verifying this with actual students is not how we believe programming should be run. When we set out to create our program, we realized that we needed input from our Neurodivergent students to ensure that the program was designed properly and to get maximum buy-in from the student body (Brownlow et al., 2023; Dwyer et al., 2023; Gillespie-Lynch et al., 2017). Our initial plan was for co-creation, wherein the board and researchers contribute equally (or close to equally) to the development of the materials (Brandsen & Honingh, 2018). However, as the process commenced, engagement of the advisory board was lower than anticipated, so co-creation was not feasible; consultation would be a more appropriate description of our board's involvement (Keating, 2021).

In our case, we found limitations in our budget and timeline that may be alleviated in other contexts and allow for more co-creation. The Tufts project timeline was relatively short, with a few months dedicated to developing the materials and running the workshop series, and the benefit of a pre-existing needs assessment. Depending on the available staffing to run such a project, careful co-creation, refinement, implementation, and evaluation could be better achieved with a yearlong process. Budget considerations are also particularly important to consider when determining student input and the demand placed on advisory board members; if financial compensation for their time and expertise is not feasible, some campuses may be able to offer independent study credit, applied experience hours, or other professional experience documentation as a potential benefit. It is particularly important to avoid asking the board to work additional time without compensation, as it is often the case that marginalized individuals are asked or expected to take on unpaid work in advocacy and research to support their communities (Black et al.,

2013; Dwyer et al., 2023; Fundación Indígena [FSI] & Kothari, 2008). In our case, because our program was the basis of a PhD dissertation (Dufresne, 2024) and was not run by a campus office, we had minimal budgetary support; the entire program, including guest speaker fees and compensation for research activities, cost just over $1000. As such, we had limitations to how much we expected our advisory board to work to ensure they were properly compensated for their time.

These factors (budget, timeline, and collaborators' capacity) are consistent with challenges to participatory research with Neurodivergent populations found in the literature (den Houting et al., 2021; Fletcher-Watson et al., 2019), so it is particularly important for program developers to proactively address them. One suggestion is to offer advisors an additional hourly rate (or course credit, applied experience hours, etc.) for ongoing writing and editing of materials in replacement of or in addition to advisory board meetings. This method has been seen in other studies (Brownlow et al., 2023; Han et al., 2024) and could allow for the advisory board members to have more say when changes inevitably need to be made mid-program.

Collaboration Across Campus: Considerations for Partnerships

One surprising finding from our experience creating this program was the variation in responses from different campus departments, which speaks to the contextual factors (net vulnerability) that students are experiencing. As mentioned earlier, Tufts does not have a disability-specific identity center and most of the accessibility center's work is focused on providing accommodations and academic support for students, so there is no centralized entity directing programming for Neurodivergent students. As such, we carefully considered which campus departments would be most important to collaborate with, and these decisions were supported by our advisory board. Some departments were very excited to partner with us and think creatively about how to tailor their information and resources specifically to Neurodivergent students. Others were less open-minded and preferred to provide written resources or share their contact information to connect with students individually. Our experience leads us to a few recommendations for others looking to engage in this type of work:

Listen to the Students

We found that our students, both in the pre-program planning and on the advisory board, had a very good sense of which departments were most challenging and which were the easiest to work with, which mapped on to our experiences working with those departments. In developing supports for a specific institution, it is important to consider whether departments may be able to provide the information that program developers are looking for, or if that topic requires thinking more creatively about how to get students information without putting them in the middle of a particularly convoluted or difficult system.

Get Higher-Ups Involved

Generally speaking, directors and department chairs were more receptive to our outreach than individual employees. This approach is advantageous, as higher-ups tend to have a better sense of who might be most interested in, best positioned to, and has the bandwidth to collaborate. Reaching out to supervisors initially allowed us to connect with the folks who were most enthusiastic about partnering with us.

Consider a Neutral Party in the Service Delivery

When debriefing with our participants after the workshop series had finished, we discussed replicating the series and if students thought that it should be owned and run by any particular department. Our students shared that they appreciated that the series was run by a "neutral" third party who collaborated with campus partners as opposed to having the entire program run by a certain office, as they feel siloing the program can lead to a biased approach. By incorporating "experts" from different departments, students receive the most up-to-date, specialized information about the various topics from the person or people best positioned to discuss them. Additionally, having a neutral facilitator allows for more frank discussions about challenges without concern that students' opinions will color any future interactions with specific campus departments.

Adaptation and Replicability - Potential Continued Impact of the Series

We hope that with resources like this book, more college campuses will be empowered to develop programming for Neurodivergent students in ways that are most relevant to their student population and their campus environment. While our pilot was not able to explicitly capture longer term use of stable coping responses or stage-specific coping outcomes (per PVEST), there are some findings from the literature that provide support for promising future effects of the workshop series and offer opportunities for further development and study.

One study by Rowe and colleagues (2020) looking at longer term effects of participating in a support program for Autistic students found that students who were involved in the program had a higher rate of returning to college the following year than the general student population. Newman and colleagues (2019) found that students with learning disabilities who utilized available support at their institution (e.g., use of a writing program) with or without accommodations had 27-30% higher graduation rates than those who received no support. Similar improvements in higher education outcomes (e.g., persistence, degree completion) have been found for other minority groups (e.g., students of color, first generation students) when students are involved in culturally specific supportive programming at the undergraduate and graduate level (DeRuy, 2016; O'Bryant & Schaffzin, 2017; Tovar, 2015). Additionally, Neurodivergent students who have "found their people" and made supportive social connections experience more psychosocial success in higher education, such as developing confidence and a positive sense of self and finding ways to positively contribute to their community (Accardo et al., 2019; Irvine & MacLeod, 2022). Thus, participation in programming like our pilot (a support in and of itself), and potential engagement in additional supports introduced during the program, could have positive effects on the participants' long-term outcomes.

There is more work to be done, however, before rolling out our workshop series to a wider audience. As mentioned earlier in the chapter, we followed recommendations from the British Medical Research Council on evaluating complex interventions (Skivington et al., 2021), the first stage of which is feasibility testing. We are planning for another round of feasibility testing currently, which we would recommend to anyone attempting to create their own program. The next stage of study should be a more comprehensive evaluation, during which the focus shifts from estimating objective effectiveness of the intervention's primary outcome (i.e., whether people gained relevant coping mechanisms) to identifying broader outcomes of the intervention in real-world contexts (Skivington et al., 2021). Our pilot examined preliminary perceived impact, but only through retroactive reflection from the participants. Expanding the program evaluation to include objective measures of impact would strengthen the argument for its efficacy. These measures could capture both immediate changes (from reactive coping processes, e.g., pre-post measures on aspects like confidence and competence with the topics, acute anxiety, acute coping mechanisms and utilization, and social connections) and more longitudinal outcomes (or stable coping responses, e.g., long-term coping mechanism use, retention and degree completion rates, service utilization rates, psychosocial changes). It would be beneficial in this development process to conduct follow-up assessments or interviews with the pilot participants to understand the longer-term effects the program had on their experience (e.g., whether they have referenced or used any of the strategies they learned during the workshops). Understanding more about the participants' experiences following the series would help to identify areas to explore in future assessments and which measures to develop or adapt.

The final stage in the MRC's guidelines is implementation, which may take the form of "transferability into different contexts" (Skivington et al., 2021, p. 7). Although the workshop series was designed for Tufts students, we created the overall framework for easy adaptation for use at other colleges and universities, particularly those that do not have robust support for Neurodivergent students available. For adaptation, it would be important to convene an advisory board at the institution to decide whether the topics and materials in this curriculum make sense for the institution's student population and how they may need to be adapted. For example, if the university has a higher commuter population, there may not be as much of an emphasis on student organizations, and it may be more useful to focus on social opportunities and resources off-campus. However, the topics (self-advocacy and disclosure, accessing accommodations, social life and community, executive functioning and self-care, and housing/living on their own) are fairly universal to college students, particularly Neurodivergent students (Accardo et al., 2019; Flegenheimer & Scherf, 2022; Lei et al., 2020). Most colleges and universities also have similar campus partners to the offices involved in the pilot (e.g., an entity that handles student accommodations, a counseling center) who could be recruited to participate in providing a workshop series tailored to that institution.

CONCLUSION

There is still much work to be done to improve the landscape of higher education for Neurodivergent students, but the program presented in this chapter shows the efficacy of investing in supports to foster students' success and is a promising first step in making higher education more accessible. This workshop series was a relatively small pilot program, but the response from participants indicates that students respond to this type of programming and are looking for more of it to address the challenges that they are experiencing in higher education settings. Continuing to offer workshops where Neurodivergent students can learn about resources and strategies can lead to more effective skill-building and reduce some of the negative outcomes for this population. Neurodiversity is an important component of equity, inclusion, and justice work that is often overlooked (Scheef et al., 2020), and while colleges and universities are working to dismantle systemic inequality, students are in need of support to access spaces that have not been (as successfully) accessed by Neurodivergent students.

Aside from continuing to offer programming like this workshop series, what became clear from this study was the need for higher education institutions to provide more support overall to their Neurodivergent students. Clearer communication across the board about expectations of students, availability of resources (and how to access these resources), and opportunities for engagement with peers will allow students to more equitably participate in campus life. More information and instruction on specific strategies like executive functioning and self-care supports can build an individual's capacity for positive coping strategies. Additionally, offering neurodiversity-specific instruction or navigation on topics like future employment and engaging with faculty would augment existing programming in a way that is more accessible to Neurodivergent students. This workshop series helped to bridge some of the gaps that Neurodivergent students face in higher education, but it was only a small part of what would be needed to improve systems. It is up to higher education institutions to see the value of Neurodivergent student success and take larger steps to facilitate it.

POSITIONALITY STATEMENT

While we are non-neurodivergent, White, cisgender women, we use a neurodiversity-affirming framework in our study of Neurodivergent presentations and interactions with Neurodivergent people and carefully consider the effects of intersectional identities in our work. To combat our biases, we strive to ensure that our work is informed by actual Neurodivergent youth and adults. Neurodiversity (and disability in general) is one of the few remaining fields that is primarily studied by people outside of the community; but this is changing, and we have realized that there is no ethical way to continue this work without authentic partnerships with Neurodivergent people. We utilize the information we have been generously given by Neurodivergent people and our privileged positions as academics to join in advocacy efforts and ensure that Neurodivergent voices are represented and heard.

In our work, we have seen the impact of quality, comprehensive support on a young person's self-defined success and their outlook on their context. However, we recognize that most often in the context of neurodivergence, the onus is placed on the individual to learn and adapt to their surroundings. Due to the newness of conversations around neurodiversity at our university, our workshop program did not attempt to disrupt the status quo, but rather to support students in accessing systems the way they currently exist, which we recognize is not enough to truly create more equitable practices. While our goal is that collaborating with Neurodivergent students *and* larger campus communities can contribute to a more inclusive culture in higher education, the primary goal of this program was to address gaps in knowledge of and access to information and support for students as a first step. We hope that future work replicating, adapting, and expanding our efforts will further these efforts in new settings.

CASE STUDIES AND DISCUSSION QUESTIONS

Case Study 1: Cam's Story

A student's residential advisor (RA) has reached out to you for advice about one of the sophomore students on their floor, "Cam", who has disclosed that they are Autistic and have ADHD. Cam is consistently attending their classes but is not registered for academic accommodations and has shared that they are behind on a number of assignments due to their executive dysfunction. Cam shared that their grades have historically been good, but they feel like they can't keep up with the demands of college and are burning out. As a result, Cam has dropped out of the student groups they had been in the previous year and doesn't spend much time outside of their dorm room. The RA is concerned about Cam's mental health and is worried about Cam's isolation, signs of depressive symptoms, and how overwhelmed they appear. They have not had an openly Neurodivergent student on their floor before and don't know what to recommend to Cam.

Questions

For both academics and social/student life, consider the following:

1. What resources are available to Cam on your campus? Generally, and for Neurodivergent students specifically?
2. How do students access these supports, and how is this information shared with students? Particularly for services that require a referral, how user-friendly are these referral processes?
3. How might you empower Cam (or support the RA in empowering Cam), to access these resources and strengthen their coping responses?

Case Study 2: Sky's Story

"Sky", a first year student in your work study program, comes to you and shares that they believe they are Neurodivergent and are looking into getting a formal neuropsychological assessment. They share that they have historically had trouble meeting people and making connections, as they don't feel like they make a good first impression. They have tried making conversation with other students in their classes and on their dorm floor, but these interactions don't seem to go past a short conversation. Sky is looking for other Neurodivergent students to connect with, for both peer support and social opportunities, but doesn't know where to start.

Questions

1. Do student-driven spaces exist for Neurodivergent students on your campus?
2. If so, what do these spaces look like and how do students get connected with them?
3. If not, how could you support Sky and/or other students in creating authentic spaces for Neurodivergent students to connect with one another? Consider aspects such as leveraging existing resources, space, budget, and accessibility.

ACKNOWLEDGEMENTS

The authors thank Sara K. Johnson, Laura Crane, Brett Ranon Nachman, and Kristina Aikens for their editorial support with the Dufresne (2024) dissertation manuscript, on which this chapter was largely based. We would also like to thank our pilot advisory board, campus partners, and workshop participants for their time and perspectives. The "Navigating Tufts for Neurodivergent Students" pilot workshop series and evaluation were funded by the Tufts University Graduate Student Research Competition.

REFERENCES

Accardo, A. L., Bean, K., Cook, B., Gillies, A., Edgington, R., Kuder, S. J., & Bomgardner, E. M. (2019). College access, success and equity for students on the autism spectrum. *Journal of Autism and Developmental Disorders, 49*(12), 4877–4890. DOI: 10.1007/s10803-019-04205-8 PMID: 31482372

Adam, M. (2021). *A grounded theory of overcommitment in undergraduate college students* (Doctoral dissertation, Florida Atlantic University). https://www.proquest.com/docview/2621326323/abstract/3B0BDB12600C4E3EPQ/1

Aguilar, O., & Lipson, S. K. (2021). A public health approach to understanding the mental health needs of college students with disabilities: Results from a national survey. *Journal of Postsecondary Education and Disability, 34*(3), 273–285. https://eric.ed.gov/?id=EJ1325421

Aladin, S., Smith, T., Dufresne, S., & Crehan, E. T. (2022, April 14). *Increasing accessibility at Tufts for neurodiverse individuals.* Poster presented at the 29th Annual Fred Rothbaum Student Presentation Day, Medford, MA.

Anderson, A. H., Stephenson, J., & Carter, M. (2017). A systematic literature review of the experiences and supports of students with autism spectrum disorder in post-secondary education. *Research in Autism Spectrum Disorders, 39*, 33–53. DOI: 10.1016/j.rasd.2017.04.002

Ardeleanu, K., Steinberg, H., Garfield, T., Voltaire, S., Shea, L., Brown, M., Chvasta, K., & Tan, C. D. (2024). Self-identification of autism: Why some autistic adults lack a clinical diagnosis and why this matters for inclusion. *Autism. Autism, 13623613241297222*, 13623613241297222. Advance online publication. DOI: 10.1177/13623613241297222 PMID: 39552426

Armstrong, T. (2010). *Neurodiversity: Discovering the extraordinary gifts of autism, ADHD, dyslexia, and other brain differences*. ReadHowYouWant.com.

ASAN. (2013). *Navigating college: A handbook on self advocacy written for autistic students from autistic adults*. The Autistic Press.

Bakker, T., Krabbendam, L., Bhulai, S., & Begeer, S. (2019). Background and enrollment characteristics of students with autism in higher education. *Research in Autism Spectrum Disorders, 67*, 101424. Advance online publication. DOI: 10.1016/j.rasd.2019.101424

Beck, T. J. (2023). Neurodivergent culture and embodied knowledge beyond neoliberal identity politics. *Culture & Psychology*, Article 1354067X231191489. DOI: 10.1177/1354067X231191489

Berg, L. A., Jirikowic, T., Haerling, K., & MacDonald, G. (2017). Navigating the hidden curriculum of higher education for postsecondary students with intellectual disabilities. *The American Journal of Occupational Therapy, 71*(3), 7103100020. Advance online publication. DOI: 10.5014/ajot.2017.024703 PMID: 28422626

Black, K. Z., Hardy, C. Y., De Marco, M., Ammerman, A. S., Corbie-Smith, G., Council, B., Ellis, D., Eng, E., Harris, B., Jackson, M., Jean-Baptiste, J., Kearney, W., Legerton, M., Parker, D., Wynn, M., & Lightfoot, A. (2013). Beyond incentives for involvement to compensation for consultants. *Progress in Community Health Partnerships, 7*(3), 263–270. DOI: 10.1353/cpr.2013.0040 PMID: 24056508

Brandsen, T., & Honingh, M. (2018). Definitions of co-production and co-creation. In Brandsen, T., Steen, T., & Verschuere, B. (Eds.), *Co-production and co-creation: Engaging citizens in public services*. Routledge. DOI: 10.4324/9781315204956-2

Bronfenbrenner, U. (1977). Toward an experimental ecology of human development. *The American Psychologist, 32*(7), 513–531. DOI: 10.1037/0003-066X.32.7.513

Brown, S. A., Silvera-Tawil, D., Gemeinboeck, P., & McGhee, J. (2016). The case for conversation: A design research framework for participatory feedback from autistic children. *OzCHI '16: The 28th Australian Conference on Computer-Human Interaction*, 605–613. DOI: 10.1145/3010915.3010934

Brownlow, C., Martin, N., Thompson, D.-M., Dowe, A., Abawi, D., Harrison, J., & March, S. (2023). Navigating university: The design and evaluation of a holistic support programme for autistic students in higher education. *Education Sciences, 13*(5), 521. Advance online publication. DOI: 10.3390/educsci13050521

Butcher, L., & Lane, S. (2024). Neurodivergent (autism and ADHD) student experiences of access and inclusion in higher education: An ecological systems theory perspective. *Higher Education*. Advance online publication. DOI: 10.1007/s10734-024-01319-6

Caldora, J. B.II, & Coghill, E. M. H. (2020). Self advocacy. In Coghill, E. M. H., & Coghill, J. G. (Eds.), *Supporting neurodiverse college student success: A guide for librarians, student support services, and academic learning environments* (pp. 8–22). Rowman & Littlefield.

Chiwandire, D., & Vincent, L. (2019). Funding and inclusion in higher education institutions for students with disabilities. *African Journal of Disability*, *8*(0), 336. Advance online publication. DOI: 10.4102/ajod.v8i0.336 PMID: 30899686

Clouder, L., Karakus, M., Cinotti, A., Ferreyra, M. V., Fierros, G. A., & Rojo, P. (2020). Neurodiversity in higher education: A narrative synthesis. *Higher Education*, *80*(4), 757–778. DOI: 10.1007/s10734-020-00513-6

Coghill, E. M. H., & Coghill, J. G. (2020). *Supporting neurodiverse college student success: A guide for librarians, student support services, and academic learning environments*. Rowman & Littlefield.

College Autism Network. (n.d.). *Autism-specific College Support Programs (ASPs)*. Retrieved March 5, 2024, from https://can.softr.app/

Cox, B. E., Edelstein, J., Brogdon, B., & Roy, A. (2021). Navigating challenges to facilitate success for college students with autism. *The Journal of Higher Education*, *92*(2), 252–278. DOI: 10.1080/00221546.2020.1798203

Cox, B. E., Thompson, K., Anderson, A., Mintz, A., Locks, T., Morgan, L., Edelstein, J., & Wolz, A. (2017). College experiences for students with Autism Spectrum Disorder: Personal identity, public disclosure, and institutional support. *Journal of College Student Development*, *58*(1), 71–87. https://muse.jhu.edu/article/646663. DOI: 10.1353/csd.2017.0004

Crane, L., Hearst, C., Ashworth, M., & Davies, J. (2023). Evaluating the online delivery of an autistic-led programme to support newly diagnosed or identified autistic adults. *Autism & Developmental Language Impairments*, *8*, 1–9. DOI: 10.1177/23969415231189608 PMID: 37529634

Crane, L., Hearst, C., Ashworth, M., Davies, J., & Hill, E. L. (2021). Supporting newly identified or diagnosed autistic adults: An initial evaluation of an autistic-led programme. *Journal of Autism and Developmental Disorders*, *51*(3), 892–905. DOI: 10.1007/s10803-020-04486-4 PMID: 32266684

Crehan, E. T., Phillips, A., Ngo, A., Donaghue, A., Bartlett, N., Rothstein, D., & Dufresne, S. (in preparation). What's autism and neurodiversity got to do with it? How liberal arts campuses in the US are (or are not) discussing invisible disabilities. *Eliot Pearson Department of Child Study & Human Development. Tufts University.*

Crompton, C. J., Hallett, S., Ropar, D., Flynn, E., & Fletcher-Watson, S. (2020). 'I never realised everybody felt as happy as I do when I am around Autistic people': A thematic analysis of Autistic adults' relationships with autistic and neurotypical friends and family. *Autism, 24*(6), 1438–1448. DOI: 10.1177/1362361320908976 PMID: 32148068

den Houting, J. (2019). Neurodiversity: An insider's perspective. *Autism, 23*(2), 271–273. DOI: 10.1177/1362361318820762 PMID: 30556743

den Houting, J., Higgins, J., Isaacs, K., Mahony, J., & Pellicano, E. (2021). 'I'm not just a guinea pig': Academic and community perceptions of participatory autism research. *Autism, 25*(1), 148–163. DOI: 10.1177/1362361320951696 PMID: 32854511

DeRuy, E. (2016, March 23). How to graduate more black students. *The Atlantic.* https://www.theatlantic.com/education/archive/2016/03/how-to-graduate-more-black-students/475077/

Dexter, S., Grace, K., Quinnell, S.-L., Surrey, A., & Crane, L. (2024). Towards 'a level playing field': A participatory study of autistic university students' experiences with academic support in England. *International Journal of Disability Development and Education, 72*(1), 26–41. DOI: 10.1080/1034912X.2024.2317475

Dijkhuis, R., de Sonneville, L., Ziermans, T., Staal, W., & Swaab, H. (2020). Autism symptoms, executive functioning and academic progress in higher education students. *Journal of Autism and Developmental Disorders, 50*(4), 1353–1363. DOI: 10.1007/s10803-019-04267-8 PMID: 31939082

Dufresne, S. R. (2024). *Navigating Tufts for Neurodivergent Students: Developing, implementing, and evaluating a workshop series at a U.S. university* [Doctoral dissertation, Tufts University]. ProQuest Dissertations & Theses Global. https://www.proquest.com/docview/3059316104/abstract/EA60821E016B4156PQ/1

DuPaul, G. J., Franklin, M. K., Pollack, B. L., Stack, K. S., Jaffe, A. R., & Gormley, M. J. Anastopoulos, A. D., & Weyandt, L. L. (2018). Predictors and trajectories of educational functioning in college students with and without attention-deficit/hyperactivity disorder. *Journal of Postsecondary Education and Disability, 31*(2), 161–178. https://pmc.ncbi.nlm.nih.gov/articles/PMC6586431/

DuPaul, G. J., Gormley, M. J., Anastopoulos, A. D., Weyandt, L. L., Labban, J., Sass, A. J., Busch, C. Z., Franklin, M. K., & Postler, K. B. (2021). Academic trajectories of college students with and without ADHD: Predictors of four-year outcomes. *Journal of Clinical Child and Adolescent Psychology*, *50*(6), 828–843. DOI: 10.1080/15374416.2020.1867990 PMID: 33529049

DuPaul, G. J., Weyandt, L. L., O'Dell, S. M., & Varejao, M. (2009). College students with ADHD: Current status and future directions. *Journal of Attention Disorders*, *13*(3), 234–250. DOI: 10.1177/1087054709340650 PMID: 19620623

Dupree, D., Spencer, T. R., & Spencer, M. B. (2015). Stigma, stereotypes and resilience identities: The relationship between identity processes and resilience processes among Black American adolescents. In Theron, L. C., Liebenberg, L., & Ungar, M. (Eds.), *Youth Resilience and Culture: Commonalities and Complexities* (pp. 117–129). Springer Netherlands., DOI: 10.1007/978-94-017-9415-2_9

Dwyer, P., Mineo, E., Mifsud, K., Lindholm, C., Gurba, A., & Waisman, T. (2023). Building neurodiversity-inclusive postsecondary campuses: Recommendations for leaders in higher education. *Autism in Adulthood: Challenges and Management*, *5*(1), 1–14. DOI: 10.1089/aut.2021.0042 PMID: 36941859

Elmore, K., Saia, T., & Thomson, E. A. (2018). *Special feature: An introduction to disability cultural centers in U.S. higher education, part I.* AHEAD - Association on Higher Education And Disability. https://www.ahead.org/professional-resources/publications/hub/hub-nov-2018/hub-nov-2018-special-feature-disability-cultural-centers

Eng, S., & Onysko, M. (2025, March 25). Tufts accepts 10.5% of applicants to the Class of 2029. *The Tufts Daily*. https://www.tuftsdaily.com/article/2025/03/tufts-accepts-105-of-applicants-to-the-class-of-2029

Evans, D., Granson, M., Langford, D., & Hirsch, S. (2023). Autism spectrum disorder: Reconceptualising support for neurodiverse students in higher education. *Journal of Higher Education Policy and Management*, *45*(2), 243–257. DOI: 10.1080/1360080X.2023.2180168

Fabri, M., Andrews, P. C. S., & Pukki, H. K. (2016). Using design thinking to engage autistic students in participatory design of an online toolkit to help with transition into higher education. *Journal of Assistive Technologies*, *10*(2), 102–114. DOI: 10.1108/JAT-02-2016-0008

Flegenheimer, C., & Scherf, K. S. (2022). College as a developmental context for emerging adulthood in autism: A systematic review of what we know and where we go from here. *Journal of Autism and Developmental Disorders, 52*(5), 2075–2097. DOI: 10.1007/s10803-021-05088-4 PMID: 34060001

Fletcher-Watson, S., Adams, J., Brook, K., Charman, T., Crane, L., Cusack, J., Leekam, S., Milton, D., Parr, J. R., & Pellicano, E. (2019). Making the future together: Shaping autism research through meaningful participation. *Autism, 23*(4), 943–953. DOI: 10.1177/1362361318786721 PMID: 30095277

Fundación Indígena [FSI], & Kothari, B. (2008). Rights to the benefits of research: Compensating indigenous peoples for their intellectual contribution. *Human Organization, 56*(2), 127–137. DOI: 10.17730/humo.56.2.j63678502x782100

Gelbar, N. W., Shefyck, A., & Reichow, B. (2015). A comprehensive survey of current and former college students with Autism Spectrum Disorders. *The Yale Journal of Biology and Medicine, 88*(1), 45–68. https://pmc.ncbi.nlm.nih.gov/articles/PMC4345538/ PMID: 25745374

Gillespie-Lynch, K., Bublitz, D., Donachie, A., Wong, V., Brooks, P. J., & D'Onofrio, J. (2017). "For a long time our voices have been hushed": Using student perspectives to develop supports for neurodiverse college students. *Frontiers in Psychology, 8*. Advance online publication. DOI: 10.3389/fpsyg.2017.00544 PMID: 28458645

Gillespie-Lynch, K., Daou, N., Obeid, R., Reardon, S., Khan, S., & Goldknopf, E. J. (2021). What contributes to stigma towards autistic university students and students with other diagnoses? *Journal of Autism and Developmental Disorders, 51*(2), 459–475. DOI: 10.1007/s10803-020-04556-7 PMID: 32504342

Hamilton, L. G., & Petty, S. (2023). Compassionate pedagogy for neurodiversity in higher education: A conceptual analysis. *Frontiers in Psychology, 14*, 1093290. Advance online publication. DOI: 10.3389/fpsyg.2023.1093290 PMID: 36874864

Han, E., Scior, K., Grace, K., Heath, E., Dufresne, S., & Crane, L. (2024). 'Who, When, How to Share': Pilot study of a new disclosure decision-making programme for autistic adults. *Autism, 28*(8), 2090–2104. Advance online publication. DOI: 10.1177/13623613231221685 PMID: 38339979

Hillier, A., Goldstein, J., Tornatore, L., Byrne, E., & Johnson, H. M. (2019). Outcomes of a peer mentoring program for university students with disabilities. *Mentoring & Tutoring, 27*(5), 487–508. DOI: 10.1080/13611267.2019.1675850

Hilton, S. (2023, September 25). The net of overcommitment: How we keep each other overburdened. *The Wesleyan Argus*. https://wesleyanargus.com/2023/09/25/the-net-of-overcommitment-how-we-keep-each-other-overburdened/

Hope, E. C., & Spencer, M. B. (2017). Civic engagement as an adaptive coping response to conditions of inequality: An application of Phenomenological Variant of Ecological Systems Theory (PVEST). In Cabrera, N. J., & Leyendecker, B. (Eds.), *Handbook on Positive Development of Minority Children and Youth* (pp. 421–435). Springer International Publishing., DOI: 10.1007/978-3-319-43645-6_25

Hotez, E., Shane-Simpson, C., Obeid, R., DeNigris, D., Siller, M., Costikas, C., Pickens, J., Massa, A., Giannola, M., D'Onofrio, J., & Gillespie-Lynch, K. (2018). Designing a summer transition program for incoming and current college students on the autism spectrum: A participatory approach. *Frontiers in Psychology*, *9*, 46. DOI: 10.3389/fpsyg.2018.00046 PMID: 29487547

Irvine, B., & MacLeod, A. (2022). What are the challenges and successes reported by Autistic students at university? A literature review. *Good Autism Practice, 23*(1), 49–59. https://discovery.ucl.ac.uk/id/eprint/10157822/1/GAP_Spring_2022_ARTICLE_6_%28IRVINE_MACLEOD%29.pdf

Jackson, P. (1968). *Life in classrooms*. Teachers College Press.

Jobe, L. E., & Williams White, S. (2007). Loneliness, social relationships, and a broader autism phenotype in college students. *Personality and Individual Differences*, *42*(8), 1479–1489. DOI: 10.1016/j.paid.2006.10.021

Keating, C. T. (2021). Participatory autism research: How consultation benefits everyone. *Frontiers in Psychology*, *12*, 713982. DOI: 10.3389/fpsyg.2021.713982 PMID: 34504463

Kuder, S. J., Accardo, A., & Woodruff, J. (2021). *College success for students on the autism spectrum: A neurodiversity perspective*. Stylus Publishing, LLC.

Lawson, J. (2010). An investigation into behaviours which challenge at university: The impact of neurotypical expectations on Autistic students. *Good Autism Practice, 11*(1), 45–51. https://citeseerx.ist.psu.edu/document?repid=rep1&type=pdf&doi=ccb1d460781375d98835c76525c4e6fac3c87d37#page=46

Lei, J., Calley, S., Brosnan, M., Ashwin, C., & Russell, A. (2020). Evaluation of a transition to university programme for students with Autism Spectrum Disorder. *Journal of Autism and Developmental Disorders*, *50*(7), 2397–2411. DOI: 10.1007/s10803-018-3776-6 PMID: 30315485

Lewis, L. F. (2016a). Exploring the experience of self-diagnosis of Autism Spectrum Disorder in adults. *Archives of Psychiatric Nursing*, *30*(5), 575–580. DOI: 10.1016/j.apnu.2016.03.009 PMID: 27654240

Lewis, L. F. (2016b). Realizing a diagnosis of Autism Spectrum Disorder as an adult. *International Journal of Mental Health Nursing*, *25*(4), 346–354. DOI: 10.1111/inm.12200 PMID: 26940281

Locke, J., Osuna, A., Myrvold, R. J., & Closson, J. S. (2023). Supporting Autistic college students: Examining the Mentoring, Organization and Social Support for Autism Inclusion on Campus (MOSSAIC) program. *Journal of Autism and Developmental Disorders*. Advance online publication. DOI: 10.1007/s10803-023-05969-w PMID: 37017864

Lucas, R., & James, A. I. (2018). An evaluation of specialist mentoring for university students with Autism Spectrum Disorders and mental health conditions. *Journal of Autism and Developmental Disorders*, *48*(3), 694–707. DOI: 10.1007/s10803-017-3303-1 PMID: 28918532

McKee, T. E. (2017). Peer relationships in undergraduates with ADHD symptomatology: Selection and quality of friendships. *Journal of Attention Disorders*, *21*(12), 1020–1029. DOI: 10.1177/1087054714554934 PMID: 25359763

McLeod, J. D., Meanwell, E., & Hawbaker, A. (2019). The experiences of college students on the autism spectrum: A comparison to their neurotypical peers. *Journal of Autism and Developmental Disorders*, *49*(6), 2320–2336. DOI: 10.1007/s10803-019-03910-8 PMID: 30734173

Morton, T. R., & Parsons, E. C. (2018). #BlackGirlMagic: The identity conceptualization of Black women in undergraduate STEM education. *Science Education*, *102*(6), 1363–1393. DOI: 10.1002/sce.21477

Nachman, B. R. (2020). Enhancing transition programming for college students with autism: A systematic literature review. *Journal of Postsecondary Education and Disability*, *33*(1), 81–95.

Nachman, B. R., McDermott, C. T., & Cox, B. E. (2022). Brief report: Autism-specific college support programs: Differences across geography and institutional type. *Journal of Autism and Developmental Disorders*, *52*(2), 863–870. DOI: 10.1007/s10803-021-04958-1 PMID: 33770324

Nadeau, K. (2006). *Survival guide for college students with ADHD or LD*. Magination Press.

National Center for Education Statistics [NCES]. (2017). *Bachelor's degree attainment at first institution through June 2017 by disability* (Beginning Postsecondary Students: 2012/2017). https://nces.ed.gov/datalab/powerstats/71-beginning-postsecondary-students-2012-2017/percentage-distribution

Naylor, C. (2023). *'Much better set up to do my best work': What does 'neurodiversity-affirming practice' mean to the autistic community?* [Thesis, University of Nottingham]. https://eprints.nottingham.ac.uk/76179/

NCLD. (2023, March 30). *Remove barriers for college students with disabilities by supporting the RISE Act.* National Center for Learning Disabilities. https://www.ncld.org/news/policy-and-advocacy/bi-partisan-rise-act-opens-new-doors-for-students-with-disabilities/

Newman, L., Madaus, J. W., Lalor, A. R., & Javitz, H. S. (2019). Support receipt: Effect on postsecondary success of students with learning disabilities. *Career Development and Transition for Exceptional Individuals, 42*(1), 6–16. DOI: 10.1177/2165143418811288

Newman, L., Wagner, M., Cameto, R., Knokey, A.-M., & Shaver, D. (2010). Comparisons across time of the outcomes of youth with disabilities up to 4 years after high school: A report of findings from the National Longitudinal Transition Study (NLTS) and the National Longitudinal Transition Study-2 (NLTS2). In *National Center for Special Education Research.* National Center for Special Education Research. https://eric.ed.gov/?id=ED512149

O'Bryant, J. M., & Schaffzin, K. T. (2017). First-generation students in law school: A proven success model. *Arkansas Law Review, 70*(4), 913–958. https://heinonline.org/HOL/LandingPage?handle=hein.journals/arklr70&div=36&id=&page=

Overton, G. L., Marsà-Sambola, F., Martin, R., & Cavenagh, P. (2024). Understanding the self-identification of autism in adults: A scoping review. *Review Journal of Autism and Developmental Disorders, 11*(4), 682–702. DOI: 10.1007/s40489-023-00361-x

Ozaki, C. C., Olson, A. B., Johnston-Guerrero, M. P., & Pizzolato, J. E. (2020). Understanding persistence using a Phenomenological Variant of Ecological Systems Theory. *Community College Review, 48*(3), 252–276. DOI: 10.1177/0091552120906884

Patton, L. D. (Ed.). (2023). *Culture centers in higher education: Perspectives on identity, theory, and practice.* Routledge. DOI: 10.4324/9781003443971

Rando, H., Huber, M. J., & Oswald, G. R. (2016). An academic coaching model intervention for college students on the autism spectrum. *Journal of Postsecondary Education and Disability, 29*(3), 257–262. https://files.eric.ed.gov/fulltext/EJ1123790.pdf

Raymaker, D., & Nicolaidis, C. (2013). Participatory research with autistic communities. In J. Davidson & M. Orsini (Eds.), *Worlds of Autism* (pp. 169–188). University of Minnesota Press.

Reeble, C. J., Lefler, E. K., Abu-Ramadan, T., Bodalski, E. A., & Canu, W. H. (2023). Social support in college students with ADHD symptoms: Quantity beats quality in moderating impairment. *Journal of College Student Psychotherapy, 0*(0), 1–22. DOI: 10.1080/87568225.2023.2202351

Rosenau, K. A., Hotez, E., Fernandes, P., Gomez, C., Eagan, K., Shea, L., & Kuo, A. (2023). Anxiety and depression in autistic college students: The freshman survey results. *Cureus, 15*(3), e35820. Advance online publication. DOI: 10.7759/cureus.35820 PMID: 37033553

Rowe, T., Charles, T., & DuBose, H. (2020). Supporting students with ASD on campus: What students may need to be successful (Practice Brief). *Journal of Postsecondary Education and Disability, 33*(1), 97–101. https://files.eric.ed.gov/fulltext/EJ1273702.pdf

Salusky, I., Monjaras-Gaytan, L., Ulerio, G., Forbes, N., Perron, G., & Raposa, E. (2022). The formation and role of social belonging in on-campus integration of diverse first-generation college students. *Journal of College Student Retention: Research, Theory & Practice. Article, 15210251221092709*. Advance online publication. DOI: 10.1177/15210251221092709

Sarrett, J. C. (2018). Autism and accommodations in higher education: Insights from the autism community. *Journal of Autism and Developmental Disorders, 48*(3), 679–693. DOI: 10.1007/s10803-017-3353-4 PMID: 29243099

Scheef, A., Caniglia, C., & Barrio, B. L. (2020). Disability as diversity: Perspectives of institutions of higher education in the U.S. *Journal of Postsecondary Education and Disability, 33*(1), 49–61. https://files.eric.ed.gov/fulltext/EJ1273652.pdf

Shattuck, P. T., Narendorf, S. C., Cooper, B., Sterzing, P. R., Wagner, M., & Taylor, J. L. (2012). Postsecondary education and employment among youth with an autism spectrum disorder. *Pediatrics, 129*(6), 1042–1049. DOI: 10.1542/peds.2011-2864 PMID: 22585766

Skivington, K., Matthews, L., Simpson, S. A., Craig, P., Baird, J., Blazeby, J. M., Boyd, K. A., Craig, N., French, D. P., McIntosh, E., Petticrew, M., Rycroft-Malone, J., White, M., & Moore, L. (2021). A new framework for developing and evaluating complex interventions: Update of Medical Research Council guidance. *BMJ (Clinical Research Ed.)*, *374*, 2061. Advance online publication. DOI: 10.1136/bmj.n2061 PMID: 34593508

Southon, C. (2022). The relationship between executive function, neurodevelopmental disorder traits, and academic achievement in university students. *Frontiers in Psychology*, *13*, 958013. Advance online publication. DOI: 10.3389/fpsyg.2022.958013 PMID: 36118426

Spencer, M. B. (2006). Phenomenology and ecological systems theory: Development of diverse groups. In Damon, W., & Lerner, R. (Eds.), *Theoretical models of human development* (6th ed., pp. 829–893). Handbook of child psychology. John Wiley & Sons Inc.

Steinberg, L. D. (2022). *Adolescence* (13th ed.). McGraw Hill.

Stice, L. V., & Lavner, J. A. (2019). Social connectedness and loneliness mediate the association between autistic traits and internalizing symptoms among young adults. *Journal of Autism and Developmental Disorders*, *49*(3), 1096–1110. DOI: 10.1007/s10803-018-3812-6 PMID: 30406911

Stowers, S. (2022, June 4). *Types of neurodiversity and how to design learning experiences for them*. eLearning Industry. https://elearningindustry.com/types-of-neurodiversity-and-how-to-design-learning-experiences-for-them

Sturm, A., Huang, S., Bal, V., & Schwartzman, B. (2024). Psychometric exploration of the RAADS-R with autistic adults: Implications for research and clinical practice. *Autism*, *28*(9), 2334–2345. DOI: 10.1177/13623613241228329 PMID: 38305196

Thompson, A. C., & Lefler, E. K. (2016). ADHD stigma among college students. *Attention Deficit and Hyperactivity Disorders*, *8*(1), 45–52. DOI: 10.1007/s12402-015-0179-9 PMID: 26135022

Tovar, E. (2015). The role of faculty, counselors, and support programs on Latino/a community college students' success and intent to persist. *Community College Review*, *43*(1), 46–71. DOI: 10.1177/0091552114553788

Tufts, O. I. R. (2023a). *First Year Experience Survey 2023* (Tufts University Office of Institutional Research). Tufts University.

Tufts, O. I. R. (2023b). *Sophomore Experience Survey 2023* (Tufts University Office of Institutional Research). Tufts University.

UC Academic Senate. (2021). *Recommendations for making UC a more welcoming place for neurodivergent students*. University of California. https://senate.universityofcalifornia.edu/_files/reports/mg-mb-recs-neurodivergent-students.pdf

US News & World Report. (2025). The best national universities in America. *US News & World Report*. https://www.usnews.com/best-colleges/rankings/national-universities?_sort=rank&_sortDirection=asc

Van Hees, V., Moyson, T., & Roeyers, H. (2015). Higher education experiences of students with Autism Spectrum Disorder: Challenges, benefits and support needs. *Journal of Autism and Developmental Disorders*, *45*(6), 1673–1688. DOI: 10.1007/s10803-014-2324-2 PMID: 25448918

Wallerstein, N., Duran, B., Oetzel, J. G., & Minkler, M. (2018). *Community-based participatory research for health: Advancing social and health equity* (3rd ed.). Wiley.

White, S. W., Richey, J. A., Gracanin, D., Coffman, M., Elias, R., LaConte, S., & Ollendick, T. H. (2016). Psychosocial and computer-assisted intervention for college students with autism spectrum disorder: Preliminary support for feasibility. *Education and Training in Autism and Developmental Disabilities*, *51*(3), 307–317. https://pmc.ncbi.nlm.nih.gov/articles/PMC5241080/pdf/nihms836993.pdf PMID: 28111607

Woo, B., Fan, W., Tran, T. V., & Takeuchi, D. T. (2019). The role of racial/ethnic identity in the association between racial discrimination and psychiatric disorders: A buffer or exacerbator? *SSM - Population Health*, *7*, 100378. DOI: 10.1016/j.ssmph.2019.100378 PMID: 30923732

Wright, E., Smith, R., Vernon, M., Wall, R., & White, L. (2021). Inclusive, multi-partner co-creation for the teaching of special educational needs and disabilities in higher education. *Journal of University Teaching & Learning Practice*, *18*(7), 25–40. DOI: 10.53761/1.18.7.3

Youngblood, I. I. J.II, & Spencer, M. B. (2002). Integrating normative identity processes and academic support requirements for special needs adolescents: The application of an identity-focused cultural ecological (ICE) perspective. *Applied Developmental Science*, *6*(2), 95–108. DOI: 10.1207/S1532480XADS0602_5

ADDITIONAL READING

ASAN. (2013). *Navigating college: A handbook on self-advocacy written for autistic students from autistic adults*. The Autistic Press.

Coghill, E. M. H., & Coghill, J. G. (2020). *Supporting neurodiverse college student success: A guide for librarians, student support services, and academic learning environments*. Rowman & Littlefield.

Rigler, M., Rutherford, A., & Quinn, E. (2015). *Developing identity, strengths, and self-perception for young adults with Autism Spectrum Disorder: The BASICS College Curriculum*. Jessica Kingsley Publishers.

Rigler, M., Rutherford, A., & Quinn, E. (2015). Independence, social, and study strategies for young adults with autism spectrum disorder: The BASICS College Curriculum. Jessica Kingsley Publishers.

Chapter 4
Social Work Principles That Promote Neurodivergent Learner Success

Tulare Williams Park
https://orcid.org/0000-0002-9092-5968
Commonwealth University of Pennsylvania, USA

Steven M. Granich
https://orcid.org/0000-0002-7947-422X
Commonwealth University of Pennsylvania, USA

Carol Rogers-Shaw
https://orcid.org/0000-0003-0550-290X
University of Dayton, USA

ABSTRACT

This chapter describes how principles used in the practice of professional social work have a unique role to play for higher education faculty and staff who work with Neurodivergent students. Social work principles can provide a strong foundation for assisting Neurodivergent students in meeting their academic and social goals. Theoretical frameworks such as the person-in-environment and ecological perspectives, a strengths-based approach, advocacy, and allyship are described. Case studies illustrate collaborative strategies for the classroom and campus-based support for Neurodivergent students that improve their college experiences and support their persistence.

DOI: 10.4018/979-8-3693-8920-1.ch004

INTRODUCTION

In colleges and universities across the United States, Neurodivergent students need support to be successful, both in and outside the classroom. The transition to postsecondary education, whether for recent high school graduates or for adult learners returning to college, is an exciting time filled with promise; it is also a period of significant change requiring time management, organization, communication, and adaptation skills. For the increasing number of Neurodivergent students entering higher education, the barriers to persistence in college are more significant (Clouder et al., 2020; Hotez et al., 2022; Kuder et al., 2023) than for their neuromajority peers. In higher education, the focus on deficits instead of strengths undermines students' success (Clouder et al., 2020). Serious thought and effort must be made to create a supportive environment for Neurodivergent learners. Using strategies such as universal design to better promote equity and incorporate diverse learning styles in the classroom is critical (Spaeth & Pearson, 2023; Dwyer et al., 2023).

The social work profession has a history of advocating for different groups in the community, working toward systemic change and social justice (Bliss & Ginn, 2021). Social workers have been crucial advocates and participants in movements for civil, women's, LGBTQ+, and disability rights. They have worked to reduce poverty and provide more mental health services for individuals and communities. This legacy of advocacy can be the foundation for greater acceptance of difference and inclusion of Neurodivergent postsecondary learners (Freddolino et al., 2004).

Schelbe (2022) argued that neurodiversity is a social justice issue because it is important to identify and apply resources to address obstacles hindering Neurodivergent individuals. Ignoring neurodiversity results in injustice for Neurodivergent individuals. Social work recognizes disability within a social context, consistent with the social and relational models of disability (Haegele & Hodge, 2016; Thomas, 2004); for example, Schelbe (2022) stated, "the roles social workers play in addressing [neurodiversity] fall into the categories of identifying risk, referring, educating, and advocating" (p. 275). These practices involve getting to know and better understand the student, collaborating with them to determine how best to address their needs, advocating for the removal of barriers to their academic success, and educating other university personnel.

Neurodiversity has been recognized as a new cultural competency in social work (Terry, n.d.). Social work as a discipline provides principles on which to build supportive practices that make postsecondary education a friendlier environment for Neurodivergent individuals. Social work and education are both professions that seek to improve the lives of those within their care; working collaboratively with other professionals, they focus on promoting wellbeing and meeting social and educational needs. There are trained social workers on most college and university campuses in the United States serving as excellent resources for faculty, staff, administrators, and students (Naasko, 2022). They may be found in the Disability Resources Office (DRO), student affairs, career services, counseling and advising, wellness and health centers, the dean's office, and social work and teacher education departments. They should be invited to join collaborative groups to support Neurodivergent students as their expertise is valuable.

There are many similarities between social workers and educators. They both offer counseling, provide resources, educate, and practice advocacy. With empathy and patience, they both use highly developed interpersonal communication, problem-solving, and cultural competency skills to enhance the welfare of others. These similarities can be instructive because the principles of social work can be used effectively by non-social workers in education.

In this chapter, we describe how principles used in the practice of professional social work have a unique role to play for higher education administrators, faculty, and staff who work with Neurodivergent students. Theoretical frameworks such as the person-in-environment (Germain, 1973) and ecological perspectives (Bronfenbrenner, 1994), a strengths-based approach using biopsychosocial assessment, (Engel, 1977), advocacy (Freddolino et al., 2004), and allyship (Bourke, 2020; Williams & Sharif, 2021), can inform the design of educational and social supports for Neurodivergent students, resulting in greater success and improved wellbeing.

Zastrow et al. (2019) described several theories as important in social work as a helping profession. First, the person-in-environment perspective sees the individual as interacting with various systems in the environment. Next, the ecological perspective views the person as one of multiple parts of the family, community, and other social entities, all of which influence the others. Additionally, the strength-based approach focuses on the assets and abilities of the individuals being served. Finally, addressing social problems through advocacy is a foundational element of social justice embedded in the practice of social work; and allyship sparks collaboration among diverse groups and individuals to increase socially just practices (Zastrow et al., 2019). Each of these perspectives represents a view of the student as both an individual and part of a broader social context and community. When college administrators, professors, and staff view neurodiversity in this more positive, strengths-focused way, they can become more willing to learn about and incorporate targeted interventions to reduce academic barriers for Neurodivergent learners.

PERSON-IN-ENVIRONMENT PERSPECTIVE

A major perspective which informs the social work profession is person-in-environment. Person-in-environment (PIE) is a way to understand an individual and the challenges in their life within the context where those challenges happen, such as in their community, family, workplace, school, etc. (Kondrat, 2013; Rogers, 2022). The PIE perspective began with Germain (1973) who explained that it highlights how both the person and the environment influence each other.

The PIE perspective grew out of the historical roots of the social work profession, where the poor environmental conditions of communities led to the Settlement House movement. In settlement houses, "university-educated and socially motivated" volunteers lived and often conducted research about those in poverty, mostly in urban communities, with the goal of fostering relationships among community members, educating them, and assisting them to meet their basic needs (Hansan, 2011, para. 11). A criticism of settlement houses was that they had no particular way of accomplishing their goal and instead became focused on advocacy for improving structural social conditions, rankling the status quo (Gitterman et al., 2021). This criticism led to the creation of casework as a social work practice.

Casework, first championed by Mary Richmond (1917) and the Charity Organization Society movement, was a method created to respond to critics and legitimize social work as a profession; it aimed to transition from community advocacy to practice with individuals and a more systemic approach, similar to how the medical profession provided care to people after assessment and diagnosis (Gitterman et al., 2021). In the decades since casework was introduced, it has become integral to social work practice and has grown in scope to include services provided to the individual and family by agencies, with attention to the functioning of the agency itself, in addition to clinical diagnostic practice (Gitterman et al., 2021). At the same time, the social work profession has maintained its focus on the importance of advocacy for improving structural social conditions through macro practice which promotes change within organizations and communities (Koenig et al., 2020).

Bureaucratic organizations and social networks are part of a person's environment, and social workers practice at multiple levels within these environments: micro (individual/family), mezzo (groups), and macro (organizations and communities) (Suppes & Wells, 2018). *Practice* refers to the ways in which social workers attempt to resolve issues and accomplish goals set forth by the profession as well as by their clients or client systems (Suppes & Wells, 2018). The PIE perspective illuminates how people are influenced by and have influence on their environment; it extends across all levels of practice and social workers must understand this influence (Koenig et al., 2020; Kondrat, 2013).

Three components of the PIE perspective that inform and guide social work practice include "(a) changing the individual in relation to the social environment, (b) changing the social environment in relation to the individual, or (c) both in relation to their interaction" (Kondrat, 2013, para. 7). Social workers use a specific process to practice ethically and competently, often known as the change process or intervention process; this includes engaging, assessing, intervening, and evaluating practice with individuals, families, groups, organizations, and communities, according to standards set forth by the National Association of Social Workers' Code of Ethics (NASW, 2021) in the United States.

In U.S. colleges and universities who train students to become social workers, educators must ensure that students learn and demonstrate mastery of "social work competencies" and practice "behaviors" specified in the Educational Policy and Accreditation Standards of the Council on Social Work Education (CSWE, 2022, p. 8). These competencies and behaviors include advancing human rights and equity, using evidence to inform practice and practice to inform research, and effectively using the change process. In both clinical and macro social work practice, the PIE perspective is useful in understanding the social context of a client or system. If the PIE perspective is applied to the higher education context, it can lead to heightened understanding of the complex interplay of the institutional and individual factors which influence Neurodivergent learners' experiences. With this understanding, faculty, staff, and administrators can work together to build better methods and systems to engage with Neurodivergent students, assess their challenges and barriers individually and systemically, provide support and intervention to resolve issues, and evaluate the effectiveness of these practices on students' persistence and success.

ECOLOGICAL PERSPECTIVE

Another social work perspective that is more macro-focused is the ecological perspective, which grew from Urie Bronfenbrenner's ecological systems theory (1994), and was a response to criticism that the PIE perspective is often more focused on the individual (micro) level and their interaction with the environment. Bronfenbrenner, a psychologist, argued that social science research typically studied children in an unnatural environment rather than in their home, school, and community settings. He claimed that researchers did not account for nor consider how this affected children and, subsequently, the study's findings (1974). He developed his ecological systems theory based on this view.

Ecological systems theory was built on the PIE perspective, going beyond understanding how people and environments influence each other; instead, the aim was "to understand and explain human learning and development through how individuals interact with and are influenced by interrelated systems within their environments" (Butcher & Lane, 2024, p. 4). The ecological perspective illustrates how individuals are always interacting with multiple systems in their environment which also interact with each other. It is therefore impossible to view individuals' challenges as solely within themselves, or solely the domain of the environment;

challenges and barriers must be viewed from the lens of the interaction and influence of multiple small systems within the larger environment.

Carel Germain (1973) was instrumental in building on Bronfenbrenner's theory and translating it to social work practice. Later writing with Alex Gitterman, Germain developed the "Life Model of Social Work Practice", an ecological perspective which has evolved since its initial development to include the following purpose encompassing both micro and macro levels:

> *...improve the level of fit between people and their environments, especially between human needs and environmental resources. In providing direct services to individuals, families, groups, and communities, the social work purpose is to help clients mobilize and draw on personal and environmental resources to (1) eliminate or alleviate life stressors and the associated stress, and (2) influence social and physical environmental forces to be responsive to people's needs. (Gitterman et al., 2021, p. 83)*

In social work practice based on the Life Model, collaboration between practitioners and people with whom they work is paramount and is supported by four phases of systematic work together on an issue, including "preparatory, initial, ongoing, and ending" phases (Gitterman et al., 2021, p. 108). This process helps people to analyze their life experiences and resolve challenges.

The ecological perspective has important applications to work with Neurodivergent individuals. Mandy (2023) described how the ecological perspective's recognition of the interplay between individual and environment reflects a shift in approach to understanding autism, particularly for researchers. Instead of a "pathology approach," the ecological perspective is a "neurodiversity approach...with an emphasis on seeing neurodivergence as difference rather than disorder and centering autistic perspectives in research and practice" (Mandy, 2023, pp. 1853-1854). By understanding neurodiversity as interplay between person and environment, it becomes possible to see that environments are not always accessible to everyone, including educational environments. It is those environmental barriers in colleges and universities which must be changed so that *all* people can live, work, and learn there.

PIE AND ECOLOGICAL PERSPECTIVES: CONNECTIONS IN EDUCATION

Often, environmental and systemic factors in postsecondary education are problematic and can create barriers that are disadvantageous to Neurodivergent learners (Cox et al., 2021). For example, the medical model of disability, a perspective prevalent in postsecondary education, is deficit-based, and views neurodiversity as a problem with the individual based on their diagnosis (Farrant et al., 2022). This model places the responsibility for success in the college environment on the student and their ability to overcome their learning challenges. Subsequently, colleges and universities require disclosure of diagnosis and demand students provide medical or other assessment documentation to receive reasonable accommodations, such as extended time to take exams, or use of note-taking services or software (Clouder et al., 2020). Providing academic accommodation is a *reactive* response to a student's learning needs, rather than a *proactive* one. Putting in place accommodations after a student has disclosed is a systemic reaction to the disclosure process. It can also occur in response to negative student outcomes if they choose to disclose when they are already struggling academically. Rather than a reactive, deficit-focused practice, a proactive design that anticipates how to provide an accessible learning environment for the wide variety of learning differences is better aligned with the PIE and ecological perspectives.

Transition to College

Supporting Neurodivergent students in postsecondary education often involves building on connections between the PIE and ecological perspectives and what they reveal about students' experiences. This is particularly important as students transition to college from high school or adult endeavors and responsibilities. PIE and ecological perspectives must be considered in determining how best to provide both access and inclusion for Neurodivergent students within the context of the classroom, public spaces, and the social environment. Implementing Universal Design for Learning (UDL) (CAST, 2018) in course design and instructional strategies, creating sensory-friendly spaces and activities on campus, and matching incoming students with mentors are proactive, strength-based measures that positively support all students.

Using the PIE and ecological perspectives can inform how we view the ways collegiate faculty and staff interact with Neurodivergent students and with each other when the student transitions from high school or employment to college. Just as social workers must consider clients' contexts and the systems involved, university personnel must do the same to maximize the persistence of students. The context of a Neurodivergent college student's life involves their family, university, and community systems, and subsets within each of these systems. In the university system, there are subsystems for student onboarding, orientation, instruction, and engagement among others.

Mandy (2023) described how an ecological perspective can inform changes to the educational environment to make it socially more welcoming and less stigmatizing to Autistic students. This could be accomplished through university transition-to-college programs which build community, offer mentoring, and provide neurodiversity education to faculty, staff, and students on campus, such as the Dub-C Autism Program at West Chester University in Pennsylvania (West Chester University, n.d.).

Inclusivity and Accessibility

Neurodivergent learners can experience disadvantages with inclusivity and accessibility that are built into the higher education system. Rigidity in policies and processes including course design, instruction, examination procedures, disclosure processes, and eligibility for support can be marginalizing and detrimental (Butcher & Lane, 2024). One study illuminated several "micro-systems" that demonstrate critical interaction between students and their environment that have reciprocal effects, including "curricula, assessments, teachers, [other] students, spaces, support, RAPs [reasonable adjustment plans], and student clubs and associations" (Butcher & Lane, 2024, p. 16). Moreover, the researchers found that students' neurodiverse identities, their disclosure decisions and experiences, and their level of connectedness to others affected and was affected by these environmental systems. The PIE and ecological perspectives can create an openness for university personnel to understand diverse identities and consider the environment in which people live and learn as they create processes and procedures. These two perspectives integrate the micro, mezzo, and macro levels in social work; this can be applied systemically and collaboratively in a university setting to assist faculty, staff, and students to enhance the growth and education of Neurodivergent students.

Students are someone's family members, parents, and employees, in addition to being learners. These different aspects of identity must be understood for all learners, but neurodiversity is an additional aspect that must be understood in the college context. We must think about how to make changes when a component of the environment that is disadvantageous to Neurodivergent learners, students with disabilities, and others is recognized. We must integrate neurodiversity as an aspect of diversity in general and work to proactively promote inclusivity and accessibility through design of programs, classroom learning environments, online learning environments, and physical spaces on campus. Supporting a Neurodivergent student takes collaboration that leverages their strengths and involves the student, faculty, and staff on campus.

STRENGTH-BASED APPROACH

A strength-based approach moves away from attention only on problems; it does not focus on the individual as the center of the problem and the only source of a resolution. Instead, it is oriented toward the growth and development of the whole person (Weick et al., 1989). In the late 1980s and early 1990s, the strength-based approach in social work began with case management for mental health clients and then expanded to others (Saleebey, 1996). Strength-based practices have been found useful with clients with severe mental illness, as well as in managing the difficulties of the elderly, those living in poverty, and individuals experiencing substance abuse (Rapp et al., 2005).

According to Weick and colleagues (1989), when social workers looked beyond a client's symptomology and worked with the client on finding productive employment that met the client's aspirations (Weick et al., 1989), this strength-based approach was effective. A study about case management serving people with severe mental illnesses revealed that centering the social environment rather than the pathology of the clients was also successful (Rapp & Chamberlain, 1985). This strength-based case management model concentrated on finding resources for the client to be effective in achieving their goals. The case management interventions focused on the everyday aspects of life such as housing, health, recreation, and other social needs. Rapp et al. (2005) distinguished 6 aspects of the strength-based approach including: the client will set goals with the social worker; there is a systematic plan for assessment which focuses on the client's current situation; the environment is seen as a wellspring of resources; there are methods for identifying client strengths and resources; there is an instillation of hope when building professional relationships; and clients making their own decisions is respected. The authors argued that strength-based social work requires concrete criteria to determine if it can be accurately labeled as strength-based.

Moore (2022), who utilized a strength-based relationship and reciprocity approach, supported similar principles when working with the elderly. The Care Act (2014) in the United Kingdom (UK) requires social workers to consider the strengths of each person. It shows the shift away from a needs-based assessment to a strength-based assessment which is necessary for a trusting and supportive relationship between the social worker and the client. Moore (2022) believed in five elements similar to those of Rapp et al. (2005) including: the emphasis is on strengths rather than deficiencies; there is a model of growth for the client; the relationship between the social worker and the client is the key to success; within a trusting relationship, the client directs the process of change; and community is an important part of the change process.

The broad scope of strength-based practices is relevant to working with Neurodivergent people. For example, the three conversations approach used with the elderly in the UK could be applied to Neurodivergent students in higher education (Cole, 2016). This approach is geared toward utilizing the resources within the person and within the community. The first conversation focuses on the individual's assets and connecting to services such as discussing the tutoring center or a peer tutoring program with a Neurodivergent student. The second conversation addresses emergency needs when the individual is facing a crisis, such as identifying assistance for a Neurodivergent student in danger of failing a class. The third conversation makes a plan for long term support such as guiding a student through the process of attaining a formal diagnosis and disclosing to the Disability Resources Office (DRO) to receive accommodations. Asset mapping, one tool of strength-based practice, is the process of identifying individual and community resources which can assist a person on a daily basis. Asset mapping creates a visual representation of an individual's knowledge bases, skills, talents, available resources, and support networks (Caiels et al., 2021). Neurodivergent students can work with university social workers, the DRO staff, faculty members, and mentors to map their assets and discuss how these strengths can be used effectively to achieve success academically and socially.

Social work from a strength-based perspective requires knowledge of neurodiversity and co-occurring challenges in the postsecondary setting. Eki and Isaksoon (2013) discussed strategies to help individuals with ADHD become successful as adults. For people with ADHD, organized and communal activities can be helpful in gaining success in work and academics. These events can assist individuals in identify resources; a panel discussion on neurodiversity can explain the role of the DRO in supporting Neurodivergent students; an award ceremony can acknowledge the strengths of Neurodivergent students; and a student organized board game night can provide social interactions without sensory challenges present at a loud crowded sporting event or a dance party with flashing lights and a large number of participants.

A history of negative experiences resulting in low self-esteem and low self-efficacy can be mitigated using effective resources to move a person toward a strength-based perspective. One can then begin to think positively about one's life experience. It is important to understand that for Neurodivergent adults complications can be met with strength and resilience. Neurodivergent learners may have ADHD, dyslexia, and autism, among other cognitive differences. Challenges for these learners could include academic underperformance, interpersonal issues, and problems with substance abuse and mental health (Custodio et al., 2024); however, they also exhibit valuable strengths. For example, learners with ADHD can demonstrate strong social and communication skills, excellence in creative pursuits, and empathic and compassionate personalities (Hotez et al., 2022). For individuals with dyslexia, reading may be a challenge; however, a strength-based lens can reveal that they have excellent three-dimensional spatial reasoning and pattern detection. Their creativity may be enhanced by divergent thinking, and they may have superior problem-solving skills (Eide & Eide, 2023). While individuals with autism may experience stigma due to their neurodiverse traits such as non-majority social interaction, their strengths may include focused interests, systems thinking, consistent honesty, or perfect pitch along with many others (Woods & Estes, 2023). It is essential that Neurodivergent students recognize their superior skills in some areas to manage the challenges in others.

Family, peers, participants in their support networks, or faculty members can encourage students to use their assets. Two methods which could provide guidance are the "SPELL framework (Structure, Positive approaches and expectations, Empathy, Low arousal, and Links), and "person-centered active support" (Caiels et al., 2021, p. 418). The SPELL framework helps illuminate things students find interesting, as well as their talents, to assist with learning and development. Person-centered active support is similar, but includes scaffolding areas of challenge. These methods are broadly applicable, including for adults in college.

Hamilton and Petty (2023) argued that Neurodivergent students can be assisted in achieving higher education goals through "compassionate" approaches such as universal design and a strength-based perspective. Neurodivergent students come to universities from environments which have often been exclusive of them. Universal design allows the student flexibility and choice in their learning process. Farrant et al. (2022) posited that to create a friendly environment for Neurodivergent students and a more stress-free approach to teaching, the classroom should consider the learning needs of *all* students by using neurodiverse language, employing extensions for assignment deadlines, offering different types of study such as both full-time and part-time programs in face-to-face and virtual settings, providing clear instructions and expectations, and utilizing peer support. These techniques enable Neurodivergent students to approach learning through their assets rather than their deficits.

It is clear that Neurodivergent students succeed in higher education with a supportive and collaborative environment as they share their successes and participate in a collaborative community (Onwumelu, 2024). Morin and Kirchner-Morris (2023) recommended team teaching as a valuable method for working with Neurodivergent students. A strength-based perspective helps campus stakeholders with a compassionate view collaborate where the students can grow and develop as participants on the team, adapting a positive perspective of growth and development.

A Biopsychosocial Model of Assessment for Strength-based Social Work Practices

The biopsychosocial model originated with Engel in the 1970s (Engel, 1977). A biopsychosocial model posits that nature and nurture interact with each other (Cooper et al., 2012). Bisman (2001) defined the biopsychosocial model in social work: "biological information of family and individual medical history, psychological data covering the intrapsychic and personality factors, and social information about social supports and community resources" (p. 4). Stone et al. (2007) saw the reciprocity between the social and biological aspects of the biopsychosocial model. The model considers that biological issues seemingly have a social and psychological component. This leads the social worker to assess situations in a broad perspective and look for biological, psychological, and social factors that are influencing what is deemed an individual problem.

The use of a biopsychosocial method is very helpful for assessment in social work because it gives a comprehensive view of the person. Gale (2022) detailed the aspects of completing a biopsychosocial assessment as first reviewing any prior information and exercising care if the information is deficit based. Then the social worker conducts a face-to-face interview with the client and observes the client's interactions in their natural environment. It is vital to obtain information from collateral sources such as friends, family, and other people of importance, and then utilize standardized instruments for assessment. Assessing risk factors including medical history and any mental health or substance abuse history is crucial. This approach gives the social worker a comprehensive view from different perspectives to provide interventions in collaboration with the client. This same model is useful for assessing and supporting Neurodivergent learners in postsecondary education to identify challenges and strengths.

Given that neurodiversity is biologically based and affected by social and psychological factors, the biopsychosocial model more fully explains neurodiversity. Biological aspects are important because medical and genetic factors can have a significant effect on an individual's functional abilities. Understanding human behavior means discerning the interaction between the mind and body and the social and psychological environment (Burns et al., 2019). Engaging and working with Neurodivergent people can be facilitated by utilizing this biopsychosocial approach. Conducting a thorough biopsychosocial assessment will help determine what past factors influence current functioning. A Neurodivergent student can better understand themselves within the context of their social environment through this process (Doyle, 2020; Farrant et al., 2022). Understanding the medical, educational, family, and mental health histories of a Neurodivergent student enables the student and the DRO to derive interventions that support their growth and development.

A social worker with familiarity of the biopsychosocial model can be a key collaborator in supporting Neurodivergent students. With a very thorough biopsychosocial assessment, a social worker can give input to a collaborative team to come up with a student-centered plan for support. The student and their support network can assess their progress toward goals on an ongoing basis. This model leads the social workers and other members of the university team to a holistic approach to meeting the needs of Neurodivergent students.

ADVOCACY

Advocacy plays an important role in the history of social work dating back to the 18th and 19th centuries. The profession of social work grew out of the need to address "social problems" through advocacy efforts for marginalized individuals and communities (Bliss & Ginn, 2021, p. 432). Jane Addams, one of the architects of the Settlement House movement in the U.S. in the late 1800s, advocated politically to improve urban conditions and equitable opportunities for the urban poor and immigrants (Fabricant & Fisher, 2008). Addams also wrote about and worked extensively on international peace efforts and later won the Nobel Peace Prize (Alonso, 1995).

As expressed by Schneider (2008) and colleagues, "social work is the one profession that has acknowledged, decade after decade, a healthy tension between individual needs and the policies of the larger society" (para. 2) which leads social workers to become advocates on micro and macro levels. This principle of social justice is one of the core values that the social work profession has embedded (National Association of Social Workers, 2021). Social workers advocate for people to become empowered to improve their own social functioning and obtain resources and support. There are many ways that social workers advocate for individuals; Freddolino et al. (2004) stated that advocacy is an important aspect of social work, but it varies in its delivery.

Within the profession, portrayals of social work advocacy involve system level (e.g., case and class advocacy), type of service (e.g., family service, case management), form of advocacy (e.g., legislative advocacy, whistle blowing, rights representation), social reaction to recipients (e.g., people who experience oppression and people who are considered to be vulnerable), and diagnostic category of recipients (e.g., people with mental illness, people coping with HIV/AIDS) (Freddolino et al., 2004, p. 119).

The literature about advocacy points to several ways that social workers and others engage with social justice challenges at various levels. tefani (2023) stated that advocacy is part of macro social work practice, which involves advocating for systemic-level social justice and social change. Addams and the Settlement House movement embodied macro social work advocacy, also known as "cause advocacy" (Gasker, 2023, p. 522). In contemporary society, examples of macro social work practice include leadership within non-profit organizations, providing testimony in front of legislatures, writing issue briefs for publication, running for office, working in political campaigns, lobbying legislators, community organizing, and coalition work. Using these social work practices would be valuable in the advocacy of the neurodiversity movement.

Dalrymple and Boylan (2016) described the need for advocacy at the micro or mezzo level in the context of an individual, family, or group of people without power needing support to negotiate complex health and social welfare systems. This is known as "case advocacy" (Gasker, 2023, p. 522), and its history can be traced back to Mary Richmond and the Charity Organization Society movement, which focused on providing therapeutic and support services to individuals through casework (Gitterman et al., 2021). Today, these services are more commonly known as case management and clinical practice. For example, social workers provide inpatient and outpatient psychotherapy, case management support, and linkage to resources to obtain food, shelter, health and mental health care, and other needs. Advocacy can be the purpose of an agency, or the social worker may individually initiate advocacy; however, self-advocacy is often at the beginning, because people must be willing to participate in the process of getting their needs met in collaboration with social workers. Self-advocacy is also a key element of Neurodivergent student success (Park et al., 2023; Rogers-Shaw et al., 2023).

Advocacy in Relationship to Postsecondary Education

Collaborative efforts among students, faculty, staff, and administrators are critical for student success in postsecondary educational settings; the social work profession's model of advocacy for both systemic change and meeting individual needs can inform these collaborations. As students transition to college, they must develop greater self-advocacy skills to successfully navigate the initial transition, as well as the subsequent years of study until graduation (Rogers-Shaw et al., 2023). For adult learners returning to college, they must also become self-advocates as they acclimate to the environment and balance their educational and life responsibilities (Bergman, 2021). Communicating with faculty and staff to ask for resources and support is a necessary self-advocacy skill. In turn, university personnel can advocate for students on a macro level by making the environment accessible and inclusive and providing those resources and support, such as mentoring, advising, tutoring, using technological tools, and building community.

The growth of self-advocacy among people with disabilities has become a powerful movement which has led to the international recognition of how individuals with differences have been marginalized and has led to the passage of U.S. civil rights laws protecting individuals with disabilities from discrimination, and allowing greater participation in higher education (Shallish, 2015). However, when students face a university environment which is not friendly and supportive of neurodiversity or other differences, they continue to experience barriers to access and success.

Being an Advocate for Neurodivergent Learners in Postsecondary Education

Often, the only obvious advocates for Neurodivergent students on campus are the students themselves, the staff who work for the DRO and neurodiversity-specific support programs, and individuals who have personal experience with or knowledge of neurodiversity. Neurodiversity must be recognized broadly in the university community as an aspect of intersectional identity and difference, and not something a person must change to fit into the environment. Advocates for inclusivity, support, and funding among administrators, provosts, and presidents are needed to make a lasting difference in the university community.

Anicha and colleagues (2024) described five initiatives university leaders can undertake to advance social justice related to disability and difference, such as ensuring that all differences are proactively included in policy, procedure, and change initiatives for physical and online spaces, as well as in communications (e.g. universal design). These researchers noted that each of these initiatives "will call for cross-institutional collaboration and long-term work-plans in order to create meaningful change for disability equity" (Anicha et al., 2024, p. 17).

Using the principles of advocacy championed by the social work profession, university faculty, staff, and administrators can specifically address exclusion and marginalization of Neurodivergent learners. At the macro level, university leaders and personnel can advocate with legislators and grantors for funding that can be used to promote access to college through TRIO programs (Council for Opportunity in Education, n.d.) and neurodiversity-specific programming; they can create community-building initiatives and train faculty and staff about Neurodivergent students' experiences. These efforts should be undertaken in collaboration with Neurodivergent students, who can choose to lend their expertise and voice. Faculty, staff, and administration can work together to create university procedures that prioritize communication of academic and co-curricular information in multiple modalities (print, learning management system announcements, websites, and social media), and design sensory-friendly spaces and dining options on campus.

At the mezzo and micro levels, methods of advocacy can be wide-ranging. Partnerships between social work department faculty and students and neurodiversity advocates could produce training materials and toolkits about neurodiversity for the various audiences on campus. Individuals who live, work, and learn on campus can become educated about the unique aspects of neurodiversity (Anicha et al., 2024); this knowledge can aid in advancing inclusion for everyone, as well as combating ableism in the community, through advocacy and allyship.

ALLYSHIP

An ally is a member of a dominant group, with a level of authority, power, and privilege that enables them to support those in a marginalized group and fight against oppressive systems; allies are part of an ingroup whose members promote fairness that supports those in the outgroup (Bourke, 2020; Williams & Sharif, 2021). An ally engages in social justice work to "individually, and collectively, push back while drawing on their positions rooted in power and privilege" (Bourke, 2020, p. 181). Allies who have an individual relationship with a member of an oppressed group can provide personal support. An ally can be someone who speaks out and advocates for marginalized individuals, takes action to change a system that discriminates, and works to dismantle power structures that oppress. The reasons for becoming an ally vary, including positive views of marginalized individuals and groups, connection to a particular individual in one of these groups, or the opportunity to enact social justice values (Bourke, 2020; Jenkins 2009; LeMaire et al., 2020; Pietri et al., 2024). Allyship can be meaningful or merely performative (Nixon, 2019).

Meaningful allyship increases "inclusion and acceptance, effectively challenging bias, empowering the recipient, and advocating for them" (Collier-Spruel & Ryan, 2024, p. 83); it provides a sense of psychological safety and diminishes the anxiety experienced by marginalized individuals. Effective allyship should intentionally focus on the experiences and voices of those to whom the support is directed rather than on the ally's behavior. In the practice of social work and education, active listening is required to be an effective ally (Collier-Spruel & Ryan, 2024; Dahunsi, 2024).

Performative allyship occurs when a nonmarginalized individual, someone who is neuromajority for example, offers superficial support that is not truly beneficial to a Neurodivergent individual and might even cause harm; a performative ally is motivated by the rewards of their allyship such as recognition or increased personal standing obtained by supporting others. An example of performative allyship could be posting support for a cause on social media without taking any significant action and then bragging about that support (Kalina, 2020; Kutlaca & Radke, 2023). Effective allyship requires a long term commitment; one cannot be an ally only when it is convenient. Performative allyship excuses individuals from making that commitment; it is exemplified in individuals who claim to be allies yet still hold marginalized individuals responsible for the inequality they face and argue that individuals, rather than social structures and institutional systems, must change to eliminate inequality (Kalina, 2020; Sumerau et al., 2021).

Allyship is not effective if the purported ally does not acknowledge their own privilege and bias and does not understand the differences between themselves and those who are marginalized. An ally who does not have the skills to appropriately support those victimized by stigma and exclusion and whose offer of support is condescending and dependency-oriented is ineffective (Collier-Spruel & Ryan, 2024; Kalina, 2020). Performative allyship has become commonplace, although effective allyship is still an important tool for supporting Neurodivergent students on college campuses.

Effective Allyship in Social Work & Education

Social workers and educators have engaged in allyship in many contexts where allies work to understand the theoretical foundation of allyship and endeavor to apply the theory to social justice practices (Bennett & Carlson-Manathara, 2024; Kickett et al., 2024). Individuals may pursue careers in social work and/or education because they have an identity within a marginalized group and understand the challenges that brings, they may have close associates in this position who they care about, and they may desire a career that can make a difference in others' lives. Alternatively, their experiences of privilege may have led them to recognize "how privilege and oppression interact and shape social work practice and faculty–student engagement in the classroom" (Goode et al., 2021, p. 43), leading to a desire to fight against oppression as they acknowledge that social workers and teachers have a responsibility to work towards social justice.

Social workers and postsecondary professionals working with Neurodivergent students face a "key challenge in … moving beyond performative and superficial efforts and representations to deeper, more nuanced, and more action-focused and impactful social justice work" (Bennett & Carlson-Manathara, 2024, pp. 6-7). Social work and education are viewed as caring professions and reflexivity is an important component in this work. Promoting the idea of critical reflexivity, Bennett & Carlson-Manathara (2024) argued that allies need to think about their own biases and how they affect ally relationships and the practice of social justice advocacy; an awareness of one's position in power structures then becomes visible and allows for significant change to disrupt systems of power. True allies "take responsibility for their learning and yet recognize their own ignorance and limitations of understanding" Bennett & Carlson-Manathara, 2024, p. 6).

Recognizing and naming actions and structures that marginalize individuals and groups is the first step to becoming an ally (Goode et al., 2021). Education on effective allyship should include increasing self-awareness through reflexive practices and generating new knowledge of what allyship is and how to practice it in a meaningful way. Important elements include examining how one's own strengths and privileges can be used to enhance allyship. Using appropriate language and guiding others in its use is one example. Offering hands-on experiences, intergroup dialogue, and discussion of creative scenarios can teach effective allyship skills (Craig et al., 2022; Goode et al., 2021; LeMaire et al., 2020; Williams & Sharif, 2021).

Allies of Neurodivergent students should listen to them and ask what support they want. They should learn about neurodiversity and seek out Neurodivergent colleagues who can be an asset as a mentor for a neuromajority ally. Allies should speak up, even if what one has to say will be uncomfortable for others to hear. For example, do not back down from supporting Neurodivergent students because others who have diminished and stigmatized these students would not like to hear they have committed microaggressions. Allies should read materials on bias or attend a workshop on equity or a training session on cultural competency. They might join an organization focused on diversity where they can come together with others who have similar goals.

Allies recognize expertise in others and value it and promote it to limit power differentials. They intentionally recruit diverse individuals for their own groups and organizations, thereby creating more inclusive environments. Allies know when not to speak, especially when one's privilege often puts them in a position where their voice is valued. Allies amplify the voices of marginalized individuals rather than speaking themselves (LeMaire et al., 2020). An individual may see themselves as an ally, but if marginalized people do not view them that way, then they are not effective in the ally role. Neurodivergent students often do not see others like themselves in academic settings; therefore, their challenges to fit in and thrive may preclude success. Effective allies can be crucial in bringing about change on campus and creating a more inclusive environment (LeMaire et al., 2020, p. 6).

Neurodivergent students are not completely homogenous; they have differences due to the characteristics of their neurodiverse diagnoses and differences in the way their neurodivergence is affected by their body and/or their environment (Wolbring & Lillywhite, 2023, p. 3). Therefore, they have different needs for an ally to consider. Social work practices create an awareness of power imbalances and both social workers and postsecondary institution faculty, staff, and administration have a responsibility to work toward shifting these power structures if they are to provide meaningful and effective alliances across neurotypes (Gillespie-Lynch et al., 2020).

Being an Ally for Neurodivergent Learners in Postsecondary Education

There are several places in postsecondary education where allyship can make a substantial difference, including research, teaching, and mentoring (LeMaire et al., 2020, p. 11). Researchers should include members of marginalized groups on research teams, particularly Neurodivergent scholars and students when working on neurodiverse topics; however, "researchers must also be cautious to avoid tokenizing collaborators with marginalized identities" (LeMaire et al., 2020, p. 13); their participation must be significant and valued.

Faculty members can become allies by using inclusive course design and diverse course material that includes marginalized voices. Applying the elements of UDL is one method for creating inclusive classrooms. Caring faculty allies can model effective allyship by revealing a desire to continue to learn through training in accessible course design and materials, attending professional development workshops on neurodiversity and available supports for Neurodivergent students, and paying attention to appropriate terminology and word choices. They can acknowledge their own biases as they come up during class and interact with students in multiple ways such as recorded and transcribed lectures, group activities, one-on-one tutoring, mentoring, and email communications (LeMaire et al., 2020; Park et al., 2023; Rogers-Shaw et al., 2023).

Allies committed to supporting others can provide peer, faculty, and staff mentorship opportunities that assist Neurodivergent students in integrating into college life. Mentors can point out opportunities and bring Neurodivergent students into a network of supporters. Marginalized individuals often have difficulty in finding mentors who understand their neurodiversity so formal and structured college mentor programs are important, as is a mentor's commitment to guiding students through significant transitions. An ally who is skilled at mentoring can provide students with necessary knowledge of university systems and policies, organizations and activities of interest, and academic resources. No matter what form of allyship is pursued, it can have a lasting effect on marginalized individuals.

Allies can offer powerful support for Neurodivergent students through peer friendships, instructor/tutor/DRO academic support, and staff interventions. Creating effective cross-campus allyship requires collaborative efforts to grow awareness of neurodiversity through campus-wide education efforts, stressing the importance of authentic ally motivation (Radke et al., 2020) rather than making minimal performative efforts. Participating in activities to support Neurodivergent students such as inclusive social interactions, developing campus networks of students, faculty, staff, administrators, departments and organizations that come together to support Neurodivergent students, and building inclusive programming are ways to be allies (Pietri et al., 2024).

A significant problem for Neurodivergent students who may not easily find and develop relationships with allies is that they may need to spend time away from neuromajority allies, no matter how well-intentioned they are (Gillespie-Lynch et al., 2020). Power imbalances can be lessened when Neurodivergent students are involved in allyship. Peer allyship is an important factor in creating inclusive opportunities; "[p]articipatory approaches, and approaches solely led by Neurodivergent people can begin to address concerns about power and representation within the neurodiversity movement while shifting public understanding" (Gillespie-Lynch et al., 2020, p. 189).

Allyship does not work towards a cure that erases neurodiverse characteristics; however, it advocates for changes within the systems and structures of society and individualized support to address personal challenges through strengths (Gillespie-Lynch et al., 2020). Campus spaces for collaboration bring together both Neurodivergent individuals and neuromajority people.

USING SOCIAL WORK APPROACHES IN COLLABORATIVE POSTSECONDARY TEAMS

Social workers must collaborate with a host of other professionals including service providers, government agencies, and educational institutions. They must develop collaborative relationships with clients who may struggle with mental health issues or learning disabilities as well as interact with their families and caregivers. Creating genuine partnerships is a daily part of their practice (Whittington, 2023). It is valuable to recognize that there is interdependence between individuals and specific groups on campus who share the same goals of supporting Neurodivergent students in achieving success. Just as flexibility and reflection are important factors in academic assistance to Neurodivergent students, they are also elements of a strong collaborative team (Bronstein, 2003). While campus stakeholders may have personal commitments and similar objectives to creating a positive inclusive campus environment for Neurodivergent students, the foundation of their caring attitude may vary; effective collaborative teams need to be clear about roles and objectives to move campus entities toward the goal of Neurodivergent student success and belonging (Hesjedal et al., 2015). The underlying principles of the practice of social work offer models of collaboration that can guide campus teams.

Collaboration through Person-in-Environment & Ecological Perspectives

Preparation for transitioning into the workplace after graduation provides an opportunity for collaboration that considers PIE and ecological perspectives. Challenges to successful employment involve several specific contexts including the DRO, the career services office, departments related to career fields, neurodiverse student organizations, on campus job locations, community businesses offering internships, college fairs, and workplaces. Steps that need to be developed to support Neurodivergent students seeking post graduation success should begin while the individual is a student. The DRO and career services can work with neurodiverse student organizations and departments related to career fields to develop workshops and job fairs that enhance career skill development and expand knowledge of career opportunities in a variety of fields. Resume writing, interviewing techniques, and career exploration strategies are examples of possible workshop topics. Career services and the DRO can reach out to campus departments offering on-campus jobs and community businesses interested in hiring student interns to create on-ramps for Neurodivergent students. Community connections with career services can bring career specialists to campus as guest speakers and mock interview participants. In this way businesses, campus offices, and social networks can support Neurodivergent students on micro, mezzo, and macro levels.

Strengths-Based Collaborative Advocacy

Strengths-based collaborative advocacy needs to be focused on what Neurodivergent students can do and do well. Neurodivergent program award ceremonies, newsletters with stories highlighting Neurodivergent student successes, and presentations on neurodivergent strengths emphasize talents. They can be organized by DRO staff, Neurodivergent student organizations, and student affairs professionals. Workshops and professional development for faculty and university staff can be designed and implemented by the DRO, the school of education, and Neurodivergent students, sharing ways to use specific neurodiverse strengths in classrooms and student organizations.

Collaborative planning and executing college disability days with dedicated events that raise awareness about disability issues, celebrate the contributions of people with disabilities, and promote inclusive environments on college campuses can educate and empower both students and faculty, increasing their disability awareness, their understanding of access, and their knowledge of student rights. In these endeavors, it is important to include panel discussions, film screenings, training workshops, performances, poetry readings, art exhibits, guest speakers, and student story sharing. Highlighting online publications like the Invisible Disability Project, campus examples of universal design, promoting YouTube Channels and videos like Ask an Autistic (where one person answers questions about what it's like for her to live with autism), The Tommy Edison Experience (where one person uses humor to answer popular questions about living without sight), A Day Through a Deaf Person's Eyes (where people share different aspects of their life while Deaf), and Disability, the Truth (a video that interviews people to hear their insights on disability) (Burgstahler, 2024) can be valuable contributions. Planning of awareness events must not promote ableist views, nor be condescending. Resources to ensure appropriate content include: What are Alternatives to Disability-Related Simulations to Promote Disability Awareness? (Burgstahler, 2024) and the Disabilities,

Opportunities, Internetworking, and Technology (DO-IT) Center (University of Washington, n.d.).

Using a Biopsychosocial Model of Assessment as a Collaborative Tool

While research has documented the growing number of students with disabilities in postsecondary education, a lack of disclosure prevents an accurate rate of disability presence (Aquino et al., 2025). Many Neurodivergent students may not disclose through the formal documented disability process and so do not receive accommodations although they may disclose informally to peers, faculty, or university staff with whom they interact. In most cases, the current disclosure process relies on a medical diagnosis that focuses on biology and is less attentive to the social and psychological components of neurodiversity. Working collaboratively, campus stakeholders can provide a more comprehensive description of Neurodivergent students on campus based on their interactions with those who do not disclose but are perceived to have learning challenges or those who disclose informally; colleges and universities can decrease ableism through training in more inclusive policies, practices, and services that support all students (Aquino et al., 2025).

By developing a broader view of neurodiversity through collaborative team discussions and collaborative research projects designed to discover the needs of the informally disclosed or undisclosed Neurodivergent students on campus, faculty and staff training can be designed and implemented to better meet the needs of these Neurodivergent students. Teaching and learning centers, the DRO, faculty governance organizations, the provost's office, and academic departments can increase professional development opportunities on the implementation of UDL in course design, instruction, and assessment so that the needs of all students can be better supported. Student affairs professionals, the DRO, resident life staff, and mental health counselors can work together to incorporate social activities and spaces that meet the needs of diverse students. Administrators can work with the DRO and faculty to "regularly evaluate the effectiveness of accommodations and ensure that policies support flexible and student-centered approaches to disclosure" (Aquino et al., 2025, p. 12). Simplifying the disclosure process and highlighting academic supports that do not require a formal disclosure, such as tutoring centers, peer tutoring, and formalized study groups can address the needs of all students, including those who do not disclose their neurodivergence. Exploring the expansion of these options is a valuable task that can result from evaluations of current student supports.

Allied Collaboration

In building collaborative groups across campus, there are some significant recommendations that should be emphasized. Use appropriate terminology, listening for how Neurodivergent individuals identify themselves and using those words to describe them while recognizing the broad range of terms Neurodivergent individuals choose for themselves. As an ally, one should argue that neurodivergence is a difference, not a tragedy to be corrected, acknowledging that all people have strengths and weaknesses. Remember that Neurodivergent individuals are experts on neurodiversity, yet Neurodivergent students are not all alike; show understanding that neurodiversity includes students with autism and ADHD, but that there are many other diagnoses under the neurodiversity umbrella. Emphasize the need for systems and structures to change rather than Neurodivergent individuals (Gensic & Brunton, 2022).

Avoid judging competence based on one's closeness to neuroconformity. Share authentic stories and amplify the voices of Neurodivergent individuals rather than sharing overcoming stories that offer simplistic and condescending one-size-fits-all solutions. Include Neurodivergent students in group activities such as research, program design, planning education and awareness events, and developing campus organizations that support neurodiversity. Reach out and talk with Neurodivergent people about their experiences, work with organizations that support neurodiversity, stay informed about changes in the field, acknowledge past errors and move forward, aiming to become more enlightened (Gensic & Brunton, 2022).

It is important to realize that research and advocacy can spread misconceptions and stigmatize individuals if there is a lack of understanding of the intricacies of neurodiversity. Collaborative research teams, consisting of faculty from different departments, practitioners from a variety of programs, and students who are neurodivergent and neuromajority, are an effective means of allyship. These teams should recruit widely through varied methods to ensure the participant population is diverse and use inclusive data collection and analysis methods. They can connect stakeholders across campus and contribute valuable knowledge to the field of inclusion and neurodiversity (Gillespie-Lynch et al., 2020; LeMaire et al., 2020).

The type of research conducted can also develop allyship as action research which is intended "to improve the lives of those it was meant to impact. The mission of action research is to extend research beyond publication into implementing strategies that directly and positively impact others as opposed to contributing to theory alone" (LeMaire et al., 2020, p. 13), thus moving allyship to the action stage. Participatory research studies reflect effective allyship as they share power in equitable ways, involving participants in decision-making. They build trust and base the research objectives on shared goals (Gillespie-Lynch et al., 2020), fostering effective alllyship. Social workers have valuable knowledge of working together to improve lives and educators can learn from their theories and practices.

CONCLUSION

Neurodivergent learners frequently enter college having encountered many challenging educational experiences in their primary and secondary school careers (Connolly et al., 2023; Shepherd et al., 2024; Wiener & Daniels, 2016), thereby beginning with a preconceived idea that it will continue to be a place filled with barriers. Clouder et al. (2020) described the challenges Neurodivergent students often face when they enter higher education, which leads them to struggle with specific issues in the academic environment. These obstacles can include emotional distress and the struggle to maintain emotional wellbeing, social isolation from peers, lack of academic support, and difficulty coping with the academic environment. Coupled with potentially negative past experiences, adjustment to the postsecondary setting can be fraught for Neurodivergent learners.

Bureaucratic systems of the university can also be difficult to navigate and can create barriers to success for all learners, including Neurodivergent students (Farrant et al., 2022; Kuder et al., 2023). Students may not have awareness and understanding of university policies and procedures, such as how to make decisions about course or semester withdrawals. Learners may also lack understanding of university policies on requesting an incomplete grade which allows more time to complete a course after the end of a semester, or policies about options to repeat classes in which they performed poorly.

Social work literature and theory is highly instructive in working with and teaching Neurodivergent learners, faculty, staff, and administrators in college and university settings. Through our review of the concepts of person-in-environment and ecological perspectives, a strength-based approach, advocacy, and allyship, we have illustrated how educators can shift their work with students from a focus on overcoming deficits to one of leveraging and building on strengths. The examples of collaborative practices delineated above and visible in the case studies provide guidance for increasing effective neurodivergent student support. As more collaborations are developed across campus offices and stakeholders in colleges and universities, the elimination of unnecessary barriers and systemic inequities for Neurodivergent learners in the higher education environment become more achievable.

CASE STUDIES AND DISCUSSION QUESTIONS

Case Study 1: Biopsychosocial Assessment Model

Leo is a first-year college student at a four-year university who is undecided on a major program of study. He is taking a variety of courses during his first semester, one of which is an introduction to social work course. About a month into the semester, Leo's social work professor notices that he has not attended class or completed assignments for the last two weeks. The professor contacts Leo via email, asking how Leo is doing, and expressing concern about his wellbeing since he hasn't been in class. The professor asks if Leo would like to schedule a meeting to talk about the class and how she can support him to get back on track. Leo replies that he has been feeling overwhelmed and agrees to meet with the professor.

During the meeting, Leo discloses that he was diagnosed with ADHD while in high school and has been having difficulty with concentrating during class and while doing homework. He shared that his attendance in most classes has been poor the last few weeks, and he has begun avoiding his assignments. He feels guilty, embarrassed, and scared to approach his other professors. Leo's professor shared with him that many students experience challenges during the transition to college, and his professors would likely be supportive if he reached out to them. They talked with Leo about what he might want to say to them. He wrote an email draft while in their office and agreed to send it later that evening. The professor also introduced Leo to student support resources on campus and encouraged him to contact some offices which could offer immediate help: the disability resources office, the student learning center, and the counseling center. Leo agreed to contact these offices, and to keep the social work professor informed about how he was doing. Leo was able to make connections with on-campus support offices and learned some strategies to better manage his concentration, focus, and time management. His class attendance and assignment completion began to improve, and he expressed to his social work professor that he felt like he now had a "network" of people in his corner.

Questions

1. How did the professor use the elements of the biopsychosocial assessment model to help understand Leo and the areas to prioritize in connecting him to resources?
2. How can faculty, student learning center staff, and other student support staff connect with each other to better understand how to support students like Leo?
3. How can faculty and staff learn social work principles that can help them support Neurodivergent students?

Case Study 2: Strengths-Based Model

Morgan is a psychology major in her second year of college. She is a member of the honors program at her college and has consistently earned high grades in her courses. She has a few friends she's made through the honors program but often does not attend program events or large gatherings. This semester, she is taking a world politics course which meets in-person twice a week. The format of the course is primarily Socratic; the professor engages students in question-and-answer discussions during classes, based on their readings or on current world events in the news. Readings are shared with students through the university's online learning management system, but assignment instructions are provided in class verbally or on handouts. The class grades are based on written exams only, taken in class, in addition to participation during class meetings.

Morgan met with her advisor and during the meeting stated that she is very frustrated with her world politics class. She disclosed that she understands the discussions during class but stated that she has no idea how to study for an exam based on class discussions. Morgan said that she attempts to take notes but that the discussions are "all over the place," and that information and expectations "are not written down, only talked about in class." She explained that she prefers written information and directions instead of verbal ones because "things are not going to change when they're written down." She reported that she got a D on the first exam and is worried about failing the course. The advisor asked Morgan about how she handled challenging assignments and courses in the past and reminded her that she can use those skills again. She reminded her that she has had to learn new skills before and that navigating this course will require her to learn additional skills.

Morgan's advisor suggested that Morgan should reach out to her world politics professor to schedule a meeting to talk about her difficulties with the class and ask for guidance. She also referred her to meet with the student learning resource center and to request a tutor. The advisor also informed Morgan about the disability resources office (DRO), where she could choose to pursue academic accommodations if she wanted to do so. Morgan disclosed that she is Autistic but has never needed academic support in school before; the support she received was related to social skills, and she hasn't used that since elementary school. The advisor described to Morgan that the DRO offers more than academic accommodations such as peer connection opportunities with other Autistic students, if she would find that helpful. Morgan decided to first meet with her professor and the student learning center, and to keep in touch with the advisor for the next few weeks to discuss her progress.

Questions

1. In what ways did the advisor use a strengths-based approach to help Morgan?
2. How can the connection to peers potentially be a benefit to Morgan? How would this connection benefit *all* students?
3. In what ways could the student learning resource center and disability resources office partner with advisors and professors to increase knowledge of strengths-based approaches when working with students?

Case Study 3: Advocacy

Antonia is an adult learner in her thirties who has returned to college to pursue an online social work degree. She has two young children and is working full-time while attending college. She has spent many years working as a direct support professional in a group home for individuals with intellectual disabilities and is motivated to advance her career. She knows that she can complete her degree but has always struggled with reading textbooks as quickly as other students and with comprehending what she reads. During an online biology class in her first semester, Antonia found herself falling behind in reading the textbook chapters each week and in remembering the terminology she read. She performed poorly on the first two weekly quizzes. In a panic, she reached out to her biology professor, who video-conferenced with Antonia and gave her guidance about how to use the course materials to supplement her reading. In addition, the biology professor demonstrated how to use the built-in "read aloud"/text-to-speech features of the electronic textbook, which is accessible through the university's learning management system (LMS). The professor also referred Antonia to the Disability Resources Office (DRO) for a consultation.

Antonia video-conferenced with the DRO director and disclosed that she had been diagnosed with dyslexia as an elementary school student. She was given extra time to take tests and quizzes during her high school years, but she often felt embarrassed and that it was a hassle to go to a separate room for tests, so she stopped using the extra time during her sophomore year of high school. Antonia and the DRO director collaborated to develop a plan of support, including implementation of academic accommodations. The DRO director connected Antonia with the student learning resource center to learn study strategies and locate a tutor. They also planned that Antonia would talk regularly with the DRO director and with her biology professor during online office hours. After two more weeks, Antonia reported to the DRO director that she had learned a great deal about how to study more effectively and was making positive progress. Her regular video meetings were very helpful in keeping her accountable and helping her feel more confident as an adult learner.

Questions

1. University efforts to make sure students are treated equitably and feel like they belong often overlook individuals with disabilities. How can college faculty and staff become culturally competent regarding ability status and neurodiversity?
2. In what ways can university personnel work together to ensure that learning environments are designed to work well for the diverse needs of *all* learners?

REFERENCES

Alonso, H. H. (1995). Nobel peace laureates, Jane Addams and Emily Greene Balch: Two women of the Women's International League for Peace and Freedom. *Journal of Women's History*, *7*(2), 6–26. DOI: 10.1353/jowh.2010.0337

Anicha, C. L., Aragon, C., Bilen-Green, C., Blaser, B., & Burgstahler, S. (2024). A continuum of actions you can take now to ADVANCE disability equity: A report from the field. *Advance Journal (Corvallis, Ore.)*, *4*(2), 1–32. DOI: 10.5399/osu/ADVJRNL.4.2.9

Aquino, K. C., Cook, K. D., & Bittinger, J. (2025). A national look at shifts in disability self-identification for students enrolled in higher education. *AERA Open*, *11*, 23328584251322511. DOI: 10.1177/23328584251322511

Bennett, M., & Carlson-Manathara, E. (2024). Introducing the special theme issue: Examining allyship with Indigenous peoples. *Canadian Social Work Review*, ●●●, 5–18. DOI: 10.7202/1114538ar

Bergman, M. (2021). Adult learners in higher education. In Rocco, T. S., Smith, M. C., Rizzi, R. C., Merriweather, L. R., & Hawley, J. D. (Eds.), *Handbook of adult and continuing education* (20th ed., pp. 266–274). Stylus Publishing. DOI: 10.4324/9781003447849

Bisman, C. D. (2001). Teaching social work's bio-psycho-social assessment. *Journal of Teaching in Social Work*, *21*(3–4), 75–89. DOI: 10.1300/J067v21n03_07

Bliss, D. L., & Ginn, H. (2021). Expanding presence of social work advocacy on the national stage. *Journal of Social Work Education*, *57*(3), 432–444. DOI: 10.1080/10437797.2019.1671266

Bourke, B. (2020). Leaving behind the rhetoric of allyship. *Whiteness and Education*, *5*(2), 179–194. DOI: 10.1080/23793406.2020.1839786

Bronfenbrenner, U. (1974). Developmental research, public policy, and the ecology of childhood. *Child Development*, *45*(1), 1–5. DOI: 10.2307/1127743

Bronfenbrenner, U. (1994). Ecological models of human development. In Husen, T., & Postlethwaite, T. (Eds.), *The International Encyclopedia of Education* (2nd ed., Vol. 3, pp. 1643–1647). Pergamon.

Bronstein, L. R. (2003). A model for interdisciplinary collaboration. *Social Work*, *48*(3), 297–306. DOI: 10.1093/sw/48.3.297 PMID: 12899277

Burgstahler, S. (2024). *What are alternatives to disability-related simulations to promote disability awareness?* University of Washington, DO-IT (Disabilities, Opportunities, Internetworking, and Technology) Center. https://www.washington.edu/doit/what-are-alternatives-disability-related-simulations-promote-disability-awareness#:~:text=Another%20way%20to%20do%20this,for%20her%20live%20with%20autism

Burns, A., Dannecker, E., & Austin, M. J. (2019). Revisiting the biological perspective in the use of biopsychosocial assessments in social work. *Journal of Human Behavior in the Social Environment*, *29*(2), 177–194. DOI: 10.1080/10911359.2018.1500505

Butcher, L., & Lane, S.Butcher & Lane. (2024). Neurodivergent (Autism and ADHD) student experiences of access and inclusion in higher education: An ecological systems theory perspective. *Higher Education*, •••, 1–21. DOI: 10.1007/s10734-024-01319-6

Caiels, J. C., Milne, A., & Beadle-Brown, J. (2021). Strengths-based approaches in social work and social care: Reviewing the evidence. *Journal of Long-Term Care*, *401-402*, 401–422. Advance online publication. DOI: 10.31389/jltc.102

Center for Applied Special Technology (CAST). (2018). *Universal Design for Learning Guidelines* version 2.2. http://udlguidelines.cast.org

Clouder, L., Karakus, M., Cinotti, A., Ferresya, M. V., Fierros, G. A., & Rojo, P. (2020). Neurodiversity in higher education: A narrative synthesis. *Higher Education*, *80*(4), 757–778. DOI: 10.1007/s10734-020-00513-6

Cole, A. (2016). The 'three conversations' model: turning away from long-term care. *The Guardian*. https://www.theguardian.com/social-care-network/2016/nov/01/the-three-conversations-model-turning-away-from-long-term-care

Collier-Spruel, L. A., & Ryan, A. M. (2024). Are all allyship attempts helpful? An investigation of effective and ineffective allyship. *Journal of Business and Psychology*, *39*(1), 83–108. DOI: 10.1007/s10869-022-09861-9

Connolly, S. E., Constable, H. L., & Mullally, S. L. (2023). School distress and the school attendance crisis: A story dominated by neurodivergence and unmet need. *Frontiers in Psychiatry*, *14*, 1237052. Advance online publication. DOI: 10.3389/fpsyt.2023.1237052 PMID: 37810599

Cooper, P. C., Bilton, K., & Kakos, M. (2012). The importance of a biopsychosocial approach to interventions for SEBD. In Daniels, H., Cole, T., & Visser, J. (Eds.), *The Routledge International Companion to Emotional and Behavioural Difficulties*. Routledge.

Council for Opportunity in Education. (n.d.). *COE and TRIO programs*. https://coenet.org/coe-and-trio-programs/

Council on Social Work Education. (2022). *Educational policy and accreditation standards for baccalaureate and master's social work programs*. https://www.cswe.org/accreditation/policies-process/2022epas/

Cox, B. E., Edelstein, J., Brogdon, B., & Roy, A. (2021). Navigating challenges to facilitate success for college students with autism. *The Journal of Higher Education*, *92*(2), 252–278. DOI: 10.1080/00221546.2020.1798203

Craig, S. L., Gardiner, T., Eaton, A. D., Pang, N., & Kourgiantakis, T. (2022). Practicing alliance: An experiential model of teaching diversity and inclusion for social work practice and education. *Social Work Education*, *41*(5), 801–819. DOI: 10.1080/02615479.2021.1892054

Custodio, R. J. P., Hengstler, J. G., Cheong, J. H., Kim, H. J., Wascher, E., & Getzmann, S. (2024). Adult ADHD: It is old and new at the same time - what is it? *Reviews in the Neurosciences*, *35*(2), 225–241. DOI: 10.1515/revneuro-2023-0071 PMID: 37813870

Dahunsi, O., Robinson, N., Parks, C., & Nittrouer, C. (2024). How a DEI climate can enable allies and support people who are neurodivergent. In Patton, E., & Santuzzi, A. M. (Eds.), *Neurodiversity and Work: Employment, Identity, and Support Networks for Neurominorities* (pp. 207–230). Springer. DOI: 10.1007/978-3-031-55072-0_10

Dalrymple, J., & Boylan, J. (2016). Effective advocacy in social work. *Sage*.

Doyle, N. (2020). Neurodiversity at work: A biopsychosocial model and the impact on working adults. *British Medical Bulletin*, *135*(1), 108–125. DOI: 10.1093/bmb/ldaa021 PMID: 32996572

Dwyer, P., Mineo, E., Mifsud, K., Lindholm, C., Gurba, A., & Weisman, T. (2023). Building neurodiversity-inclusive postsecondary campuses: Recommendations for leaders in higher education. *Autism in Adulthood: Challenges and Management*, *5*(1), 1–14. DOI: 10.1089/aut.2021.0042 PMID: 36941859

Eide, B. L., & Eide, F. F. (2023). *The dyslexic advantage (revised and updated): Unlocking the hidden potential of the dyslexic brain*. Penguin.

Eki, A., & Isaksoon, G. (2013). How adults with ADHD get engaged in and perform everyday activities. *Scandinavian Journal of Occupational Therapy*, *20*(4), 282–291. DOI: 10.3109/11038128.2013.799226 PMID: 23713791

Engel, G. L. (1977). The need for a new medical model: A challenge for biomedicine. *Science*, *196*(4286), 129–136. DOI: 10.1126/science.847460 PMID: 847460

Fabricant, M., & Fisher, R. (2008). *Settlements and neighborhood centers. Encyclopedia of Social Work*. Oxford University Press. https://www.oxfordreference.com/view/10.1093/oi/authority.20110803100457433

Farrant, F., Owen, E., Hunkins-Beckford, F. L., & Jacksa, M. (2022). Celebrating neurodiversity in higher education. *The Psychologist*, *35*, 2–3. https://www.bps.org.uk/psychologist/celebrating-neurodiversity-higher-education

Freddolino, P. P., Moxley, D., & Hyduk, C. (2004). A differential model of advocacy in social work practice. *Families in Society*, *85*(1), 119–128. DOI: 10.1606/1044-3894.241

Gale, L. (2022). Biopsychosocial-spiritual assessment: An overview. *Social Work Practice & Skill.* Cinahl Information Systems. https://www.ebsco.com/sites/g/files/nabnos191/files/acquiadam-assets/Social-Work-Reference-Center-Skill-Biopsychosocial-Spiritual-Assessment.pdf

Gasker, J. (2023). *Generalist social work practice* (2nd ed.). Sage.

Gensic, J., & Brunton, J. (2022). *The actually autistic guide to advocacy: Step-by-step advice on how to ally and speak up with autistic people and the autism community*. Jessica Kingsley Publishers. https://www.google.com/books/edition/The_ActuallyAutistic_Guide_to_Advocacy/7RJJEAAAQBAJ?hl=en&gbpv=1&dq=neurodiversity+allyship&pg=PP1&printsec=frontcover

Germain, C. B. (1973). An ecological perspective in casework practice. *Social Casework*, *54*(6), 323–330. DOI: 10.1177/104438947305400601

Gillespie-Lynch, K., Dwyer, P., Constantino, C., Kapp, S. K., Hotez, E., Riccio, A., DeNigris, D., Kofner, B., & Endlich, E. (2020). Can we broaden the neurodiversity movement without weakening it? Participatory approaches as a framework for cross-disability alliance building. In Carey, A. C., Ostrove, J. M., & Fannon, T. (Eds.), *Disability alliances and allies: Opportunities and challenges* (pp. 189–223). Emerald Publishing Limited. DOI: 10.1108/S1479-354720200000012013

Gitterman, A., Knight, C., & Germain, C. B. (2021). *The life model of social work practice: Advances in theory and practice* (4th ed.). Columbia University Press.

Goode, R. W., Cowell, M., McMillan, D., Van Deinse, T., & Cooper-Lewter, C. (2021). Preparing social workers to confront social injustice and oppression: Evaluating the role of social work education. *Social Work*, *66*(1), 39–48. DOI: 10.1093/sw/swaa018 PMID: 32793955

Haegele, J. A., & Hodge, S. (2016). Disability discourse: Overview and critiques of the medical and social models. *Quest*, *68*(2), 193–206. DOI: 10.1080/00336297.2016.1143849

Hamilton, L. G., & Petty, S. (2023). Compassionate pedagogy for neurodiversity in higher education: A conceptual analysis. *Frontiers in Psychology*, *14*, 1–9. DOI: 10.3389/fpsyg.2023.1093290 PMID: 36874864

Hansan, J. E. (2011). Settlement houses: An introduction. *Social Welfare History Project*. https://socialwelfare.library.vcu.edu/settlement-houses/settlement-houses/

Hesjedal, E., Hetland, H., & Iversen, A. C. (2015). Interprofessional collaboration: Self-reported successful collaboration by teachers and social workers in multidisciplinary teams. *Child & Family Social Work*, *20*(4), 437–445. DOI: 10.1111/cfs.12093

Hotez, E., Rosenau, K. A., Fernandes, P., Eagan, K., Shea, L., & Kuo, A. A. (2022). A national cross-sectional study of the characteristics, strengths, and challenges of college students with Attention Deficit Hyperactivity Disorder. *Cureus*, *14*(1), e21520. DOI: 10.7759/cureus.21520 PMID: 35223296

Jenkins, T. (2009). A seat at the table that I set: Beyond social justice allies. *About Campus: Enriching the Student Learning Experience*, *14*(5), 27–29. DOI: 10.1002/aca.305

Kalina, P. (2020). Performative allyship. *Technium Social Science Journal, 11*, 478. https://heinonline.org/HOL/Page?collection=journals&handle=hein.journals/techssj11&i

Kickett, G., Hendrick, A., & Young, S. (2024). Ally work at the intersections: Theorising for practice and practicing for theory. In Baines, D., Rasool, S., Harms-Smith, L., Muñoz-Arce, G., & Noble, C. (Eds.), *The Routledge International Handbook of Feminisms in Social Work* (pp. 485–497). Routledge. DOI: 10.4324/9781003317371-48

Koenig, T., Spano, R., & Thompson, J. (2020). Human behavior theory for social work practice. *Sage (Atlanta, Ga.).*

Kondrat, M. E. (2013). *Person-in-environment. Encyclopedia of Social Work*. National Association of Social Workers Press and Oxford University Press. DOI: 10.1093/acrefore/9780199975839.013.285

Kuder, S. J., Accardo, A., & Woodruff, J. (2023). *College success for students on the autism spectrum*. Taylor & Francis. DOI: 10.4324/9781003443452-2

Kutlaca, M., & Radke, H. R. (2023). Towards an understanding of performative allyship: Definition, antecedents and consequences. *Social and Personality Psychology Compass, 17*(2), e12724. DOI: 10.1111/spc3.12724

LeMaire, K. L., Miller, M., Skerven, K., & Nagy, G. A. (2020). Allyship in the academy. *Susan Bulkeley Butler Center for Leadership Excellence and ADVANCE Working Paper Series, 3* (1), 6-26. https://www.purdue.edu/butler/documents/5-WPS_Spring-2020_Allyship-in-the-Academy.pdf

Mandy, W. (2023). The old and the new way of understanding autistic lives: Reflections on the life of Donald Triplett, the first person diagnosed as autistic. *Autism, 27*(7), 1853–1855. DOI: 10.1177/13623613231194476 PMID: 37665266

Moore, T. (2022). Relationships and reciprocity: Where next for strengths-based social work in adult social care? *Journal of Social Work Practice*, *36*(4), 451–463. DOI: 10.1080/02650533.2022.2119946

Morin, A., & Kirchner-Morris, E. (2023) Is your school welcoming to neurodiverse students? *The Learning Professional, 44*(5), 46-48. https://learningforward.org/journal/reaching-all-learners/is-your-school-welcoming-to-neurodiverse-students/

Naasko, R. T. (2022). *The social work role in higher education: A systematic review.* [Doctoral dissertation University of Alabama]. UA Repository. https://ir-api.ua.edu/api/core/bitstreams/0e0782f3-0f2f-40b6-8e32-9d8f3e9b9f91/content

National Association of Social Workers. (2021). *Code of ethics.* https://www.socialworkers.org/About/Ethics/Code-of-Ethics/Code-of-Ethics-English

Nixon, S. A. (2019). The coin model of privilege and critical allyship: Implications for health. *BMC Public Health, 19*(1), 1637. DOI: 10.1186/s12889-019-7884-9 PMID: 31805907

Onwumelu, R. (2024) How you can support Neurodiverse students at Xavier. *Xavier University* https://www.xavier.edu/now/2024/how-to-support-neurodiverse-students

Park, T., Sheward, K., & Rogers-Shaw, C. *(2023).* Tips for supporting students with social skill, mental health & communication disabilities in digital settings. *eLearn. 5*(2023). https://dl.acm.org/doi/fullHtml/10.1145/3596691.3596515

Pietri, E. S., Moser, C. E., Derricks, V., & Johnson, I. R. (2024). A framework for understanding effective allyship. *Nature Reviews Psychology*, *3*(10), 1–15. DOI: 10.1038/s44159-024-00359-0

Radke, H. R., Kutlaca, M., Siem, B., Wright, S. C., & Becker, J. C. (2020). Beyond allyship: Motivations for advantaged group members to engage in action for disadvantaged groups. *Personality and Social Psychology Review*, *24*(4), 291–315. DOI: 10.1177/1088868320918698 PMID: 32390573

Rapp, C. A., & Chamberlain, R. (1985). Case management services for the chronically mentally ill. *Social Work*, *30*(5), 417–422. https://www.jstor.org/stable/23714362. DOI: 10.1093/sw/30.5.417 PMID: 10273981

Rapp, C. A., Saleebey, D., & Sullivan, W. P. (2005). The future of strength based social work. *Advances in Social Work*, *6*(1), 79–90. DOI: 10.18060/81

Richmond, M. E. (1917). *Social diagnosis*. Russell Sage Foundation. DOI: 10.2307/3406141

Rogers, A. T. (2022). *Human behavior and the social environment: Perspectives on development and the life course* (6th ed.). Routledge. DOI: 10.4324/9781003195542

Rogers-Shaw, C., Park, T. W., & Mohney, K. D. (2023). Strategies for supporting learners with disabilities in postsecondary education. *New Horizons in Adult Education and Human Resource Development*, *35*(4), 199–207. DOI: 10.1177/19394225231189136

Saleebey, D. (1996). The strengths of perspective in social work practice: Extensions and cautions. *Social Work*, *41*(3), 296–305. DOI: 10.1093/sw/41.3.296 PMID: 8936085

Schelbe, L., Pryce, J., & Gaab, N. (2022). Dyslexia in the context of social work: Screening and early intervention. *Families in Society*, *103*(3), 269–280. DOI: 10.1177/10443894211042323

Schneider, R., Lester, L., & Ochieng, J. (2008). *Advocacy. Encyclopedia of Social Work*. Oxford University Press., https://www-oxfordreference-com.proxy-commonwealthu.klnpa.org/view/10.1093/acref/9780195306613.001.0001/acref-9780195306613-e-10

Shallish, L. (2015). "Just how much diversity will the law permit?": The Americans with Disabilities Act, diversity and disability in higher education. *Disability Studies Quarterly*, *35*(3). Advance online publication. DOI: 10.18061/dsq.v35i3.4942

Shepherd, J., Sutton, B., Smith, S., & Szlenkier, M. (2024). "Sea-glass survivors:" Autistic testimonies about education experiences. *British Journal of Special Education*, *51*(2), 142–155. DOI: 10.1111/1467-8578.12506

Spaeth, E., & Pearson, A. (2023). A reflective analysis on how to promote a positive learning experience for neurodivergent students. *Journal of Perspectives in Applied Academic Practice*, *11*(2), 109–120. DOI: 10.56433/jpaap.v11i2.517

Ştefani, S. C. (2023). The role of advocacy in social work practice. *Social Work Review / Revista de Asistenta Sociala*, 4, 77–86. http://www.swreview.ro/index.pl/the_role_of_advocacy_in_social_work_practice

Stone, S., Austin, M. J., Berzin, A., & Taylor, S. (2007). Exploring the knowledge base of human behavior and the social environment using the concept of reciprocity. *Journal of Human Behavior in the Social Environment*, *16*(3), 89–106. DOI: 10.1300/10911350802107769

Sumerau, J. E., Forbes, T. D., Denise, E. J., & Mathers, L. A. (2021). Constructing allyship and the persistence of inequality. *Social Problems*, *68*(2), 358–373. DOI: 10.1093/socpro/spaa003

Suppes, M. A., & Wells, C. C. (2018). *The social work experience: A case-based introduction to social work and social welfare* (7th ed.). Pearson.

Terry, K. (n. d.) *Neurodiversity: The new cultural competency in social work education*. University of Saint Thomas. https://www.nacsw.org/Convention/Resources2018/TerryKNeurodiversity.pdf

The Care Act (2014). The National Archives of the United Kingdom. https://www.legislation.gov.uk/ukpga/2014/23/contents

Thomas, C. (2004). Rescuing a social relational understanding of disability. *Scandinavian Journal of Disability Research*, *6*(1), 22–36. DOI: 10.1080/15017410409512637

University of Washington. (n.d.). *About/overview*. Disabilities, Opportunities, Internetworking, and Technology (DO-IT) Center. https://www.washington.edu/doit/about/overview

Weick, A., Rapp, C., Sullivan, W. P., & Kisthardt, W. (1989). A strengths perspective for social work practice. *Social Work*, *34*(4), 350–354. https://www.jstor.org/stable/23715838. DOI: 10.1093/sw/34.4.350

West Chester University. (n.d.). *Dub-C Autism program (D-CAP)*. https://www.wcupa.edu/deputy-provost/dcap/

Whittington, C. (2023). Collaboration and partnership in context. In Cree, V. E., & McCulloch, T. (Eds.), *Social Work* (pp. 240–246). Routledge. DOI: 10.4324/9781003178699-46

Wiener, J., & Daniels, L. (2016). School experiences of adolescents with Attention-Deficit/Hyperactivity Disorder. *Journal of Learning Disabilities*, *49*(6), 567–581. DOI: 10.1177/0022219415576973 PMID: 25795542

Williams, M., & Sharif, N. (2021). Racial allyship: Novel measurement and new insights. *New Ideas in Psychology*, *62*, 100865. DOI: 10.1016/j.newideapsych.2021.100865

Wolbring, G., & Lillywhite, A. (2023). Coverage of allies, allyship and disabled people: A scoping review. *Societies (Basel, Switzerland)*, *13*(11), 241. DOI: 10.3390/soc13110241

Woods, S. E. O. N., & Estes, A. (2023). Toward a more comprehensive autism assessment: The survey of autistic strengths, skills, and interests. *Frontiers in Psychiatry*, *14*, 1264516. DOI: 10.3389/fpsyt.2023.1264516 PMID: 37867767

Zastrow, C., Kirst-Ashman, K., & Hessenauer, S. (2019). *Understanding human behavior and the social environment* (11th ed.). Cengage.

ADDITIONAL READING

Burns, A., Dannecker, E., & Austin, M. J. (2019). Revisiting the biological perspective in the use of biopsychosocial assessments in social work. *Journal of Human Behavior in the Social Environment*, *29*(2), 177–194. DOI: 10.1080/10911359.2018.1500505

Freddolino, P. P., Moxley, D., & Hyduk, C. (2004). A differential model of advocacy in social work practice. *Families in Society*, *85*(1), 119–128. DOI: 10.1606/1044-3894.241

Lambert, C. P., & Siegel, D. H. (2018). Social workers in higher education: New roles, new opportunities. *Social Work Today, 18*(5), 16-20. https://www.socialworktoday.com/archive/SO18p16.shtml

Saleebey, D. (1996). The strengths of perspective in social work practice: Extensions and cautions. *Social Work*, *41*(3), 296–305. DOI: 10.1093/sw/41.3.296 PMID: 8936085

Salisbury, Y., Foster, R., Hill, S., & Buck, G. (2024). Neurodiverse inclusive social work education considered through a student partnership. *Social Work Education*, 1–16. Advance online publication. DOI: 10.1080/02615479.2024.2378915

Chapter 5
Creating Inclusive University Experiences: A Bio-Ecological Perspective

Aoife Mary Lynam
https://orcid.org/0000-0002-5984-8941
Trinity College Dublin, Ireland

Conor McGuckin
https://orcid.org/0009-0001-1090-3057
Trinity College Dublin, Ireland

Jennifer M. Banks
https://orcid.org/0000-0001-8439-952X
Trinity College Dublin, Ireland

Marie Devitt
Trinity College Dublin, Ireland

Michael Shevlin
Trinity College Dublin, Ireland

Des Aston
Trinity College Dublin, Ireland

Barbara Ringwood
https://orcid.org/0000-0003-3676-5593
Trinity College Dublin, Ireland

Emer Murphy
https://orcid.org/0009-0001-3785-6641
Trinity College Dublin, Ireland

Sadbh Feehan
Trinity College Dublin, Ireland

Owen Barden
Trinity College Dublin, Ireland

Vivian Rath
https://orcid.org/0009-0005-1124-366X
Trinity College Dublin, Ireland

John Kubiak
Trinity College Dublin, Ireland

Angela Mazzocco
Trinity College Dublin, Ireland

Jill Woodnutt
Trinity College Dublin, Ireland

DOI: 10.4018/979-8-3693-8920-1.ch005

ABSTRACT

This chapter explores the development of inclusive university experiences for learners with intellectual disabilities (ID) at Trinity Centre for People with Intellectual Disabilities (TCPID) in Ireland. The TCPID model is holistic, incorporating both educational and work readiness components that empower students to make informed decisions about their future. Through the lens of Bronfenbrenner's bio-ecological systems theory, the chapter examines how social and environmental systems impact the experiences, development, and outcomes of college students with ID. At each level of the bio-ecological systems model, TCPID is a model of inclusive practice, challenging traditional barriers in higher education, workplaces, and society and sets a standard for equity and empowerment. TCPID is more than a program; it is an environment that nurtures "learning without limits" and celebrates each student's potential. The chapter provides practical insights and strategies for international higher education institutions seeking to enhance inclusivity and collaboration in supporting students with ID.

INTRODUCTION

This book explores neurodiversity as a framework for valuing different ways of thinking and being, and in this chapter we argue that intellectual disability must be included within this framework. Recognising intellectual disability as part of neurodiversity is essential to addressing the systemic exclusion and inequities faced by this often-overlooked group, particularly in education and other domains of social participation. In essence, the neurodiversity movement recognises and celebrates ways of thinking and being which contrast neurotypical or what are considered 'normal' ways. Given that intellectual disability is defined and diagnosed in terms of deviations from a psychometric statistical norm (i.e. average IQ test scores) there is a strong case for including it under the neurodiversity umbrella. This case is bolstered once we appreciate that many acquire additional diagnostic labels that some people might more readily associate with neurodiversity. That is to say, it is possible to have an intellectual disability and be autistic, or dyslexic, and so on. In fact, a significant issue with psychometric testing is that such tests can often fail to discriminate where one 'condition' ends and another begins, so we would be wise not to try and draw our boundaries too tightly. Between 1% and 3% of people globally are estimated to have some degree of intellectual disability (ID) (Patel et al., 2020). Yet, adults with ID remain significantly under-represented in higher education, facing far lower transition rates compared to their peers (Andresen, 2024; Banks et al., 2022; Newman et al., 2011). This disparity reflects broader societal challenges in ensuring equitable access for marginalized groups, a priority in international policy frameworks. While the specific goals of such initiatives vary across countries, a common thread is the aspiration to create inclusive educational systems that enable all individuals to thrive. However, national, and international research consistently reveals persistent barriers to achieving these aims, particularly for individuals with ID (Corby et al., 2020; Evans et al., 2017; Kimball et al., 2016; Lee & Taylor, 2022; Moriña et al., 2020).

Education is widely recognized as a fundamental human right, enshrined in Article 26 of the Universal Declaration of Human Rights (United Nations, 1948). This right includes all groups within society, including those with ID. Article 24 of the United Nations Convention on the Rights of Persons with Disabilities (UNCRPD) further reinforces that individuals with disabilities must have equal access to tertiary education and lifelong learning without discrimination (United Nations, 2006). Reports from UNESCO (2005, 2010) and the Right to Education Initiative (2022) have highlighted persistent inequalities in higher education, calling for affirmative action, flexible curricula, financial supports, inclusive pedagogy, and mentorship to address systemic exclusion. The importance of access to higher education is underscored by research showing improved employment outcomes for people with disabilities who complete further education (Migliore et al., 2009; Uditsky & Hughson, 2012; Watson et al., 2017). Yet, systemic obstacles persist. These include limited academic opportunities during secondary schooling, lack of institutional support, and low expectations surrounding the capabilities of individuals with ID (Gustavsson et al., 2021; Jacob et al., 2023; Stinnett et al., 2023).

In the Republic of Ireland, legislative and structural gaps further limit access to higher education for people with ID. While the Education for Persons with Special Educational Needs Act (2004) guarantees free primary education up to age 18, it does not ensure pathways to post-secondary or tertiary education. Existing access routes, such as the Disability Access Route to Education (DARE, 2025), cater primarily to students with specific learning difficulties who complete the traditional Leaving Certificate (final school examination when students are approximately 17–19 years old and which serves as the main route for university admission). This system excludes most students with ID who do not complete the Leaving Certificate, leaving them unable to apply through the Central Applications Office (CAO) system for a place in university (McGrath, 2023). Although many Irish institutions have independently introduced inclusive initiatives, their scope and impact vary significantly (Hart et al., 2006; Hennessy et al., 2024). The landscape remains fragmented, with equity of access dependent on the design and commitment of individual universities. However, advocacy efforts, including those of the Inclusive National Higher Education Forum (INHEF), have begun to influence national policy. The National

Access Plan 2022–2028 now specifically includes individuals with ID as a priority group (HEA, 2022), marking a significant policy shift.

This chapter contributes to the ongoing discourse on inclusive higher education by examining the Trinity Centre for People with Intellectual Disabilities (TCPID) at Trinity College Dublin (TCD) as a case study. The TCPID's Arts, Science, and Inclusive Applied Practice (ASIAP) program offers a holistic model that integrates education, personal development, and career readiness.

THEORETICAL FRAMEWORK

In this chapter, we use Bronfenbrenner's bio-ecological systems theory (1979, 1989, 2001) as the foundational lens for understanding how the development and experiences of students with ID in TCPID are shaped by their interactions within the interrelated social and environmental systems. Central to this model is the Process, Person, Context, and Time (PPCT) framework, which recognizes that human development occurs through complex and reciprocal exchanges between the individual and their surrounding environments, influenced not only by personal characteristics but also by institutional structures (i.e., TCPID), cultural attitudes, and historical change. This theoretical perspective is particularly valuable when examining the inclusive premise of TCPID, as it allows for a layered understanding of the individual and structural factors that influence access, participation, and outcomes for students with ID.

ID is best understood within the broader framework of disability, which has evolved over time from a predominantly medical model to a more comprehensive approach that integrates medical, social, and functional dimensions (Harris, 2006; Patel & Brown, 2017). The interplay between the medical and social models of disability is critical for understanding access and support for individuals with ID in higher education. The medical model conceptualizes disability because of a disease or health condition that limits an individual's capacity to meet personal and societal expectations (Harris, 2006; Patel & Brown, 2017). This model has been critiqued for its reductionist approach, focusing on clinical diagnoses and physical impairments while neglecting the sociological and psychological dimensions of disability (Baglieri, 2023). This perspective perpetuates stereotypes, framing individuals with disabilities as passive and inadequate. Conversely, the social model reframes disability as a societal issue, emphasising the need to dismantle systemic barriers and foster inclusive environments (Baglieri, 2023; Giri et al., 2022). Brisenden (1986) advocated for the empowerment of disabled individuals, highlighting the importance of autonomy and the ability to make independent choices. This perspective aligns with critiques that call for systemic changes in policy, infrastructure, and societal attitudes to support the full participation of individuals with disabilities in all aspects of society (Goodley, 2024). Programs like ASIAP operationalize these principles by integrating inclusive practices within educational and professional domains, thereby advancing equity and inclusion. By doing this, TCPID addresses individual needs while dismantling societal barriers, offering a holistic model for empowering students with ID and ensuring their meaningful inclusion in academic and professional domains (Mc Guckin & Minton, 2014; Goodley, 2024; Hayes et al., 2017).

TCPID has created an educational environment designed in alignment with Bronfenbrenner's theoretical principles. It operates across all levels of the ecological model, from the most immediate settings to the broader societal and temporal structures that shape the lives of its students, as can be seen in Figure One.

Figure 1. TCPID & Bio-Ecological Systems

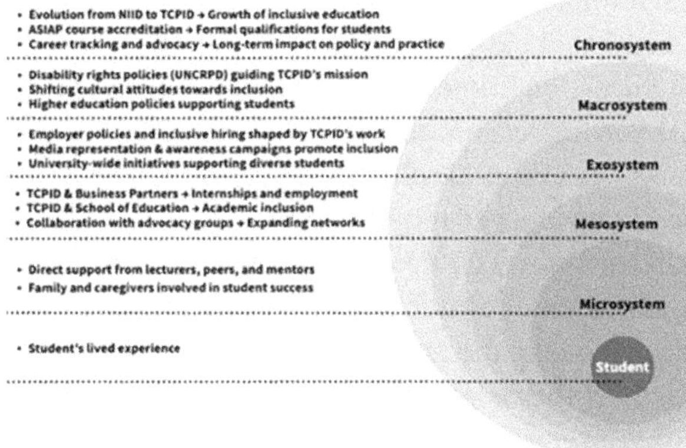

Note. The importance of the levels of the Bio-ecological Theory of Development (Bronfenbrenner, 1979, 1989) in the TCPID design is visible in the figure that identifies TCPID elements at each system level.

At the level of the microsystem, which includes the settings in which students engage in direct interactions with family members, peers, and educators (Bronfenbrenner, 1979, 1989), TCPID cultivates strong and supportive relationships that foster belonging, academic engagement, and personal development. The value of these close relationships and the critical role of family involvement and peer networks (Rosa & Tudge, 2013) in promoting success and inclusion for individuals with ID is clear. Within this immediate context, TCPID provides tailored supports such as occupational therapy, academic mentoring, co-learning opportunities, and internship (i.e., employment) all of which collaborate to empower students and increase their sense of self-efficacy.

The mesosystem, which captures the connections between different microsystems (Bronfenbrenner, 1979, 1989), is also actively developed through TCPID's work. Collaborations between families, schools, and external organisations of employment are essential in ensuring smooth transitions into higher education. Through initiatives such as transition planning, summer schools and partnerships with schools and career guidance professionals, TCPID strengthens the links between home, school, and higher education. Importantly, the program extends these connections into the professional sphere, with business partnerships that support work placements and internships. These efforts enable students to develop the confidence, skills, and networks necessary for meaningful employment, illustrating the importance of a well-connected mesosystem in shaping positive educational and professional trajectories (Ringwood et al., 2024).

Beyond these more immediate systems, the exosystem refers to the social and institutional structures that affect students indirectly, such as educational policies, community supports and national frameworks (Bronfenbrenner, 1979, 1989). In the Irish context, there have been growing efforts to develop more inclusive access routes to higher education for individuals with intellectual disabilities (Aston, 2019; Freedman et al., 2022; Grigal et al., 2012; Shevlin et al., 2020). TCPID's alignment with the Irish national qualification framework and its commitment to the principles of Universal Design for Learning ensure that its practices reflect inclusive values at an institutional level. As Quirke et al. (2024) argued, it is essential that higher education systems embed inclusive pedagogical approaches that are responsive to diverse learning needs. In this way, TCPID challenges systemic exclusion and advocates for a reimagining of what constitutes legitimate educational participation.

At the level of the macrosystem, the focus shifts to the cultural and ideological forces that influence how disability is perceived within society. Traditional deficit-based narratives have often portrayed individuals with intellectual disabilities as limited in their capacity to participate in academic and professional life. TCPID advocates for a counter-narrative that aligns with the social model of disability, which attributes barriers not to the individual but to the organization of society itself (Giri et al., 2022). By framing disability within this more inclusive and rights-based perspective, TCPID plays a role in reshaping public discourse and expectations, contributing to a broader cultural shift in how intellectual disability is understood and valued.

Finally, the chronosystem introduces the dimension of time, highlighting the importance of historical change, life transitions and evolving societal contexts (Bronfenbrenner, 1979, 1989). TCPID's work is shaped by, and responsive to, these temporal dynamics. Its development reflects broader changes in Irish and international policy, particularly the growing recognition of the rights of individuals with disabilities to access tertiary education on an equal basis. The ASIAP program's design also illustrates the shift away from a medical model of disability, which views disability as an individual deficit, towards a more holistic approach that addresses the interaction between the individual and their environment (Baglieri, 2023). This evolution is evident in the Centre's ongoing efforts to remain responsive to the changing needs of students and to influence policy and practice at a national level.

Through the application of Bronfenbrenner's bio-ecological systems theory, TCPID demonstrates how inclusive education can be understood as a dynamic and multi-dimensional process. The Centre's structure and philosophy offer a comprehensive response to the complex barriers faced by students with ID. Its practices are grounded in UDL, ensuring that curriculum content is accessible, flexible, and responsive to diverse learners (Bracken & Novak, 2019; Quirke et al., 2024; Zhang et al., 2024). Students engage in co-learning experiences with peers who are studying in other disciplines (e.g., undergraduate students in the School of English) and receive targeted academic and occupational therapy support and participate in structured employment placements through strategic business partnerships. These components collectively create an environment in which students can thrive, not only within the university but also in their future careers and communities. In TCPID, the ASIAP program was designed using the interconnected ecological systems that shape student experience and development. The TCPID model is a functioning example of how institutions can actively dismantle structural barriers, challenge cultural assumptions, and build responsive systems of support that uphold the rights and capabilities of individuals with ID. The TCPID model is further understood within the broader framework of disability in the next section.

ESTABLISHING TCPID: A MODEL FOR INCLUSION

The Trinity Centre for People with Intellectual Disabilities (TCPID) at Trinity College Dublin is a pioneering initiative that exemplifies inclusive higher education for individuals with ID. Established in 2014 within the School of Education, TCPID offers the Arts, Science, and Inclusive Applied Practice (ASIAP) program, a structured curriculum designed to provide students with a holistic educational experience. The Centre integrates academic learning with professional and social development, enabling students to achieve a nationally recognized and accredited Level 5 Certificate (this is a one-year post-secondary qualification, like an associate degree or vocational diploma in the U.S., that provides practical and academic training for entry-level jobs or further education) within Ireland's National Framework of Qualifications (NFQ). This alignment situates the program alongside mainstream academic credentials, underscoring its commitment to equity and inclusion. TCPID employs a UDL framework, ensuring accessibility and adaptability.

A key distinguishing feature of TCPID is its robust focus on work-readiness. The Centre has established partnerships with over 50 prominent businesses, many of which are international blue-chip companies, enabling students to engage in internships and work placements that are critical for their professional development. These partnerships, managed by the Centre's Business Partnership Manager and supported by an Occupational Therapy team, ensure tailored support for both students and employers. This dual focus on academic and employment pathways challenges societal perceptions of the capabilities of individuals with ID, demonstrating their potential to contribute meaningfully to the workforce. Grounded in Bronfenbrenner's (1989) bio-ecological systems theory, TCPID adopts a layered approach to student development. The theory's emphasis on the interplay of immediate, institutional, and societal systems is reflected in the Centre's design, which addresses students' needs at multiple ecological levels. Through its multifaceted, collaborative approach, TCPID exemplifies best practices in inclusive higher education. It provides a transformative educational model that not only enables students with ID to participate meaningfully in university life but also equips them with the skills and confidence to transition into independent, professionally fulfilling futures. The Centre's emphasis on academic rigour, social inclusion, and professional readiness demonstrates how higher education institutions can operationalize inclusivity in a way that benefits both individuals and society at large.

What is the ASIAP Program?

The ASIAP (Arts, Science, and Inclusive Applied Practice) program is a two-year higher education initiative by TCPID that empowers students with ID through a blend of academic, social, and professional development. Grounded in UDL, ASIAP promotes accessibility via diverse learning methods and inclusive teaching (e.g., easy-read materials, pre-recorded sessions, bridging lectures). Students engage in co-learning with peers from other disciplines throughout TCD (e.g., School of English), participate in tailored work placements, and receive holistic support including occupational therapy and mentoring. Figure 2 shows an overview of the course throughout the two years.

Figure 2. ASIAP Course Structure

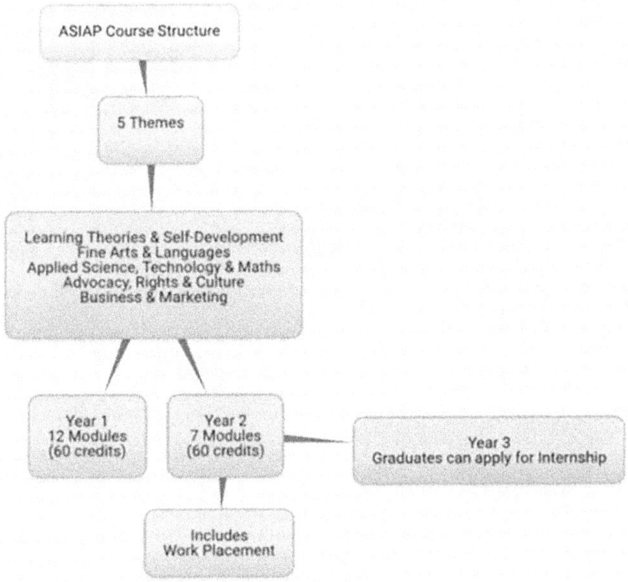

Note. The flow chart reveals not only the subject matter within the program but also the progression through both academic and workplace learning.

To support students in co-learning settings, TCPID have introduced "bridging lectures." These are "bite-sized" sessions designed to address specific content, texts, themes, or concepts that students may need to understand before attending larger tutorials or lectures with their undergraduate peers. These bridging lectures not only equip students with foundational knowledge but also build their confidence, ensuring they can actively and meaningfully engage in academic discussions alongside their peers and lead conversations and learning.

The ASIAP program breaks down barriers to higher education and employment for people with ID, setting a standard for inclusive practice. ASIAP is structured around three phases, informed by Bronfenbrenner's bio-ecological systems theory: (i) Journey Inward; (ii) Journey Through; (iii) Journey Onward as illustrated in Figure 3.

Figure 3. The ASIAP Program

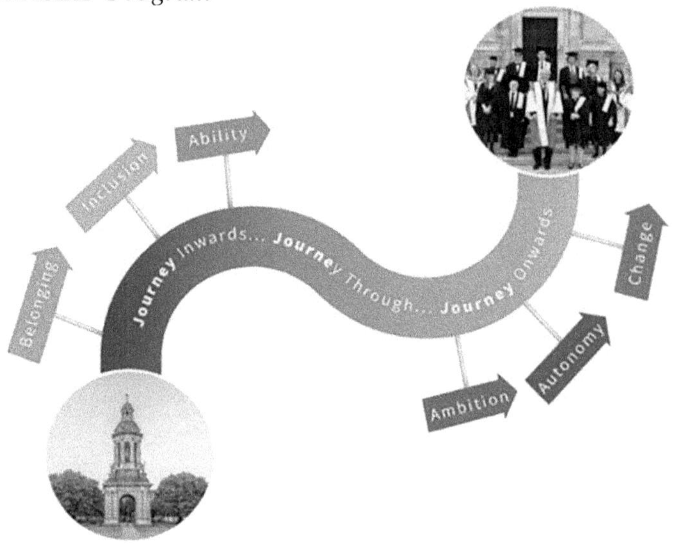

Note. Belonging, inclusion, ability, ambition, autonomy, and change are significant elements in each student's journey.

The "Journey Inward" raises national awareness of higher education options for people with ID. It includes transition planning through collaboration with families, schools, and Guidance Counsellors. Early engagement with TCPID Occupational Therapists helps families understand the program and strengthens support systems ahead of enrolment. Occupational Therapy is a professional qualification where the objective of intervention is to enable the person to perform actions they need or want to perform (AOTI, 2025; Duncan, 2021). These are generally ordinary and familiar activities that bring meaning and personal satisfaction to a person's life (Hasselkus & Dickie, 2021). In the context of university, there are several actions the student or intern must, or wants to, perform to engage with their student life or workplace.

The "Journey Through" focuses on university experience, providing a UDL-aligned curriculum, inclusive teaching, and student governance involvement. Co-learning modules with mainstream students and participation in extracurricular activities foster inclusion and independence. Occupational Therapists support students' academic progress, skills development, and preparation for employment through individual assessments and tailored interventions.

The final phase of the "Journey Onward" bridges higher education and the workforce. Students complete work placements and paid internships supported by TCPID's network of over 50 business partners. With mentoring, employer training, and ongoing support, students develop professional skills and confidence over the two years for sustainable and meaningful employment.

Bronfenbrenner's (1979, 1989) bio-ecological systems theory provides a valuable framework for analysing the Journey Inward, Journey Through, and Journey Onward phases of the ASIAP program, which support individuals with ID through interconnected systems. This is outlined in Table 1.

Table 1. The ASIAP Journey: Phases, Focus, Supports and Ecological Systems

Phase	Focus	Key Supports	Ecological Systems
Journey Inward	Awareness, aspirations, and transition planning into higher education	- National & Schools Coordinator - Open Days & Summer Schools - Family engagement - Pre-program Occupational Therapy support	Microsystem & Mesosystem
Journey Through	Participation in university life and academic, personal, and social development	- Academic modules (UDL) - Co-learning - Teaching & Learning Assistants - OTs	Microsystem, Mesosystem, & Exosystem
Journey Onward	Transition to meaningful employment and independent living	- Work placement - Graduate internships - Business partnerships - Ongoing Occupational Therapy & mentor support	Exosystem, Macrosystem, & Chronosystem

Note. The supports, built into the design of ASIAP and delivered by program, academic, and business stakeholders, align with the focus of the student journey and reflect the elements of Bronfenbrenner's (1979, 1989) bio-ecological systems, providing a model for its application to educational programs.

Each step on the student's journey reflects the collaboration between program, university, and employment entities who support the ID students. The "Journey Inward" reflects the microsystem and mesosystem by focusing on students' immediate interactions with families, educators, and Guidance Counselors, alongside initiatives such as transition planning and early engagement with Occupational Therapy, which strengthen supportive networks for successful transitions to higher education. The "Journey Through" spans the microsystem, mesosystem, and exosystem, encompassing students' interactions with teaching staff, peers, and learning assistants, while fostering inclusion through co-learning and participation in extracurricular activities. Institutional policies grounded in UDL and Equality, Diversity, and Inclusion (EDI) exemplify exosystemic influences, ensuring accessibility and academic quality. The "Journey Onward" demonstrates exosystem and macrosystem engagement by leveraging business partnerships to facilitate work placements and internships, addressing systemic employment barriers, and promoting cultural shifts in workplace attitudes.

Occupational Therapists within TCPID play a critical role in supporting students' academic engagement, skill development, and transition to employment. They conduct individual assessments to identify students' strengths, challenges, and support needs, informing tailored interventions. Occupational Therapists facilitate transition planning, self-regulation strategies, and independent skills, ensuring students can navigate university life both during the ASIAP program and for two years following graduation as they enter employment. They collaborate with teaching staff, learning assistants, and business partners to implement inclusive practices, adapt learning materials, and support work placements. By addressing cognitive, social, and environmental barriers, they enable students to develop the skills, confidence, and autonomy required for meaningful participation in higher education and employment.

Community partnerships within the TCPID are vital for enhancing employability, fostering social inclusion, and bridging the gap between higher education and the workforce. These partnerships were established through strategic collaboration with businesses, advocacy groups, and educational institutions, ensuring sustainable and meaningful engagement for students with ID. The TCPID Business Partnerships Program facilitates student work placements, graduate internships, guest lectures, and tailored workshops, providing real-world learning experiences. Partnerships were cultivated through network-building, awareness initiatives, and peer support among corporate stakeholders, reinforcing the importance of inclusive employment. By integrating mentorship, employer training, and workplace accommodations, these partnerships not only expand opportunities for TCPID graduates but also contribute to shifting societal perceptions of individuals with ID in professional settings. Collectively, three phases operate across the chronosystem capturing the temporal evolution of efforts to challenge exclusionary practices and promote lasting inclusivity.

In some instances, academic staff collaborate with TCPID to prerecord concise tutorials that are integrated into the ASIAP program as preparatory teaching resources. Additionally, TCPID have created easy-read guides on topics such as the Irish legal system (e.g., TCPID have developed a pioneering and innovative Easy Read Bureau within their Research and Innovation Hub). These guides serve a dual purpose: as resources for modules like Human Rights and Disability Rights within the ASIAP program, and as preparatory materials for students with ID attending more advanced law lectures with their undergraduate peers in the School of Law.

This multifaceted approach ensures that students are well-prepared for inclusive learning environments, fostering both their academic success and confidence. By prioritizing collaboration and tailoring resources to the specific needs of students with ID, the ASIAP program exemplifies how inclusive education can be effectively implemented in higher education.

BARRIERS AND OPPORTUNITIES IN EDUCATION

Barriers to inclusion in higher education institutions for people with ID are manifold. They arise not simply in the different layers of the ecological system, but in the interactions between those layers. Barriers which are rooted in the outer layers (chronosystem and macrosystem) pervade the inner layers. In this way, deeply seated cultural values and norms are manifested in everyday encounters and experiences.

Historically, universities like Trinity College Dublin (Ireland) have been sites of privilege and power, where knowledge about intellectual disabilities was authorized by academics, not by individuals with ID themselves (Ingold, 2018). This legacy reflects broader ableist attitudes within the macrosystem, which historically positioned people with ID as subjects for care rather than candidates for meaningful educational opportunities (Barden & Walden, 2021; Goodley, 2014). Consequently, this group faces some of the poorest post-school outcomes, an issue compounded by university inclusion schemes that are often criticized as tokenistic "inclusionism" rather than transformative (Mitchell & Snyder, 2015, p. 80). Despite claims of inclusivity, many universities continue to operate within a deficit model, offering limited accommodations rather than universally designed environments. A recent United Kingdom (UK) House of Lords report reveals that disabled students are under-represented, experience high dropout rates, face mental health challenges, and encounter physical and instructional barriers (Public Services Committee, 2024). Such structural issues reinforce a mesosystem perception among families and advocates of people with ID that university is not for "people like them" (Barden, 2021).

For students who do access higher education, these perceptions persist in the microsystem, where interactions with non-disabled peers can be sites of stigma, as noted by Goffman's concept of "primal scenes" (Goffman, 1963, p. 13). The stigma is often exacerbated by the discomfort or prejudice of non-disabled individuals who may avoid such interactions (Dixon et al., 2018; Mercier & Sperber, 2018; Staniland, 2011). Jacobs et al. (2020) examined the transition from school to adult services for young people with severe ID, focusing on decision-making processes and the involvement of young people. Using an ecological framework and case studies (N=3), the research highlighted that decision-making was primarily controlled by professionals and families, with young people often marginalized due to their disabilities. Key findings indicated that resource limitations, organizational practices, and policy constraints significantly influenced transition options, often reducing the scope for choice and meaningful involvement of young people (Jacobs et al., 2020). While the practical aspects of transitions, such as identifying suitable adult services, were generally well-managed, the broader systemic context presented challenges (e.g., funding shortages and limited service availability). This created a dissonance between the policy rhetoric of person-centered care and the actual experiences of families. Jacobs et al. (2020) also revealed tensions between ideals of independence and the reality of continued dependence on care networks for individuals with ID. Although professionals and families endeavored to include young people in decisions, their involvement was largely framed by concerns for safety and well-being rather than autonomy. Thus, transitions should be viewed as ongoing processes requiring sustained collaboration across sectors, and they advocated for more robust mechanisms to involve young people in decision-making, aligned with their support needs (Jacobs et al., 2020).

Similarly, Gauthier-Boudreault et al. (2021) investigated barriers for individuals with severe to profound ID, but from the perspective of professionals when facilitating the transition to adulthood for individuals. Through interviews with professionals from the healthcare, education, and community sectors (N=7), the study highlighted several key obstacles, including the absence of clear transition markers, inadequate financial and human resources, frequent staff turnover, and the lack of a system navigator to coordinate the complex transition process (Gauthier-Boudreault et al., 2021). Professionals expressed concerns regarding the limited recognition of the rehabilitation potential of individuals with severe to profound ID and the insufficient availability of adapted transport and appropriate daily activity services. Gauthier-Boudreault et al. (2021) emphasized the need for improved intersectoral collaboration to streamline the transition process. Professionals proposed several potential solutions, such as the development of clearer role definitions, the creation of a comprehensive transition guide, and enhanced training opportunities for staff. These solutions were seen as essential to addressing many of the existing challenges, particularly in light of the limited systemic support and resource allocation currently available. The article stressed the importance of interdisciplinary action and greater collaboration across sectors to ensure a more seamless transition to adulthood for individuals with severe to profound ID (Gauthier-Boudreault et al., 2021).

Student Supports in TCPID

For the duration of the ASIAP course and subsequent internships, students receive wide ranging supports from the Occupational Therapists and the Teaching and Learning Assistant. The Teaching and Learning Assistant provides academic support to the ASIAP students and lecturers. An important aspect of this support occurs within lectures, where the Teaching and Learning Assistant provides supports, including technology support, modelling active listening and engagement in the classroom, supporting students to complete their practical work, and offering individual support with Occupational Therapy guidance.

Accessible content is crucial to students' understanding and success in higher education. UDL is applied practically within the ASIAP program through flexible and accessible teaching methods that respond to diverse learner needs. For example, academic modules integrate easy-read materials, pre-recorded tutorials, and bridging lectures to support comprehension and confidence before students join mainstream classes. Lecturers provide multiple means of engagement (e.g., choice in topics), representation (e.g., visual aids, simplified texts), and expression (e.g., oral, written, or visual assignments), allowing students to demonstrate knowledge in varied formats (Bray et al., 2024; Quirke et al., 2024). Importantly, TCPID advocates for an approach to UDL that goes beyond simple templates and checklists, an approach often seen in the enactment of Universal Design (UD) and UDL philosophy and principles, to one where everyone is encouraged to embed a "UDL" attitude within themselves and their practice. The Teaching and Learning Assistant collaborates with staff to ensure content is accessible and support implementation in real time. This layered approach makes learning more inclusive and fosters independence, critical thinking, and active participation across academic contexts.

Throughout the ASIAP course, students build resilience and confidence through taking responsibility and being empowered to make their own decisions. Collaboration and reflexivity are an essential part of cross-disciplinary processes when working with the students throughout the course, bringing into focus the strengths and challenges faced by each student. The Occupational Framework utilized (Fisher, 1998) and collaborated on by the Teaching and Learning Assistant is outlined in Table 2.

Table 2. The TCPID Occupational Framework

Dimension	Meaning	OT Role	TLA Role
Temporal	Student's engagement in activities across time (past, present, future).	Lead transition planning and future-oriented interventions.	Observe student routines; shares insights with OT.
Environmental	Physical/social setting and tools where tasks occur.	Assess and adapts learning environments.	Implement adaptations; provides feedback on effectiveness.
Cultural	Beliefs and values influencing task performance and participation.	Develop strategies to promote autonomy and success.	Model independence; reinforces strategies in class settings.
Societal	External systems, rules, resources, and risks that impact students.	Evaluate systemic factors (e.g., risk, supports, policy).	*Not within remit.*
Social	Relationships with peers, staff, and broader social context.	Build interpersonal skills and professional relationships.	Support classroom engagement and fosters peer interactions.
Role	Student's identity and expectations (e.g., student, intern).	Clarify and support role performance across contexts.	Flag inconsistencies in role-related behaviour (e.g., lateness).
Motivational	Interests, values, and goals driving engagement.	Identify motivators; advises on appropriate challenge levels.	Support implementation and adapts materials (e.g., Easy Read).

continued on following page

Table 2. Continued

Dimension	Meaning	OT Role	TLA Role
Capacity	Cognitive, emotional, and physical capabilities impacting performance.	Explore individual strengths and support needs; co-design accommodations to enhance participation.	*Not within remit.*
Task	Specific academic or practical tasks and their demands.	Analyse and adapt tasks; provides accommodations.	Implement and give feedback on adaptations during class.

Note. The application of Fisher, 1998 (p. 514) by TCPID delineates the collaborative work of the Occupational Therapist and the Teaching and Learning Assistant in supporting the student.

Practical Strategies for Higher Education Institutions

TCPID challenges the dominant narrative regarding people with an ID, challenging the deficit thinking and demonstrating that a more contemporary approach exists (Harris, 2006; Patel & Brown, 2017). Through the ASIAP program, UD / UDL thinking and action offers an alternative way of developing an effective person-centered education that is aimed at fundamentally shifting the deficit narrative regarding post-school outcomes for young people who have an ID that have traditionally been characterized by limited social participation, economic inactivity, and resulting poverty. Quite often, the life trajectory of these students with an ID had been decided in advance by policymakers based on a deficit/medical model perspective of these young people and their capacity (or lack of it) to function effectively within society. Enabling them to transition to a meaningful adulthood requires high quality transition services typified by high expectations, person-centered goals that encourage post-school employment or further education, and collaboration between education / community agencies designed to support these young people in their post school environments (Grigal et al., 2012).

TCPID was established in 2014 to provide a higher education program designed to enable young people who have an ID to transition to a meaningful adulthood within their local communities and wider society (Shevlin et al., 2020). Engaging this cohort of learners has traditionally been based on the mistaken belief that these learners are fundamentally incapable of learning basic concepts without considerable effort from educators. The UDL approach posits that educators need to augment individual choice and relevance along with ensuring learning materials are fully accessible to these learners. In addition, a UDL approach requires that learners are presented with different and multiple options for acquiring and demonstrating information and knowledge (Quirke et al., 2024). Learners need to be able to demonstrate their knowledge and understanding in multiple ways, often diverging from traditional formats.

Gaining employment is considered to be an important marker of the transition to adulthood for all young people. However, sustainable and supported pathways into employment for young people with an ID do not exist at a systemic level; they are confined to isolated and fragmented initiatives. TCPID has challenged this perspective through establishing a viable pathway into employment through a network of business partners who are dedicated to providing work placements, internships, and the possibility of permanent employment (Ernst & Young, 2022).

TCPID was determined to ensure that their pioneering and innovative initiative did not remain an isolated enterprise with limited impact on societal perception of provision for young people who have an ID. Rather, TCPID adopted a growth model that involved scaling deep and building a consensus across education providers and policymakers that UDL informed programs for this cohort of learners needed to be established across higher education institutions. This was exemplified by the formation of a National Forum of INHEF dedicated to supporting post-secondary opportunities for this cohort (Shevlin et al., 2020). This scaling strategy has been vindicated through the recent government initiative that established post-secondary programs for these young people across the Republic of Ireland (Higher Education Authority, 2024). This is one example of positive change rippling out through the exosystem.

Partnerships for Employment and Real-World Skills

TCPID collaborate closely with a core network of business partners who provide essential financial and practical support, helping to promote inclusion in the workplace for students and graduates who have an ID. The TCPID business partners are key to helping to create greater opportunities for meaningful employment and independent living, and also to the development of a greater sense of inclusion within society for people of all abilities (Ringwood & Devitt, 2022). The TCPID business partners network is managed by the Business Partners Manager who works very closely with the business partners to develop long-term trusted partnerships and to find suitable engagement opportunities to suit each partner.

The main engagement opportunities for TCPID business partners are: (i) student work placements (work placements for one morning per week for eight weeks starting each year in early February); (ii) guest lectures (guest lectures within some of the business modules on the ASIAP course); (iii) business partner workshops (a series of tailored workshops for students, designed with TCPID business partners that run annually throughout the month of May); and (iv) graduate internships (paid employment contracts for six months for up to 20 hours per week). In order to secure new partnerships, the TCPID Business Partnerships Manager and the TCPID Ambassador conduct meetings with interested companies, outlining the impact of the partnership program and how it helps to create significant opportunities for students and graduates to learn new skills and to explore potential workplaces for the future. These meetings also explore the importance of real and meaningful inclusion within society, which cannot be achieved without inclusive employment opportunities. Potential new partners are given the opportunity to meet with current business partners to discuss the practicalities of partnership and to explore any perceived challenges. Current TCPID partners are always willing to share their experiences and to support newer partners as needed. This peer support is a vital element of the growth and strength of the TCPID business partners' network.

A strong and collaborative network united by a shared goal has driven consistent annual growth in partner engagement, with over 93% of partners renewing their commitment each year, and many maintaining partnerships with TCPID for over six years. The partnerships are carefully nurtured through ongoing communication and bespoke engagement with each partner company. TCPID publish a twice yearly "TCPID Business Partners Update" and host an annual in-person Business Partners meeting. They also host an annual SciFest@TCPID student exhibition event in association with one of their core business partners, Abbott. The TCPID also host smaller internship workshops to encourage peer-support amongst mentors who are working to support students and graduates in the workplace.

TCPID Student Work Placements and Graduate Internships

Each work placement and graduate internship involves very close collaboration between TCPID and the business partner (Ringwood & Devitt, 2022). Figure Three illustrates what each provides.

Figure 4. TCPID and Business Partnerships

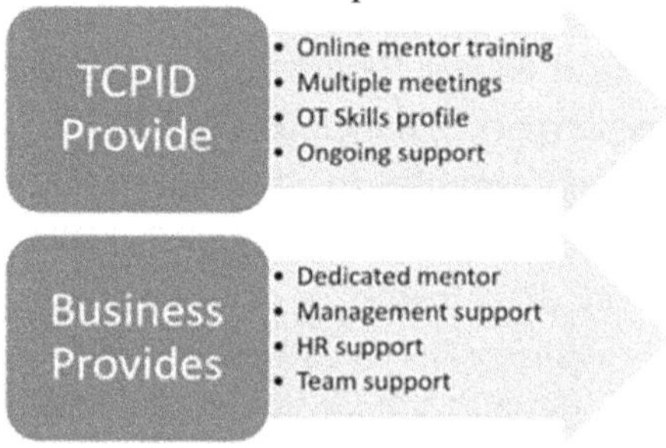

Note. This diagram of TCPID and Business Partnerships represents a model of collaboration that can be applied in other college to workplace transition programs.

Each student placement and graduate internship involves months of planning to carefully identify suitable roles and to match an individual student or graduate to each role. Multiple meetings take place with each of the business partners to fully scope-out the role and to break down the tasks that will be involved. The TCPID Business Partnerships Manager and one of the TCPID Senior Occupational Therapists then take time to match the most suitable student or graduate to each role.

TCPID works closely to support the team within each of the businesses. Training is provided in as much depth as needed for each team. This can include the TCPID Online Mentor Training program, meetings with the team, meetings with the mentor, placement and internship workshops, and accompanying support documentation as needed.

TCPID also works closely to support each of the students and graduates before and throughout their placement or internship. The TCPID Senior Occupational Therapist holds regular one-to-one meetings with each of the students and graduates to explore how they are getting on in the workplace and whether any additional support or training is needed.

The key to successful placements and internships is trust and regular communication. Where any issues arise, they can be easily resolved if TCPID are made aware of them at an early stage. The goal for all placements and internships is that they should be a positive learning experience for all involved. They should help in the development of key employment skills and in building confidence within the workplace environment.

Regular meetings are held throughout every placement and internship and a review meeting takes place once the placement or internship comes to an end. This review meeting allows the TCPID team to get detailed feedback which will help in identifying future roles for the student or graduate. In some situations, the internships may be extended, and in an ideal scenario, possibly even converted into a permanent role. Each placement and internship is a significant positive learning opportunity and does not always have to lead to permanency. In order for a permanent role to be offered, there has to be a long-term role to fit the individual at a particular time. Where this is not available, the graduate is matched to a second (or sometimes third) internship where they can further build upon the workplace skills that they have developed.

Why Inclusive Employment Matters

Participation in higher education offers transformative benefits for students with ID, including the chance to engage socially, form friendships, expand their knowledge, and explore personal interests (Alqazlan et al., 2019; Rillotta et al., 2020). TCPID have seen first-hand the importance and value of employment for graduates. Many have faced historically constrained educational and employment opportunities, which have shaped the expectations placed on them by society. Real and meaningful employment opportunities for people with an ID

> *are transforming lives - the life of the person themselves, the lives of their families, the lives of the mentors and teams within the businesses, and the lives of the wider community. Having people of all abilities in the workplace helps to create a greater reflection of the world around us and helps to encourage greater inclusion in all aspects of society. (Devitt & Ringwood, n.d., p. 29)*

It also makes good business sense as there is a huge pool of untapped talent willing and available to work, to pay taxes, and to contribute to society.

BARRIERS AND OPPORTUNITIES: STUDENT STORIES

Case Study 1 presented at the end of the chapter, shares the lived experience of a graduate from the TCPID that is conveyed entirely in their own words to preserve the authenticity and individuality of their voice. The narrative captures a rich and personal journey, tracing the graduate's educational aspirations, formative challenges, and achievements. From initial experiences in less stimulating learning environments to a growing desire for meaningful academic engagement, the graduate articulates a clear sense of ambition and self-awareness. Their story charts a determined pursuit of higher education, inspired in part by family role models and culminating in admission to Trinity College Dublin (Ireland). The account provides unique insight into the graduate's navigation of university life, from initial anxieties about fitting into the development of self-confidence, independence, and a strong sense of belonging. The story also highlights the inclusive ethos of TCPID, with tailored supports, accessible learning, and meaningful work placements contributing to a sense of empowerment and professional growth. Importantly, this unedited testimony foregrounds the graduate's voice, offering an unfiltered perspective on the impact of inclusive higher education and underscoring the transformative potential of the program for students with ID.

This case study illustrates a strong emphasis on fostering belonging through peer interaction supports within the exosystem, a particularly critical factor for marginalized groups who face disproportionate barriers to inclusion (Hurtado & Carter, 1997; Maestas et al., 2007; Strayhorn, 2012; Krause & Armitage, 2014). Family engagement also plays a pivotal role in navigating macrosystem-level barriers during transitions to higher education (Beresford, 2004; Wehman et al., 2015). Furthermore, structured work placements bridge academic and professional systems, enabling meaningful employment outcomes. While significant progress is evident, ongoing barriers underscore the need for a cohesive, ecological approach to equity and access for students with ID.

Case Study 2 demonstrates the individualized and collaborative support provided within the TCPID program to address specific learning challenges faced by a student with an ID. Drawing on Bronfenbrenner's bio-ecological systems theory, we can see in Case Study 2 the interplay between the microsystem of Clare's direct learning environment and the mesosystem of collaborative professional support, which together created a cohesive framework for addressing her needs. A cognitive assessment identified her challenges, leading to the development of a tailored Learning and Education Needs (LENS) Report to guide consistent accommodations across her modules. By breaking down Clare's goal of achieving independence with her laptop into measurable, short-term objectives, her progress was systematically supported and reassessed. This approach not only enhanced Clare's academic experience within the microsystem but also prepared her for broader societal inclusion in the exosystem of the workplace, underscoring the value of structured, multi-level interventions in fostering independence and long-term success.

Two case studies illustrate how Bronfenbrenner's (1979, 1989) bio-ecological systems theory provides a framework for understanding the multifaceted support and interactions that underpin the successful transition of graduates with intellectual disabilities (ID) into meaningful employment. In Case Study 3, Alan's experience highlights the interplay between the microsystem of his immediate work environment and the mesosystem involving the collaboration between TCPID staff, partner companies, and Occupational Therapy support. His tasks were adapted to his skills through regular, personalized interventions, demonstrating how coordinated support across these systems fosters individual growth. Adjustments to Alan's role and schedule within the exosystem of the workplace enabled him to take ownership of specific tasks, bolstering his confidence and sense of responsibility. These supports highlight Alan's agency, and the responsive adaptations made within his work environment to support his active inclusion and success.

In Case Study 4, Daniel's journey shows the developmental impact of empowering students within and across ecological systems. His initial internship provided a safe microsystem to develop confidence, skills, and self-awareness, which enabled him to articulate his career preferences. The TCPID team's active involvement in securing his second internship and preparing him for the interview reflects the mesosystem's supportive influence, bridging academic, personal, and professional environments. His successful transition to a long-term role in his preferred library setting underscores the importance of aligning individual strengths and aspirations with opportunities in the broader exosystem of the labour market. Together, these Case Studies highlight the critical role of tailored, system-level interactions in facilitating autonomy, skill development, and long-term employment success for individuals with ID. By aligning Bronfenbrenner's bio-ecological systems, TCPID ensures that its graduates can navigate interconnected personal, professional, and societal contexts.

CONCLUSION

TCPID's structure and support systems are developed in alignment with Bronfenbrenner's bio-ecological model (1979, 1989), recognizing that students' development is intricately shaped by the multiple and interconnected layers of their environment. Through this model, we see how TCPID addresses each level to create a supportive framework that not only enables students with ID to access higher education but also to thrive within it. This layered approach highlights how each ecological level contributes to creating a truly inclusive experience. By bridging gaps between these key environments, TCPID reinforces a sense of community that extends beyond the classroom, helping students with ID to feel fully integrated and respected members of the university. This interconnection fosters a cohesive support system that is essential for holistic growth. By establishing and maintaining external partnerships, TCPID opens pathways to sustainable, meaningful employment for its students.

This emphasis on work-readiness not only enhances the students' prospects but also contributes to shifting broader workplace cultures toward greater inclusivity, demonstrating the ripple effects of a well-structured exosystem. TCPID aligns with societal values and cultural shifts toward inclusivity and accessibility, reinforcing the importance of these values within its curriculum and daily practices. By embedding UD/UDL thinking and practice and aligning its qualifications with national standards, TCPID mirrors and strengthens evolving cultural attitudes that recognize the entry into the program to progression through academics, work placements, and eventual inclusion into the workforce. TCPID offers continuous support, enabling students to grow with confidence. Recognizing that development is an ongoing process, TCPID's structure supports abilities and potential of individuals with ID. This alignment with societal progress creates a positive feedback loop, in which TCPID both reflects and contributes to a broader transformation in perceptions and expectations around disability.

By guiding students through each stage, TCPID equips them with skills, resilience, and self-advocacy to navigate both university and life beyond. By addressing every layer of the ecological model, TCPID has created a dynamic and responsive environment that not only supports students academically but also empowers them to become active, valued members of their communities.

CASE STUDIES AND DISCUSSION QUESTIONS

Case Study 1: Lived Experience of a Graduate of TCPID

My name is [Mary], I live with my mam, dad, sister, younger brother and our [dog]. My parents heard about the course before I left school – they actually heard [one of the course graduates] speaking at the talk that they attended! They both thought that this would be ideal course for me when I was ready and of course they would be right!!! After I left school, I went to a center for people with Intellectual disabilities.

I found that it wasn't challenging enough for me, but it improved my independence by travelling the short distance by train every day. I really wanted to learn, because I knew I was capable of so much more, and I really love to learn about different things! So, I decided to apply for an animal care course in our local college of further education. Some of the subjects were a little bit too difficult for me, so I did as many as I could and passed the exams that I took! But I didn't feel that I achieved as much as I was capable of. I always dreamed about going to college just like my dad and sisters. In fact, my dad was one of the early students with a physical disability to attend Trinity College. So, in some way himself and my sister inspired me. [Jane] was a student at Trinity at the time too, so I got a lot of encouragement!! We went to the information day and after hearing more about the course I was determined to apply.

I will never forget the absolute joy I felt when I got my place as a student in the oldest University in Dublin. One of the hopes I had coming into TCPID was that I would meet new people and get a new perspective and be able to have the college experience. Some worries I had was I going to be able for the work and will I fit in. When I first started going to TCPID I didn't know what to expect to be honest, I was just in shock, it honestly didn't feel real. I wasn't worried per se - I was more excited to be able to study in such a historic college. I did have some challenges - for example trying to find classes; I found it quite difficult to navigate.

Some part of me was quite nervous that I wouldn't fit in but another part of me was saying why fit in when you can stand out in the crowd? I had some challenging moments but feeling included wasn't one of them, I always felt included in everything I did.

The staff in TCPID staff were so encouraging and supportive, in my learning, the programme met my needs in a lot of ways, I never felt like I was being pressured into anything. The lecturers were all so supportive in every aspect and so willing to learn from us, the students. I remember when we were doing an assessment for art history, while everyone else finished up I was the last person in the room, and I felt like I was delaying everyone, but the lecturer I had at the time, he didn't rush me, he told me that it was okay if needed some extra time, it was alright. By him saying that made me feel a lot better because knowing that it meant that I could stay at it a little bit longer meant I felt a lot more comfortable.

The course in Trinity was just a brilliant – mostly because of all the supports that are built into the course – we had occupational therapists and teachers who really understood our level of ability and made us think for ourselves. Work experience is built into the course, and we were put into jobs that were suitable for us but the employers got training in how to help us. What was great was that the work that we were given was meaningful and we learned so much. Unfortunately, Covid spoiled the end of my second year, but we learned how to communicate online and work online. When I was in TCPID I joined some societies, but the difficult thing was that most of the events were very late in the afternoon. I gained a lot of skills like: Computer skills, Time management, Social skills, Organizational skills. I used many of these skills when I was an intern and graduate even now, I used the computer skills when I had to learn how to use zoom when COVID hit, when I was in my second year we had to adapt to working from home. We had to get better at our time management.

We all got Intern jobs after graduating – I was so lucky to work in a solicitor's firm and then in TCPID in Trinity where I did my course! I was the first graduate to be employed by the Centre! I am very proud to have been made permanent at Trinity College! One of the useful pieces to help me get more confident and independent and travelling was a man named Roger from Dublin bus who guided us on what buses to get and about safe traveling. I owe him so much for making me a confident independent traveller. The course really made me feel like I could accomplish anything, it definitely made me so more confidant in myself and my independence. It also made me realize a part of myself that I didn't know before, I also found out what I really enjoyed.

My life would have been so different if I didn't have the determination to apply for the course so I'd say the course has changed my life for the better and I really hope that other students who are hopping to go and do the course can have the same determination, and I also hope that I can be a role model for them also and show them that anything is possible if you just believe in yourself.

Case Study 2: Individualized Support in TCPID

Clare is a student of the two-year higher education course (ASIAP) for people with intellectual disabilities. On commencing her course, Clare recognized very early on that her classmates were working faster than she was. They appeared to have work completed faster than her while she was still struggling with signing into her laptop. This difficulty with logging in continued as Clare was working toward recalling her password despite having the password written down. Clare recognized this difficulty herself and mentioned it to both the Teaching and Learning Assistant and the Occupational Therapist.

In the early part of the semester, Clare was supported with accessing and using her laptop in class and supported study sessions by the Teaching and Learning Assistant. The Teaching and Learning Assistant discussed these observations with the Occupational Therapist who had also observed these difficulties within modules, highlighting the benefit of cross-module support and observation in picking up challenges that students may face. Through Occupational Therapist assessment with Clare, the Occupational Therapist was able to discuss Clare's thoughts and feelings around the difficulties that she was facing with the purpose of clarifying the important aspects of university that Clare wished to focus on.

A cognitive assessment was completed with Clare which identified her challenges with attention, specifically sustained and selective attention. These challenges resulted in Clare finding it difficult to learn and recall what she was learning across her modules. The Occupational Therapist put together a Learning and Education Needs Report with Clare - identifying that she wanted to focus on becoming independent in using her laptop for learning. With Clare's consent, her Learning and Education Needs Report, which guides lecturers on the accommodations a student requires in university, was shared with both her lecturers and the Teaching and Learning Assistant.

Clare's goal was broken down into scalable achievable short-term goals that the Occupational Therapist could reassess with Clare throughout her university year. The Occupational Therapist worked with the Teaching and Learning Assistant to know how to work with Clare in the modules and supported study sessions so that there would be consistency across modules. The Occupational Therapist continued to work with Clare on extracurricular laptop work with the aim of achieving Clare's overall goal. All the work, knowledge and skill developed by Clare is captured across the two years and supports her transition into a work internship should she choose to do one.

Case Study 3: TCPID Graduate Internship

Alan (not his real name) is a graduate of the Trinity Centre for People with Intellectual Disabilities (TCPID). Alan completed a work placement as part of his course with a TCPID partner company in Dublin. This work placement was completed fully online due to the Covid pandemic. The team in the company recognized Alan's fantastic interpersonal skills and offered him the opportunity to do a six-month paid internship in their office when he completed his course.

Alan worked in a few different roles during the internship to try to figure out the best fit for his skills. Most of the computer-based tasks proved to be a challenge so the decision was made to move to a more hands-on role with the Facilities team. Alan's internship was extended, and he stayed with the company for one year. TCPID then secured another internship for Alan in a people-facing role with another partner company. Alan still needed a lot of support with some of the tasks, so they were broken down into small manageable steps by the team and the TCPID Senior Occupational Therapist, who worked onsite with Alan at regular intervals. The team then identified a regular set of tasks that needed to be done daily before the doors opened to the public. Alan was given full responsibility to do these tasks each day with a clear set of instructions and checks. This meant that his working hours had to be adjusted to do a couple of hours each day instead of fewer longer days. This new role and schedule has been a huge success and has given Alan a sense of ownership and pride in this set of daily tasks. The responsibility has helped to increase his confidence.

Case Study 4: TCPID Graduate Internship

Daniel (not his real name) is a graduate of the Trinity Centre for People with Intellectual Disabilities (TCPID). Daniel completed a work placement as part of his course with a company in Dublin. The company were very impressed with Daniel's skills and offered him a six-month internship working in their office after he completed the course. Daniel did an excellent job throughout his internship and the company was considering offering him a longer-term role. However, Daniel then expressed an interest in working in a library setting instead of in an office. Daniel would not have had the confidence to ask for this without having completed the first internship. By doing the internship he was able to recognize his own significant skills and abilities. The TCPID team managed to secure an internship for Daniel within a library setting, where the role was very suited to his personality and to his skills. The role involved interacting with lots of different people every day. Daniel did an excellent job throughout his internship and when a permanent role was advertised, Daniel's manager encouraged him to apply for it. The TCPID team helped Daniel to prepare for the interview. He was offered the permanent role after doing a really great interview. Daniel is now working in his dream job for the long-term.

Questions

1. How can higher education programs establish and embed support structures within their programs for students with ID?
2. What can Clare's (Case Study 2) lecturers do to support her challenges with selective and sustained attention?

3. How do the personalized supports provided to Alan and Daniel (Case Studies 3 and 4) reflect Bronfenbrenner's (1979, 1989) concept of the microsystem?
4. How did the personalised adaptation of Alan's work schedule and tasks contribute to his sense of autonomy and confidence (Case Study 3)?
5. What role did collaboration between the TCPID staff and the partner company play in shaping Alan's successful internship experience (Case Study 3)?
6. In what ways did Daniel's initial internship act as a developmental bridge between his academic experiences and his personal career aspirations (Case Study 4)?
7. How does Daniel's ability to express his preference for a library job reflect the impact of ecological supports on self-advocacy and long-term employment success(Case Study 4)?
8. In what ways did the interventions by the TCPID team and occupational therapists enable the graduates to build confidence and independence?
9. How do these Case Studies illustrate the importance of tailoring work roles to match individual strengths and needs?
10. How does Bronfenbrenner's (1989) mesosystem manifest in the collaboration between TCPID, Occupational Therapists, and partner companies?
11. How might universities and workplaces work together to improve long-term employment outcomes for individuals with ID?

REFERENCES

Alqazlan, S., Alallawi, B., & Totsika, V. (2019). Post-secondary education for young people with intellectual disabilities: A systematic review of stakeholders' experiences. *Educational Research Review*, *28*, 100295. DOI: 10.1016/j.edurev.2019.100295

Andresen, J. (2024). How inclusive is inclusive postsecondary education? Over-and under-representation of individuals with intellectual disabilities in postsecondary education. *Journal of Inclusive Postsecondary Education*, *5*(2). Advance online publication. DOI: 10.13021/jipe.2024.3547

Association of Occupational Therapists of Ireland (AOTI). (2025). *What is occupational therapy?* https://www.aoti.ie/what-is-ot

Aston, D. (2019). *Higher education opportunities for students with intellectual disabilities in the Republic of Ireland: A national response*. Trinity College Dublin. https://cc.careersportal.ie/mce/plugins/filemanager/files/Claire/A-National-Response%20INHEF%20Repoert.pdf

Baglieri, S. (2023). *Disability studies and the inclusive classroom. Critical practices for embracing diversity in education* (3rd ed.). Routledge.

Banks, J., Aston, D., & Shevlin, M. (2022). Falling between two stools? Post-secondary transition planning for students with intellectual disabilities in the Republic of Ireland. In *Transition programs for children and youth with diverse needs* (pp. 143–158). Emerald Publishing Limited. DOI: 10.1108/S1479-363620220000018011

Barden, O. (2021). Getting inside histories of learning disabilities. *Educational Action Research*, *29*(4), 619–635. DOI: 10.1080/09650792.2021.1899952

Barden, O., & Walden, S. J. (2021). The metanarrative of learning disability. In Bolt, D. (Ed.), *Metanarratives of disability: Culture, assumed authority, and the normative social order* (pp. 77–93). Routledge.

Beresford, B. (2004). On the road to nowhere? Young disabled people and transition. *Child: Care, Health and Development*, *30*(6), 581–587. DOI: 10.1111/j.1365-2214.2004.00469.x PMID: 15527469

Bracken, S., & Novak, K. (2019). *Transforming higher education through Universal Design for Learning. An international perspective*. Routledge. DOI: 10.4324/9781351132077

Bray, A., Devitt, A., Banks, J., Sanchez Fuentes, S., Sandoval, M., Riviou, K., Byrne, D., Flood, M., Reale, J., & Terrenzio, S. (2024). What next for Universal Design for Learning? A systematic literature review of technology in UDL implementations at second level. *British Journal of Educational Technology, 55*(1), 113–138. DOI: 10.1111/bjet.13328

Brisenden, S. J. (1986). Independent living and the medical model of disability. *Disability, Handicap & Society, 1*(2), 173–178. DOI: 10.1080/02674648666780171

Bronfenbrenner, U. (1979). *The ecology of human development: Experiments by nature and design.* Harvard University Press. DOI: 10.4159/9780674028845

Bronfenbrenner, U. (1989). Ecological systems theory. *Annals of Child Development, 6*, 187–249.

Bronfenbrenner, U. (2001). The bioecological theory of human development. In Smelser, N. J., & Baltes, P. B. (Eds.), *International encyclopedia of the social and behavioral sciences* (Vol. 10, pp. 6963–6970). Elsevier., DOI: 10.1016/B0-08-043076-7/00359-4

Corby, D., Taggart, L., & Cousins, W. (2020). The lived experience of people with intellectual disabilities in post-secondary or higher education. *Journal of Intellectual Disabilities, 24*(3), 339–357. DOI: 10.1177/1744629518805603 PMID: 30301416

Devitt, M., & Ringwood, B. (n.d.). *Business partnerships with Trinity Centre for People with Intellectual Disabilities.* Trinity College Dublin. https://www.tcd.ie/tcpid/business-partners/tcpid-business-partners-booklet-sept-2023.pdf

Disability Access Route to Education (DARE). (2025). *What is DARE?* Access College. https://accesscollege.ie/dare/

Dixon, S., Smith, C., & Touchet, A. (2018). *The disability perception gap.* Scope. https://www.scope.org.uk/campaigns/disability-perception-gap

Duncan, E. A. (2021). *Foundations for practice in occupational therapy* (6th ed.). Elsevier Health Sciences.

Education for Persons with Special Educational Needs Act. 2004. (2004). Irish Statute Book. https://www.irishstatutebook.ie/eli/2004/act/30/enacted/en/html

Ernst & Young. (2022). *Engage. enable. empower: Creating meaningful employment for persons with intellectual disabilities.* https://www.ey.com/content/dam/ey-unified-site/ey-com/en-ie/campaigns/documents/ey-ireland-engage-enable-empower.pdf

Evans, N. J., Broido, E. M., Brown, K. R., & Wilke, A. K. (2017). *Disability in higher education: A social justice approach.* John Wiley & Sons.

Fisher, A. G. (1998). Uniting practice and theory in an occupational framework. *The American Journal of Occupational Therapy*, *52*(7), 509–521. DOI: 10.5014/ajot.52.7.509 PMID: 9693695

Freedman, B., Lackey, J., & Becht, K. (2022). *Developing a college program for students with intellectual disability. Think College, 13.* University of Massachusetts Boston., DOI: 10.5014/ajot.52.7.509

Gauthier-Boudreault, C., Couture, M., & Gallagher, F. (2021). Obstacles to the transition to adulthood of people with severe to profound intellectual disability and potential solutions: Perspectives of professionals in one region of Quebec. *Journal of Intellectual & Developmental Disability*, *46*(3), 239–249. DOI: 10.3109/13668250.2021.1873753 PMID: 39818552

Giri, A., Aylott, J., Giri, P., Ferguson-Wormley, S., & Evans, J. (2022). Lived experience and the social model of disability: Conflicted and inter-dependent ambitions for employment of people with a learning disability and their family carers. *British Journal of Learning Disabilities*, *50*(1), 98–106. DOI: 10.1111/bld.12378

Goffman, E. (1963). *Stigma: Notes on the Management of Spoiled Identity*. Simon and Schuster.

Goodley, D. (2014). *Dis/ability Studies: Theorising disablism and ableism*. Routledge. DOI: 10.4324/9780203366974

Goodley, D. (2024). *Disability studies: An interdisciplinary introduction*. Sage Publications Ltd.

Grigal, M., Hart, D., & Weir, C. (2012). A survey of postsecondary education programs for students with intellectual disabilities in the United States. *Journal of Policy and Practice in Intellectual Disabilities*, *9*(4), 223–233. DOI: 10.1111/jppi.12012

Gustavsson, A., Wendelborg, C., & Tøssebro, J. (2021). Educated for welfare services—The hidden curriculum of upper secondary school for students with intellectual disabilities. *British Journal of Learning Disabilities*, *49*(4), 424–432. DOI: 10.1111/bld.12418

Harris, J. C. (2006). *Intellectual disability: Understanding its development, causes, classification, evaluation, and treatment*. Oxford University Press.

Hart, D., Grigal, M., Sax, C., Martinez, D., & Will, M. (2006). Research to practice: Postsecondary education options for students with intellectual disabilities. *Research to Practice Series, Institute for Community Inclusion, 6*(45). https://scholarworks.umb.edu/ici_researchtopractice/6

Hasselkus, B. R., & Dickie, V. (2021). *The meaning of everyday occupation* (3rd ed.). Routledge., DOI: 10.4324/9781003525035

Hayes, N., O'Toole, L., & Halpenny, A. (2017). *Introducing Bronfenbrenner: A guide for practitioners and students in early years education*. Routledge. DOI: 10.4324/9781315646206

Hennessy, T., McMahon, J., & Doody, O. (2024). How people with an intellectual disability experience inclusive third-level education: A scoping review. *British Journal of Learning Disabilities*, 1–34. DOI: 10.1111/bld.12626

Higher Education Authority (HEA). (2024). *PATH 4 Phase 2 - Course provision for students with intellectual disabilities*. Department of Further and Higher Education, Research, Innovation, and Science. https://hea.ie

Hurtado, S., & Carter, D. F. (1997). Effects of college transition and perceptions of the campus racial climate on Latino college students' sense of belonging. *Sociology of Education*, *70*(4), 324–345. DOI: 10.2307/2673270

Ingold, T. (2018). *Anthropology and/as education*. Routledge.

Jacob, S. V., Pillay, J., Adeoye, O. E., & Kelinde Oni, T. (2023). Barriers to employment of people with intellectual disability. *Work (Reading, Mass.)*, *74*(1), 207–218. DOI: 10.3233/WOR-211097 PMID: 36214017

Jacobs, P., MacMahon, K., & Quayle, E. (2020). Who decides? Transitions from school to adult services for and with young people with severe intellectual disabilities. *Disability & Society*, *35*(7), 1058–1084. DOI: 10.1080/09687599.2019.1669435

Kimball, E. W., Wells, R. S., Ostiguy, B. J., Manly, C. A., & Lauterbach, A. A. (2016). Students with disabilities in higher education: A review of the literature and an agenda for future research. In Paulsen, M. (Ed.), *Higher education: Handbook of theory and research* (pp. 91–156). Springer., DOI: 10.1007/978-3-319-26829-3_3

Krause, K. L., & Armitage, L. (2014). Australian student engagement, belonging, retention and success: A synthesis of the literature. *The Higher Education Academy, 2014*, 1-45. https://www.newcastle.edu.au/__data/assets/pdf_file/0007/558871/Australian_student_engagement_lit_syn_2.pdf

Lee, C. E., & Taylor, J. L. (2022). A review of the benefits and barriers to postsecondary education for students with intellectual and developmental disabilities. *The Journal of Special Education*, *55*(4), 234–245. DOI: 10.1177/00224669211013354

Maestas, R., Vaquera, G. S., & Zehr, L. M. (2007). Factors impacting sense of belonging at a Hispanic-serving institution. *Journal of Hispanic Higher Education, 6*(3), 237–256. DOI: 10.1177/1538192707302801

Mc Guckin, C., & Minton, S. J. (2014). From theory to practice: Two ecosystemic approaches and their applications to understanding school bullying. *Australian Journal of Guidance & Counselling, 24*(1), 36–48. DOI: 10.1017/jgc.2013.10

McGrath, J. (2023). *Curriculum, accreditation and transition pathways: Pupils with intellectual disability in special schools (Ireland)*. Trinity College Dublin https://www.tcd.ie/tcpid/assets/docs/2024/Curriculum-Accreditation-and-Transition-Pathways-Pupils-with-Intellectual-Disability-in-Special-Schools-Ireland.pdf

Mercier, H., & Sperber, D. (2018). *The Enigma of Reason. A New Theory of Human Understanding*. Penguin Books.

Migliore, A., Butterworth, J., & Hart, D. (2009). Postsecondary education and employment outcomes for youth with intellectual disabilities. *Institute for Community Inclusion, Data Note Series, 21*. https://www.communityinclusion.org/pdf/DN21.pdf

Mitchell, D. T., & Snyder, S. L. (2015). *The biopolitics of disability: Neoliberalism, ablenationalism, and peripheral embodiment*. The University of Michigan Press. DOI: 10.3998/mpub.7331366

Moriña, A., Sandoval, M., & Carnerero, F. (2020). Higher education inclusivity: When the disability enriches the university. *Higher Education Research & Development, 39*(6), 1202–1216. DOI: 10.1080/07294360.2020.1712676

Newman, L., Wagner, M., Knokey, A. M., Marder, C., Nagle, K., Shaver, D., & Schwarting, M. (2011). *The post-high school outcomes of young adults with disabilities up to 8 years after high school: A report from the National Longitudinal Transition Study-2 (NLTS-2)*. SRI International. https://eric.ed.gov/?id=ED524044

Patel, D. R., & Brown, K. A. (2017). An overview of the conceptual framework and definitions of disability. *International Journal of Child Health and Human Development, 10*(3), 247–252. https://www.proquest.com/scholarly-journals/overview-conceptual-framework-definitions/docview/1999052730/se-2

Patel, D. R., Cabral, M. D., Ho, A., & Merrick, J. (2020). A clinical primer on intellectual disability. *Translational Pediatrics, 9*(S1, Suppl. 1), S23–S35. https://tp.amegroups.org/article/view/36118/28320. DOI: 10.21037/tp.2020.02.02 PMID: 32206581

Public Services Committee. (2024). *Think work first: The transition from education to work for young disabled people.* House of Lords. https://publications.parliament.uk/pa/ld5901/ldselect/pubserv/12/12.pdf

Quirke, M., McGuckin, C., & McCarthy, P. (2024). *Adopting a UDL attitude within academia: Understanding and practicing inclusion across higher education.* Routledge. DOI: 10.4324/9781003137672

Rillotta, F., Arthur, J., Hutchinson, C., & Raghavendra, P. (2020). Inclusive university experience in Australia: Perspectives of students with intellectual disability and their mentors. *Journal of Intellectual Disabilities, 24*(1), 102–117. DOI: 10.1177/1744629518769421 PMID: 29685066

Ringwood, B., Banks, J., & Shevlin, M. (2024). Breaking new ground? An analysis of the use of embedded occupational therapy in a postsecondary education program for students with intellectual disabilities. *British Journal of Learning Disabilities, 52*(2), 422–431. DOI: 10.1111/bld.12583

Ringwood, B., & Devitt, M. (2022, October 22). *The TCPID graduate internship programme: The need for a pathway with a feedback loop to support graduates and businesses with an ever-evolving working world* [Conference proceedings]. European State-Of-The-Art Congress on Inclusive Post-Secondary Programmes for Students with Intellectual Disabilities, Salzburg, Austria. https://joinin.education/wp-content/uploads/2022/12/ESOTA-2022-conferenceproceedings.pdf

Rosa, E. M., & Tudge, J. (2013). Urie Bronfenbrenner's theory of human development: Its evolution from ecology to bioecology. *Journal of Family Theory & Review, 5*(4), 243–258. DOI: 10.1111/jftr.12022

Shevlin, M., Kubiak, J., O'Donovan, M., Devitt, M., Ringwood, B., Aston, D., & Mc Guckin, C. (2020). *Effective practices for helping students transition to work.* Oxford University Press., DOI: 10.1093/acrefore/9780190264093.013.1234

Staniland, L. (2011). *Public perceptions of disabled people. Evidence from the British Social Attitudes Survey, 2009.* Office for Disability Issues.

Stinnett, C. V., Lazo, R., & Pound, S. (2023). "Think higher. Think college." A resource guide for inclusive postsecondary education for students with intellectual disability. *Think College.* University of Massachusetts Boston. https://thinkhighered.net/uploads/TCcampaign-resource-booklet_R-fixed.pdf

Strayhorn, T. L. (2012). *College students' sense of belonging: A key to educational success for all students.* Routledge. DOI: 10.4324/9780203118924

Uditsky, B., & Hughson, E. (2012). Inclusive postsecondary education: An evidence-based moral imperative. *Journal of Policy and Practice in Intellectual Disabilities*, *9*(4), 298–302. DOI: 10.1111/jppi.12005

United Nations. (1948). *Universal declaration of human rights*. United Nations Department of Public Information. https://www.un.org/en/about-us/universal-declaration-of-human-rights

United Nations. (2006). *Convention on the rights of persons with disabilities*. https://www.un.org/development/desa/disabilities/convention-on-the-rights-of-persons-with-disabilities.html

United Nations Educational, Scientific and Cultural Organization (UNESCO). (2005). *Guidelines for inclusion: Ensuring access to education for all*. United Nations Educational, Scientific and Cultural Organization. https://unesdoc.unesco.org/ark:/48223/pf0000140224

United Nations Educational, Scientific and Cultural Organization (UNESCO). (2010). *Implementing the right to education: A compendium of practical examples*. UNESCO Education Sector. https://unesdoc.unesco.org/ark:/48223/pf0000245196

Watson, D., Lawless, M., & Maître, B. (2017). Employment transitions among people with disabilities in Ireland: An analysis of the quarterly national household survey, 2010–2015. *The Economic and Social Research Institute*. https://www.voced.edu.au/content/ngv:75674

Wehman, P., Sima, A. P., Ketchum, J., West, M. D., Chan, F., & Luecking, R. (2015). Predictors of successful transition from school to employment for youth with disabilities. *Journal of Occupational Rehabilitation*, *25*(2), 323–334. DOI: 10.1007/s10926-014-9541-6 PMID: 25240394

Zhang, L., Carter, R. A.Jr, Greene, J. A., & Bernacki, M. L. (2024). Unraveling challenges with the implementation of Universal Design for Learning: A systematic literature review. *Educational Psychology Review*, *36*(1), 35. Advance online publication. DOI: 10.1007/s10648-024-09860-7

ADDITIONAL READING

EY Playbook: Engage Enable and Empower. Trinity College Dublin. https://www.ey.com/en_ie/engage-enable-empower

Ringwood, B., Banks, J., & Shevlin, M. (2024). Breaking new ground? An analysis of the use of embedded occupational therapy in a postsecondary education program for students with intellectual disabilities. *British Journal of Learning Disabilities, 52*(2), 422–431. DOI: 10.1111/bld.12583

TCPID Business Partner Updates. Trinity College Dublin. https://www.tcd.ie/tcpid/business-partners/business-partner-updates.php

TCPID Business Partners / Graduate Internship Booklet. Trinity College Dublin. https://www.tcd.ie/tcpid/business-partners/tcpid-business-partners-booklet-sept-2023.pdf

Chapter 6
Exposing Socialization and Systemic Exclusion Barriers in UK Universities

Laura Dean
https://orcid.org/0000-0003-3642-2654
University of Sheffield, UK

ABSTRACT

This chapter examines the systemic barriers Neurodivergent students face in United Kingdom higher education, with a focus on international students from China, who often lack autism diagnoses, and female students, who are frequently underdiagnosed or misdiagnosed. It explores how financial structures, cultural expectations, and institutional policies create an environment that fosters disengagement and learned helplessness among Neurodivergent students. Drawing on Seligman's Learned Helplessness Theory, Bandura's Social Learning Theory, and Vygotsky's Sociocultural Theory, the chapter analyzes how repeated institutional failures discourage self-advocacy and reinforce disadvantage. The chapter advocates for Universal Design for Learning (UDL) as a solution to reduce the burden of self-advocacy and create more inclusive academic environments. There are recommendations for systemic reform, including culturally competent disability support, proactive outreach, and structural changes to enhance accessibility for neurodivergent students in higher education.

INTRODUCTION

Neurodivergent students face many shared barriers in higher education. However other aspects of identity, such as race, gender, and cultural background, can also

DOI: 10.4018/979-8-3693-8920-1.ch006

bring separate barriers or compound others. Intersectionality of neurodivergence with other aspects of the self can significantly shape an individual's experiences of support, inclusion, and success. For example, female Neurodivergent students or international Neurodivergent students, particularly those from cultures where disability carries stigma, can face unique diagnostic, social, and institutional challenges. These students may experience discrimination across multiple domains simultaneously, amplifying their exclusion and making it harder to access appropriate support. Neurodivergent learners are not a homogenous group, and understanding their needs requires recognizing the layered effects of intersectionality. This chapter focuses specifically on Chinese international students and female students as two groups whose intersectional identities can deepen disadvantage and contribute to systemic under recognition, misdiagnosis, and social isolation.

The discussion begins by outlining the financial and institutional structures governing disability support in UK universities, including the impact of tuition fees, funding allocations, and legislation such as the Equality Act 2010. The chapter highlights disparities in access to support, with Chinese students facing complex diagnostic processes and cultural stigmas surrounding autism, while female students struggle with societal expectations and a medical model that prioritizes male-presenting autism traits. This systemic failure in recognizing and supporting Neurodivergent students reinforces learned helplessness—where repeated obstacles lead individuals to believe that seeking support is futile.

The discussion incorporates Seligman's (1975) Learned Helplessness Theory, alongside Bandura's (1977) Social Learning Theory and Vygotsky's (1978) Sociocultural Theory, to explain how Neurodivergent students internalize systemic failures, leading to withdrawal from self-advocacy and institutional engagement. Repeated failures to access accommodations, unclear university policies, and cultural barriers to seeking support reinforce helplessness, particularly for Autistic female students, who are often conditioned to suppress their needs, and international students, who may be unfamiliar with UK disability services.

To address these challenges, the chapter advocates for the adoption of Universal Design for Learning (UDL) (CAST, 2024), which promotes accessibility by embedding flexibility into academic structures rather than requiring individual students to request accommodations. A case study demonstrates how implementing UDL in a university module significantly improved engagement and reduced the burden of self-advocacy for Autistic students.

The chapter concludes with recommendations for systemic change, including proactive outreach, culturally competent disability support, and structural reforms to ensure that Neurodivergent students can succeed without unnecessary bureaucratic barriers. By shifting from a deficit-based model to an inclusive framework, universities can create environments that support all learners, fostering equity and long-term success for Neurodivergent students in higher education and beyond.

PROBLEMS IN UK UNIVERSITY EDUCATION SYSTEMS

There are several significant systemic barriers to success for Neurodivergent students at universities throughout the UK. They include funding complications, difficulties securing employment, and navigating the university systems. Some Neurodivergent students must overcome cultural and gender-based obstacles.

Higher Education Funding for Students with Disabilities

The United Kingdom consists of four countries: Scotland, Northern Ireland, England, and Wales. While student funding varies across these regions, all UK higher education institutions (HEIs) operate within a distinct funding framework. Most funding for teaching comes from governments. The UK government handles national matters like defense, foreign policy, and taxation, while devolved governments in Scotland, Wales, and Northern Ireland oversee education, health, and transport. Scotland has the most devolved powers, followed by Wales and Northern Ireland. Funding mainly comes from the UK government via the Barnett Formula, though devolved governments can set certain taxes. Devolution is asymmetric, meaning each nation has different powers (Kelly, 2021).

Tuition fees for home students are capped at £9,250 per year at public universities, with most charging this maximum. In Scotland, the government covers tuition for Scottish students at Scottish universities, while Welsh students receive financial support reducing costs. International students pay significantly higher fees, typically £15,000 to £30,000 per year. Most UK universities are public, with only six private universities, three of which are for-profit. Private universities set their own fees but must meet regulatory standards from bodies like the Office for Students, 2022 (OfS) (Bolton, 2023).

The tuition cap for home students in England has remained at £9,250 since 2012 but does not apply to private universities. UK universities rely on tuition fees, government grants, and research funding. The UK government provides block grants through bodies such as the OfS in England, HEFCW in Wales, SFC in Scotland, and the Department for the Economy in Northern Ireland (Bolton, 2023). Research-intensive universities also receive substantial UK Research and Innovation (UKRI) funding (UK Research and Innovation, 2023).

While many universities operate on tight budgets, institutions like Oxford and Cambridge have large financial reserves due to historic endowments and land ownership. The Russell Group, a network of 24 research-intensive universities, receives a disproportionate share of research funding, benefiting from national and international grants. Teaching-focused universities, though still receiving government grants, operate with fewer resources and emphasize aspects like smaller class sizes and hands-on learning.

For home students, tuition is typically covered by income-contingent government-backed student loans, administered by the Student Loans Company (SLC). Graduates repay these loans only if their income exceeds a threshold, with repayments deducted at a fixed rate. Many students, particularly those in lower-paid sectors, never fully repay their loans, as debt is written off after 30 years (Bolton, 2023).

The UK education system includes disability legislation and funding mechanisms affecting Neurodivergent students, including those with autism, Attention Deficit Hyperactivity Disorder (ADHD), and dyslexia. The Equality Act 2010 requires institutions to make reasonable adjustments to prevent discrimination, such as extra exam time, assistive technology, and alternative assessments (Equality Act 2010). The term ‘reasonable adjustment’ is a legal one, equivalent to ‘reasonable accommodations’ in the Americans with Disability Act (1990). The Children and Families Act 2014 introduced Education, Health, and Care Plans (EHCPs) for students up to age 25 needing significant support, but many Neurodivergent students, particularly in higher education, do not qualify (Children and Families Act 2014).

Financial support for Neurodivergent students varies. Disabled Students’ Allowance (DSA) provides grants for specialist equipment, non-medical helpers, and disability-related travel. However, the application process requires medical evidence, creating barriers for students without prior formal diagnoses. International students and those from low-income backgrounds are particularly affected, as private assessments can cost over £1,000 and are often the only timely option (Doyle, 2020). Delays in securing DSA mean some students go much of the academic year without necessary support, especially in one-year master’s programmes. These funding barriers are not just procedural, they undermine equity by limiting access to essential tools, increasing the risk of academic failure, mental health struggles, and withdrawal from study.

Significant Differences in Employment Rates for Autistic Graduates

Employment outcomes for graduates in the UK vary significantly based on disability status, with Autistic graduates facing particularly pronounced challenges, with stark disparities in employment rates between non-disabled graduates, disabled graduates, and Autistic graduates (Office of National Statistics, 2022).

These differences arise due to a range of structural, social, and workplace-related factors (Bathmaker, 2015).

Graduates without disabilities tend to experience the most favorable employment outcomes in the UK. Office of National Statistics (2022) data revealed that 81.6% of non-disabled graduates are in full-time paid employment or further study within 15 months of graduation. In contrast, the employment rate for disabled graduates is lower, currently 53.5%. Among disabled graduates, Autistic graduates experience the lowest employment rates, at 29%. Autistic graduates are more likely to be unemployed or underemployed than their disabled and non-disabled peers, despite possessing equivalent or even superior academic qualifications in some cases.

Autistic individuals often gravitate toward areas of personal interest, sometimes prioritizing subject passion over market-driven employability concerns (Gelbar et al., 2014). However, Vincent and Ralston (2024) analyzed data from the Higher Education Statistics Agency (HESA) covering 1,326,416 graduates between 2012 and 2018 finding that Autistic graduates pursued a diverse range of academic programs, challenging the stereotype that they predominantly enroll in specific fields.

There are several key barriers contributing to lower employment rates for Autistic and disabled graduates. Workplace accessibility remains a significant issue, as many employers still struggle to implement effective adjustments that accommodate the needs of disabled and Neurodivergent employees. While the Equality Act 2010 mandates reasonable adjustments in the workplace, Davies et al., (2022) showed that employers often lack understanding of how to support Neurodivergent employees effectively and Autistic employees often struggle to understand what might be possible for them (Day et al., 2024). Providing flexible working arrangements, sensory-friendly workspaces, and clearer communication structures can significantly enhance workplace accessibility for Neurodivergent and disabled employees. However, the limited implementation of such adjustments places these individuals at a disadvantage. Many struggle to thrive in traditional office environments or find themselves in roles that do not align with their qualifications and skills.

A common concern among employers is the perceived cost of workplace modifications. While traditional approaches, such as clinical diagnoses and formal workplace needs assessments, can be expensive (Society of Medicine, 2022), many effective adjustments require little to no financial investment. Moreover, these accommodations often enhance productivity for all employees (McDowall et al., 2023), making them a worthwhile investment rather than an undue burden.

Bias in recruitment and selection processes also presents a substantial barrier. Many employers continue to rely on competency-based interviews and assessment centers, which often disadvantage Neurodivergent graduates. These processes frequently prioritize social communication and networking skills, which can be particularly challenging for Autistic individuals, who may struggle with non-verbal communication, small talk, or understanding unspoken expectations. As a result, highly skilled Autistic graduates may be overlooked in favor of candidates who conform more closely to neuromajority communication styles, even when their technical skills and academic achievements are strong (Austin & Pisano, 2017).

Another challenge is the lack of targeted career support available to Neurodivergent students during their time at university. While many universities provide general employability support, fewer offer tailored guidance that addresses the specific challenges faced by disabled and Neurodivergent graduates, such as deciding whether to disclose their disability to potential employers, navigating reasonable adjustments, or dealing with employer bias (Dean, 2019; Vincent & Fabri, 2020). Without structured and proactive support, Neurodivergent graduates are often left to navigate the complex transition into employment alone, increasing their risk of long-term unemployment or underemployment.

Workplace stigma and cultural expectations further compound these barriers. Many Autistic graduates report difficulties in workplace social environments due to misunderstandings or stigma surrounding autism (Bury et al., 2020; Lorenz & Heinitz, 2014). Research suggests that Autistic employees are often perceived as difficult to manage or as lacking teamwork skills, despite evidence showing that many Autistic individuals bring strong analytical abilities, attention to detail, and deep expertise in their fields (Scott et al., 2017). Workplace social expectations, such as informal networking, team-based projects, and implicit hierarchies, can create additional stress for Neurodivergent graduates, making it harder for them to integrate into workplace cultures that do not accommodate neurodiverse thinking styles.

These challenges combine to create significant disparities in employment outcomes for Neurodivergent graduates compared to their neuromajority peers. While the reasons behind these employment gaps are complex, they reflect a broader failure to create inclusive and accessible hiring processes and workplace environments (The Buckland Review of Autism Employment, 2023). The impact of these barriers is significant, not only in terms of employment rates but also in terms of career progression, job satisfaction, and financial independence for autistic and disabled graduates in the UK (The Buckland Review of Autism Employment, 2023).

Navigating Systems

The challenges faced by Autistic students in higher education highlight the crucial need for self-advocacy. While all students must learn to navigate university structures, Neurodivergent students encounter additional systemic, social, and cultural barriers that require them to proactively secure the adjustments and support they need. Universities, despite legal obligations under the Equality Act 2010, often fail to ensure accessible and straightforward accommodations, leaving Neurodivergent students with no choice but to advocate for themselves.

However, self-advocacy is particularly difficult for some Neurodivergent students. Many struggle with communication, uncertainty about institutional processes, and anxiety related to disclosure due to past negative experiences (Dean, 2019; Anderson et al., 2019). Communication difficulties inherent to autism, such as challenges with pragmatic language and interpreting social cues, further limit Autistic students' ability to effectively self-advocate (Gobbo & Shmulsky, 2012; Cai & Richdale, 2016).

Gendered socialization further exacerbates this challenge for autistic women, who are often conditioned to prioritize the needs of others over their own, making it even harder to seek necessary adjustments (Bargiela et al., 2016). Autistic women frequently face additional difficulties, including late or missed diagnoses due to gender biases in diagnostic processes which can lead to delayed recognition of their support needs (Hull et al., 2020b; Gould & Ashton-Smith, 2011).

International Autistic students, particularly those from cultures where autism carries a strong stigma, may have never been encouraged to advocate for themselves, making the UK higher education system especially challenging to navigate (Gelbar et al., 2014). Additionally, Neurodivergent students often experience isolation, anxiety, and heightened uncertainty about expectations within the higher education context, further impeding their capacity for self-advocacy (Jackson et al., 2018; Van Hees et al., 2015).

PROBLEMS SPECIFIC TO INTERNATIONAL STUDENTS

The UK is one of the most popular destinations for international students, attracting over 605,000 students from outside the UK as of the 2021/22 academic year (UKCISA, 2023). These students make up a significant proportion of the UK's higher education population, with many enrolling in postgraduate programs, particularly one-year master's degrees. Most international students come from China, India, Nigeria, the United States, and Pakistan, with Chinese students representing the largest cohort—approximately 151,690 students in 2021/22, accounting for 25% of all non-UK students (HESA, 2023).

International students in the UK tend to be concentrated in specific academic disciplines. A significant proportion, especially Chinese students, are enrolled in business, management, finance, and engineering programs (HESA, 2022). These courses often attract large international cohorts, which, while offering familiarity and a support network, can limit interaction with UK students. Many business schools have high numbers of international students, sometimes exceeding 70% of the cohort, meaning that these students often find themselves primarily socializing with peers from their home countries rather than integrating into UK student life.

This lack of social integration can lead to challenges in adapting to the academic culture and broader university experience in the UK. Unlike domestic students, who may be more accustomed to interactive learning, critical thinking exercises, and open classroom discussions, many international students come from educational backgrounds that emphasize rote learning, deference to authority, and structured assessments (Marginson, 2019). Furthermore, cultural and linguistic barriers can make it harder for international students—especially those from East Asian countries like China, South Korea, and Japan—to participate in classroom debates, social activities, and networking opportunities.

While universities have introduced initiatives to encourage intercultural exchange, many international students continue to experience academic and social isolation, particularly if they do not live in mixed accommodation or actively participate in extracurricular activities (Gu & Schweisfurth, 2015). This context is crucial when considering international Autistic students who may already struggle with social communication and self-advocacy. Given the additional challenges they face, such as navigating the UK healthcare system for an autism diagnosis or overcoming cultural stigma surrounding disability, the lack of integration into broader university life can exacerbate feelings of exclusion and hinder their access to necessary support services.

Cultural Barriers to Diagnosis and Advocacy

Cultural stigma surrounding autism in many Asian countries continues to hinder early diagnosis, self-advocacy, and social acceptance. The deeply rooted perceptions of disability, influenced by cultural, religious, and societal factors, create significant barriers for autistic individuals and their families. In many Asian cultures, traditional beliefs about disability and mental health conditions contribute to this stigma. Societal expectations emphasize conformity, collectivism, and filial responsibility, making neurodivergence particularly challenging to accept (Ng & Ng, 2022). Families often fear that an autism diagnosis will bring shame or dishonor, leading to reluctance in seeking formal a diagnosis or support (Leng et al., 2023). Confucian ideals prioritize social harmony and respect for hierarchy. Autism, which often presents with social and communicative differences, may be seen as a failure to adhere to social norms. Parents may perceive an Autistic child as reflecting poorly on their upbringing and family values. In some communities, autism is viewed as divine punishment, karmic retribution, or the result of supernatural forces (Daley, 2004). Such beliefs can prevent families from seeking medical or educational interventions, relying instead on spiritual or alternative healing practices. In many Asian societies, the medical model dominates discussions around autism, framing it as a disorder that needs to be "fixed" rather than a neurodiverse way of being (Hirota et al., 2024). This perspective reinforces the stigma and discourages acceptance of autism as part of human diversity.

This stigma significantly impacts Asian Autistic students when studying in the UK. Many Neurodivergent students arrive at university without a formal diagnosis due to cultural reluctance to seek professional assessment, leaving them without access to accommodations and support that could ease their academic experience (Rowan, 2024). Those who do have a diagnosis may still hesitate to disclose it, fearing discrimination from peers and educators, as well as judgment from their families (Chen et al., 2017). Unlike their UK counterparts, who often have prior experience navigating disability support structures, Asian students may struggle with self-advocacy. The concept of requesting accommodations can be unfamiliar or even uncomfortable for students raised in cultures where individual needs are often subordinated to group expectations (Ting and Hwang, 2009). The emphasis on academic excellence and parental expectations can further exacerbate their difficulties. In many Asian households, success in education is seen as a reflection of family honor, and any perceived struggle is often met with increased pressure rather than support (Ma et al.,2018). Consequently, Autistic students from Asian backgrounds may push themselves to mask their difficulties, leading to higher stress levels and burnout.

Among Asian students in the UK, Chinese students can face challenges due to deeply ingrained cultural attitudes toward disability and academic success. In China, autism awareness is still relatively low, and diagnoses are often avoided due to the fear of social stigma (Yu et al., 2020). The collectivist nature of Chinese society places significant emphasis on family reputation, and an autism diagnosis may be seen as a source of shame (Leng et al., 2023). As a result, Chinese students may have had little exposure to discussions about autism before arriving in the UK, making it even harder for them to seek accommodations or support services. Furthermore, Chinese students may experience higher academic pressures from family expectations, which can lead them to suppress or downplay their struggles rather than seek help.

Language and social differences present additional barriers. While many Neurodivergent students face challenges with social integration, those from Asian cultures may encounter unique difficulties due to different social norms and communication styles (Lin, 2024). Expectations around eye contact, directness, and personal space vary widely, and autistic students who already struggle with social nuances may find these cross-cultural differences even more disorienting. The lack of role models and representation in both their home countries and in the UK adds to their sense of isolation. Autistic self-advocacy movements in many Asian countries are still in their infancy, meaning that students may arrive in the UK without exposure to the idea that autism can be a positive identity rather than a condition to be hidden.

Even in the UK, the dominant narratives around autism tend to reflect Western experiences, leaving Asian students feeling excluded from mainstream discussions on neurodiversity.

Addressing these challenges requires a multi-faceted approach, including awareness campaigns, educational reforms, legal protections, and the amplification of Autistic voices in advocacy efforts. UK universities must ensure that their disability services are culturally responsive and that international Autistic students receive tailored support. Encouraging open conversations about autism within Asian communities and fostering safe spaces for disclosure can help dismantle the stigma that limits these students' potential. Only through cultural shifts and systemic support can true inclusivity and acceptance be achieved for Autistic individuals in both their home countries and their academic experiences abroad.

Accessing an Autism Diagnosis in the UK

The UK higher education system requires students to disclose their autism diagnosis to access disability accommodations, a process that presents significant barriers for many international students. The disclosure requirement means that students must have a formal diagnosis before they can request adjustments such as extended deadlines, additional support, or modifications to their learning environment. For many Asian students, especially those from China, the expectation of disclosure can be challenging due to the cultural stigma surrounding autism. Additionally, students who arrive in the UK without a diagnosis face considerable obstacles in securing timely support due to the backlog in the National Health Service (NHS) diagnostic pathway (National Autistic Society, 2021).

Obtaining an autism diagnosis in the UK is a complex and time-consuming process. The pathway typically begins with a referral from a general practitioner, who may request evidence from teachers, parents, or previous medical professionals before proceeding (NICE, 2016). Once referred, the individual must wait for an assessment by a specialist team, which often includes a clinical psychologist, psychiatrist, or speech and language therapist (Bishop-Fitzpatrick et al., 2013). Due to the high demand for autism assessments, waiting times for a diagnosis can be exceptionally long.

The Autism Act 2009 marked a significant turning point in the recognition and support of autistic adults in the UK. As the first legislation of its kind globally, it required the government to develop a national autism strategy aimed at improving diagnostic services, access to support, and public awareness. A key outcome of the Act was the establishment and expansion of adult diagnostic services across local authorities. In 2009, fewer than 50% of local authorities in England offered adult autism assessments, but by 2019, this figure had risen to 93%. This increase in services, combined with growing awareness of autism in adulthood, led to a sharp rise in diagnostic demand (National Autistic Society, 2021).

Despite these improvements, the demand for autism assessments has significantly outpaced the availability of services. According to a 2021 report by the National Autistic Society, the average waiting time for an adult autism assessment in the UK is over two years, with some individuals waiting up to four years to receive a formal diagnosis (National Autistic Society, 2021). The National Institute for Health and Care Excellence (NICE) recommends that individuals referred for an autism assessment should be seen within three months. However, data from April to December 2023 indicates that the median waiting time ranged between 218 and 306 days (approximately seven to ten months), far exceeding the recommended timeframe (UK Parliament Research Briefing, 2023).

For international students pursuing short-term studies in the UK, these prolonged waiting periods pose a significant challenge. Many arrive at university without a formal diagnosis. If they choose to seek an assessment while in the UK, they may struggle to obtain a diagnosis within the duration of their degree. Even those who secure a referral might find that the lengthy waiting times make it impractical to receive accommodations and support during their studies (Anderson et al., 2018).

The Autism Act has undeniably increased recognition and diagnosis rates, benefiting many adults who previously lacked access to assessments. However, the growing demand has highlighted systemic bottlenecks that continue to leave many individuals—particularly international students—without timely access to crucial diagnostic services and support. Addressing these challenges requires further collaborative investment in diagnostic capacity, service expansion, and greater awareness of the unique barriers faced by autistic individuals from diverse cultural backgrounds.

The structure of UK master's programs further exacerbates these challenges. Unlike in many other countries, where master's programs might last two years, UK master's degrees are generally only twelve months long (UKCISA, 2023). This condensed structure means that students must adapt quickly to academic expectations and have limited time to navigate any barriers they encounter. If an autistic student does not have pre-agreed accommodations in place at the beginning of their program, there is often insufficient time to rectify the situation before the course concludes (Adams & Brown, 2006). The intensive nature of these programs also makes it difficult for students to manage the additional stress of seeking a diagnosis and negotiating accommodations while keeping up with their academic workload (Pellicano et al., 2021).

Moreover, the UK's reliance on formal documentation as a prerequisite for support creates disparities between students who arrive with a diagnosis and those who seek one after arrival (Russell et al., 2020). For UK students who were diagnosed as children, the transition to university support services is relatively seamless, as their diagnosis is already on record. In contrast, international students who lack a prior diagnosis must first navigate an unfamiliar healthcare system, which often includes additional bureaucratic hurdles such as registering with a GP, obtaining referrals, and scheduling multiple appointments. The requirement to provide medical evidence from their home country can also be problematic, as not all countries have standardized diagnostic procedures or recognize autism in the same way as the UK does (Ng & Ng, 2022).

PROBLEMS SPECIFIC TO FEMALE STUDENTS

While international Neurodivergent students face problems due to their cultural identity, female UK college students have challenges that are reflective of their gender identity.

Underdiagnosis & Misdiagnoses of Autism in Women

Autism has long been perceived as a condition that predominantly affects males, leading to systemic underdiagnosis and misdiagnosis in women (Brickhill et al, 2023; Loomes et al., 2017). This gender disparity in diagnosis has significant implications for Autistic women, many of whom go undiagnosed until adulthood. Instead of being identified as autistic, many women receive alternative diagnoses such as anxiety, depression, or eating disorders, which can obscure their true neurological profile and prevent them from accessing appropriate support (Dean, 2019; Kentrou et al, 2024).

Research has consistently shown that autism is diagnosed later in females than in males (e.g., Cumin et al., 2021, Edgewick et al., 2021). Studies by Begeer et al. (2013), Giarelli et al. (2010), and Shattuck et al. (2009) highlighted that diagnostic tools and clinical criteria have historically been based on low masking presentations of autism, a form more often taken by males. The phenomenon of autistic females being "twice excluded," as described by Shefcyk (2015, p.132), refers to their marginalization both from the neuromajority female population and from autism research itself. Many diagnostic criteria emphasize externalized traits such as repetitive behaviors and social communication difficulties, which may be more pronounced in boys. In contrast, Autistic females often exhibit more subtle social difficulties and engage in camouflaging behaviors, consciously mimicking neuromajority peers to mask their struggles (Attwood, 2006, 2007). This ability to superficially blend in with their surroundings can result in delayed or entirely missed diagnoses.

Recent theorists have introduced terms such as "high masking" and "low masking" to describe variations in how Autistic individuals present their traits across different social and environmental contexts (e.g., Price, 2022). Masking refers to the conscious or unconscious effort to suppress or hide autistic traits to conform to neuromajority social norms. Whilst masking is not uniquely female, the tendency of Autistic women to mask their difficulties contributes to their frequent misdiagnosis with mental health conditions. Many participants in Dean's (2019) study had initially been referred for mood or anxiety disorders, a pattern reflected in broader research (Bashe & Kirby, 2005; Kopp & Gillberg, 1997; Kopp et al., 2009). Differential diagnosis rates indicate that males in the UK are diagnosed at approximately a 4.3:1 ratio relative to females, (National Autistic Society, 2023) with high masking/high-functioning Autistic women are often diagnosed later or not at all (Baio et al., 2018, Dean, 2019). Other studies have suggested that for high-functioning/high-masking individuals, the male-to-female diagnosis ratio can be as high as 10:1 (Van Wijngaarden-Cremers et al., 2014), further illustrating the underrepresentation of women in autism diagnoses. Mattila et al. (2007) reported that when diagnostic criteria are adjusted to consider autistic traits in women, the ratio of male-to-female diagnoses drops significantly, suggesting a hidden prevalence of undiagnosed autistic women (Dean, 2019; Hull et al., 2020a).

Misdiagnosis often occurs because autistic females internalize their difficulties rather than displaying externalizing behaviors. Solomon et al. (2012) found that autistic teenage girls are more likely to internalize their struggles than autistic boys or neuromajority girls, a factor that can predispose them to anxiety and depression. Mood disorders may stem from the ongoing pressure to conform to neuromajority social expectations, leading to chronic stress and eventual mental health decline. One woman in Dean's (2019) study stated, "I always felt like something was wrong with me, but every time I saw a doctor, they just told me it was anxiety. I wasn't anxious—I was overwhelmed by a world that didn't make sense to me."

Another common misdiagnosis is eating disorders, particularly anorexia nervosa. Nilsson et al. (1999) linked autism-related taste hypersensitivity to restrictive eating behaviors. While restrictive eating in Autistic individuals often stems from sensory sensitivities rather than body image concerns, clinicians may misinterpret these behaviors as indicative of an eating disorder. This is an example of diagnostic overshadowing, where the presence of one condition masks or leads to the misinterpretation of another (Reiss & Szyszko, 1983). Without recognition of underlying autism, treatment approaches may fail to address the sensory and cognitive needs of these individuals. One participant in Dean's (2019) research shared her experience of being placed in an eating disorder program: "They kept telling me I had body image issues, but I didn't. I just couldn't handle the textures of food, but nobody listened."

While initiatives like the National Autistic Society's (2022) "Now I Know" campaign aim to challenge this perception by raising awareness of late diagnoses in autistic women and non-binary individuals, significant gender disparities in autism diagnosis persist. This gender bias influences both public perception and clinical practices, leading to the misattribution of autistic traits in females as symptoms of anxiety, depression, or personality disorders. Because mental health conditions such as anxiety and depression are more frequently diagnosed in women, clinicians may default to these diagnoses rather than considering autism as a potential underlying cause. One participant in Dean's (2019) study described how she had been diagnosed with borderline personality disorder due to her struggles with emotional regulation and relationships: "It took over a decade before someone suggested I might be autistic. By then, I had been through years of therapy for a disorder I never actually had."

Many Autistic women develop coping strategies that allow them to navigate social interactions more effectively than their male counterparts. Attwood (2006) and Kopp and Gillberg (1992) described how Autistic girls may consciously imitate their peers' behaviors, facial expressions, and speech patterns to appear neuromajority, something Hull et al (2017) describe as 'social camouflaging' While this strategy helps them function in familiar environments, it places immense cognitive strain on the individual and can lead to emotional exhaustion. Additionally, these coping mechanisms often fail in unfamiliar or high-stress environments, such as when transitioning to university or the workplace, revealing the underlying difficulties that had previously been masked.

The long-term consequences of masking can be severe. Women who mask their autistic traits may experience high levels of burnout, increased risk of anxiety and depression, and difficulties in forming authentic social relationships (Hull et al., 2017). The process of masking also complicates the diagnostic journey. Clinicians may not recognize autism in individuals who have learned to suppress or compensate for their challenges, leading to years of misdiagnosis or even outright dismissal of their concerns (Lai et al., 2015; Raymaker et al., 2020).

Research has demonstrated that autistic burnout—a condition characterized by chronic exhaustion, loss of executive functioning, and reduced tolerance to stimuli—is significantly more prevalent among those who engage in high levels of masking (Raymaker et al., 2020). The inability to maintain social camouflaging long-term can lead to severe mental health consequences, including increased suicidality (Cassidy et al., 2018; Cage & Troxell-Whitman, 2019). Moreover, the experience of constantly adjusting behavior to conform to neuromajority expectations has been linked to minority stress, where Autistic individuals suffer from the cumulative effects of discrimination, stigma, and internalized pressure to fit in (Botha & Frost, 2020).

These challenges are exacerbated by the fact that many mental health professionals remain unfamiliar with the presentation of autism in women, further delaying access to appropriate diagnosis and support (Hull et al., 2017). As a result, many Autistic women are initially diagnosed with conditions such as anxiety, depression, or borderline personality disorder before receiving an autism diagnosis, if they receive one at all (Dean, 2019; Lai et al., 2015). One woman described being diagnosed with an ever-changing array of conditions from the age of thirteen, including OCD and generalized anxiety disorder. It was only after years of ineffective treatments that clinicians considered autism as a possibility (Dean, 2019). Another woman recounted a series of diagnoses, including ADHD as a child, later autism, and then a retraction of that diagnosis in favor of depression before ultimately being correctly diagnosed with classic autism (Dean, 2019).

The underdiagnosis of autism in women and the frequent misattribution of their struggles to anxiety, depression, and eating disorders illustrate the need for greater awareness of gender differences in autism presentation. Many Autistic women navigate their lives without the recognition or support they need due to societal and clinical biases. Addressing this issue requires a shift in diagnostic practices, increased awareness among clinicians, and a move away from rigid, male-centered/low-masking conceptions of autism. By acknowledging the unique ways in which autism manifests in women, researchers and clinicians can improve identification and provide more tailored support to those who have historically been overlooked.

Lack of Adjustment Leads to Self-Management

The underdiagnosis and misdiagnosis of autism in women not only delay access to appropriate support but also fundamentally shape how these individuals navigate their daily lives. Without a formal diagnosis or recognition of their autistic identity, many women grow up lacking familiarity with reasonable adjustments that could make their environments more accessible. Unlike their diagnosed male counterparts who may receive early interventions and accommodations in school, Autistic women often navigate their challenges independently. This lack of familiarity with appropriate adjustments leads to an internalized belief that they must "just try harder" rather than advocate for support (Wassell and Burke, 2022).

Research consistently highlights that undiagnosed autistic women internalize negative self-perceptions due to unrecognized difficulties. Bargiela et al. (2016) found that women frequently viewed their social challenges as personal failings rather than manifestations of autism, leading to self-blame and lowered self-esteem. Similarly, Hull et al. (2017) noted that autistic women commonly internalize their difficulties, reinforcing harmful perceptions that their struggles are due to inherent inadequacies rather than external support deficits.

Without external support or accommodations, Autistic women often develop their own coping mechanisms to navigate neuromajority environments. One of the most common strategies is masking or camouflaging, which involves mimicking neuromajority behaviors to blend in. Masking can include forcing eye contact, imitating social gestures, suppressing stimming behaviors, and carefully scripting conversations. Research by Cage and Troxell-Whitman (2019) has shown that autistic women engage in masking more frequently and intensely than autistic men, likely due to social expectations placing greater pressure on women to conform to social norms. While masking can temporarily help individuals avoid immediate social stigma, it requires significant cognitive effort and is often emotionally draining.

Participants in qualitative research by Bargiela et al. (2016) described masking as second nature—something they had been doing since childhood without recognizing its impact. One participant explained, "I just copied what everyone else did, assuming that's what everyone was doing." This illustrates how deeply ingrained masking becomes for many undiagnosed autistic women, often to the point where they struggle to separate their authentic selves from their masked personas.

Other self-management strategies identified across studies include rigid adherence to routines, overpreparation, and excessive self-monitoring. Leedham et al. (2019) found that autistic women frequently develop meticulous routines to create predictability, helping them manage uncertainty and sensory overload. However, these routines can become restrictive, causing significant distress when disrupted. Additionally, Milner et al. (2019) highlighted perfectionism as a common coping mechanism among autistic women. Their study indicated that women frequently pursue high achievements academically or professionally to compensate for perceived social inadequacies, often setting unattainably high standards that lead to increased stress and self-criticism.

The cumulative effects of lacking adjustments and relying on self-management strategies contribute significantly to burnout among autistic women. Autistic burnout, characterized by chronic physical, mental, and emotional exhaustion, has increasingly been recognized as a serious issue within the autistic community (Raymaker et al., 2020). Unlike typical occupational burnout, autistic burnout results from prolonged efforts to mask and navigate environments ill-suited to autistic needs. Symptoms include persistent fatigue unresponsiveness to rest, heightened sensory sensitivity, loss of previously mastered skills, anxiety, depression, suicidal ideation, and withdrawal from social responsibilities (Raymaker et al., 2020).

Many autistic women experience burnout in early adulthood during significant life transitions, such as starting university or entering employment, where self-management strategies become insufficient (Cage et al., 2018). These transitions often reveal the limitations of coping mechanisms, leading to a pronounced deterioration in well-being. Delayed or missed diagnoses exacerbate burnout, as women attribute their struggles to personal failures rather than recognizing them as consequences of prolonged masking and inadequate support. This self-blame can intensify distress and hinder help-seeking behavior, perpetuating a cycle of unsupported coping and burnout (Hull et al., 2020).

SOCIALIZATION CHALLENGES

Higher education institutions are structured around neuromajority social norms, placing Neurodivergent students at a significant disadvantage. Despite legal protections and institutional policies aimed at fostering inclusivity, Neurodivergent individuals frequently encounter systemic, social, and academic barriers that reinforce feelings of learned helplessness and social exclusion. These barriers are deeply rooted in socialization processes, which pressure individuals to conform to dominant social norms, leading to masking, stress, and eventual withdrawal from academic and social engagement. This section examines how Neurodivergent students are socialized into neuromajority norms and how this process exacerbates learned helplessness. It draws on Bandura's Social Learning Theory, Vygotsky's Sociocultural Theory, and Seligman's Learned Helplessness Theory to explore how institutional structures, social expectations, and repeated failures lead to disengagement and poor outcomes.

Bandura's Social Learning Theory (1977) highlights the role of observation, modelling, and reinforcement in shaping human behavior. According to this framework, individuals learn by observing others and mimicking their behaviors. Social learning occurs within a reinforcement framework, meaning that behaviors that receive positive reinforcement, such as praise or success, are more likely to be repeated, while those associated with aversive experiences or avoidance behaviors that remove discomfort are likely to be suppressed due to negative reinforcement (Bandura, 1986). Unlike punishment, which directly discourages a behavior by imposing a negative consequence, negative reinforcement involves the removal of an unpleasant stimulus when a behavior is performed, inadvertently reinforcing avoidance strategies.

In higher education, Neurodivergent students are often expected to internalize and replicate neuromajority social norms, such as engaging in collaborative learning, group participation, and networking. These behaviors are inherently socially demanding, and favor extroverted, neuromajority communication styles (Milton, 2014). When Neurodivergent students attempt to mimic these behaviors and struggle with aspects such as eye contact, small talk, or interpreting implicit social cues, they may experience aversive social feedback, such as exclusion, misunderstandings, or even direct criticism. This creates a cycle of negative reinforcement, where they withdraw from social and academic engagement to avoid further discomfort. As a result, self-doubt, anxiety, and reluctance to engage in social and academic settings become reinforced over time, ultimately discouraging participation.

This process aligns closely with masking, a phenomenon in which Autistic individuals and other Neurodivergent people consciously suppress their natural behaviors to blend into neuromajority social norms (Hull et al., 2017). While masking can sometimes facilitate temporary social acceptance, it has been linked to anxiety, depression, and emotional exhaustion (Cage et al., 2018). Many Neurodivergent students rely on masking as a coping strategy, but the cognitive effort required to maintain constant social mimicry is significant, often leading to burnout, disengagement, and, ultimately, a sense of learned helplessness. The process of masking does not only affect social interactions but also academic participation, as students may feel pressured to present themselves in ways that do not reflect their actual cognitive and sensory needs. Over time, the negative reinforcement cycle of avoidance, exhaustion, and disengagement reinforces the belief that they cannot succeed within the educational system, contributing to an internalized sense of failure and perceived inability to meet academic expectations (Cage et al., 2018; Hull et al., 2017).

By framing these experiences through Bandura's theory, it becomes evident that interventions should focus not only on skill-building but also on reducing the aversive aspects of social learning experiences for Neurodivergent students. Collaboratively creating an environment that accommodates diverse communication styles and reduces social penalties for neurodiverse behaviors can help break this cycle and encourage more authentic and sustainable engagement in higher education. Professional learning across campus can build knowledge of neurodiversity, and as faculty and staff learn to apply inclusive practices, Neurodivergent students may experience less aversive feedback.

Vygotsky's Sociocultural Theory (1978) expands on social learning by emphasizing that learning occurs through social interactions and is shaped by cultural and institutional structures. The concept of the Zone of Proximal Development (ZPD) is particularly relevant here, as it highlights the gap between what an individual can achieve independently and what they can achieve with the right support (Vygotsky, 1978). For Neurodivergent students, the lack of appropriate scaffolding and structured support within higher education prevents them from fully engaging with learning opportunities. An example is when Autistic students are given easy to implement, but ultimately ineffective accommodations such as exceptions from groupwork. It is a relatively common adjustment to let autistic students conduct group projects alone to mitigate their communication issues, but it does not support increased social engagement and is not directed at the ultimate cause of group communication issues. Using this strategy means they simply do not learn to work effectively in teams and so are disadvantaged in later job opportunities. Scaffolded opportunities to practice teamwork can be more staff intensive and so not implemented.

Most universities operate under a deficit model, expecting Neurodivergent students to adapt to neuromajority environments rather than adapting the environment to accommodate different cognitive styles. This structural exclusion reinforces learned helplessness as students repeatedly encounter unsupportive systems that fail to acknowledge their needs. When students experience repeated institutional failures, they may internalize a sense of powerlessness, which discourages them from seeking further support or attempting new strategies to overcome academic and social barriers. This lack of adaptive support can create a self-perpetuating cycle, in which students begin to believe that no matter what they do, their efforts will not lead to meaningful change.

Martin Seligman's Learned Helplessness Theory (1975) provides a framework for understanding the disengagement and withdrawal experienced by Neurodivergent students who face repeated institutional failures. Learned helplessness occurs when individuals experience persistent negative outcomes despite their best efforts, leading to passive resignation and diminished motivation (Peterson et al., 1993). In the context of UK higher education, many Neurodivergent students struggle to access accommodations due to bureaucratic hurdles such as complex Disabled Students' Allowance applications, delays in support services, and inconsistent implementation of reasonable adjustments. Even when students successfully advocate for adjustments, these accommodations are not always delivered effectively, leading to repeated disappointment. Social exclusion also plays a role in this process, as rejection from peer groups, difficulty making friends, and stigma surrounding neurodivergence can lead to avoidance of social and academic engagement. When students repeatedly attempt to access necessary support and are met with resistance or outright refusal, they may cease advocating for themselves altogether.

The process of socialization into neuromajority norms places Neurodivergent students in an impossible position. They are expected to navigate an educational system that prioritizes neuromajority styles of learning and communication while simultaneously being denied the tools and accommodations that would allow them to succeed. This often results in heightened anxiety, depression, and academic disengagement, which are strongly correlated with learned helplessness and the perception of systemic failure (Pellicano et al., 2021). The impact of this process extends beyond education, as Neurodivergent students who internalize feelings of helplessness may struggle with self-advocacy in professional and social settings after graduation.

The pressure to conform to neuromajority norms is particularly damaging in its reinforcement of masking and emotional exhaustion. Masking is often viewed as a necessary strategy for survival in higher education, particularly for Autistic students who are expected to suppress stimming behaviors, force eye contact, and engage in neuromajority social scripts despite discomfort. Participation in group discussions and networking events may be encouraged, even when these environments are overwhelming or inaccessible. Research has shown that masking can lead to withdrawal from higher education (Cage et al., 2018; Cassidy et al., 2018). Many Neurodivergent students experience long-term mental health consequences due to the overwhelming demand to conform (Mandy, 2019).

Institutional structures play a significant role in reinforcing learned helplessness among Neurodivergent students. Many university policies fail to provide accessible learning environments, which further discourages engagement. Rigid assessment methods such as timed exams, oral presentations, and traditional essay formats disproportionately disadvantage students with executive functioning or communication challenges. The lack of inclusive teaching strategies means that many lecturers rely on implicit social cues when delivering content, making it difficult for autistic students to interpret unspoken expectations. Furthermore, institutional processes for requesting accommodations are often unclear, inconsistent, and emotionally taxing, which serves as another barrier to accessing support (Anderson et al., 2018).

Addressing these challenges requires a fundamental shift toward inclusive education that prioritizes accessible learning environments, flexible assessments, and proactive institutional support. Without these structural changes, Neurodivergent students will continue to experience systemic exclusion and disadvantage, reinforcing cycles of learned helplessness and disengagement that extend beyond university into professional and personal life. Collaborative strategies can support the shift toward inclusivity of all students.

OVERCOMING CHALLENGES

Ensuring equitable access to education for Neurodivergent students, including those with autism, ADHD, dyslexia, and dysgraphia for example, requires intentional structural changes and proactive support systems. The challenges outlined in the previous sections demonstrate the gaps in policy, funding, and cultural understanding that can disadvantage these students. To address these issues, universities must adopt comprehensive strategies that emphasize early intervention, universal design principles, and student self-advocacy. It is essential to move away from a model that places the burden on students to seek and justify accommodations, shifting instead toward an approach where accessibility is built into the educational environment from the outset (AHEAD, 2021).

One of the primary barriers Neurodivergent students face in higher education is the requirement for formal diagnosis before they can access accommodations. The diagnostic process is often time-consuming, expensive, and difficult to navigate, particularly for international students or those from underrepresented backgrounds (Irvine & MacLeod, 2022). Many students who would benefit from support fall through the cracks, unable to access necessary adjustments due to bureaucratic obstacles (Anderson et al., 2018). Universities must shift from a deficit-based model, where accommodations are only provided to students with a medical diagnosis, to a proactive support framework that prioritizes accessibility for all (AHEAD, 2021).

This shift requires a cultural change within higher education, ensuring that Neurodivergent students do not need to prove they are "deserving" of support but instead are given equal opportunities to engage with learning in ways that work for them.

A key component of this approach is outreach initiatives that help students recognize and articulate their needs before they reach a crisis point. Many Neurodivergent students struggle with self-advocacy, particularly if they come from cultures where asking for help is stigmatized (Ng & Ng, 2022). Through collaboration across campus, universities can address this by providing workshops and resources before students arrive on campus, educating them about available support services and how to access accommodations. Online modules and mentorship programs that connect new students with experienced Neurodivergent peers can help ease the transition and create a sense of community from the outset (Gurbuz et al., 2019). Additionally, faculty and staff must receive training on neurodivergence, helping them recognize signs that a student may need support and equipping them with strategies to adapt teaching methods to accommodate different learning styles (Gibson, 2012). Professors should understand that flexibility in assessment, participation, and deadlines benefits all students, not just those with formal diagnoses. These trainings can be designed and created collaboratively with academic departments throughout the university. Learning together through these workshops can instigate collaboration on strategies for faculty to apply their new knowledge.

Beyond outreach, institutions must create safe spaces for self-advocacy and peer support. Many Neurodivergent students are socialized into believing that accommodations are an unfair advantage rather than a tool for equity (Brown & Leigh, 2020). Creating dedicated spaces and activities where students can meet others with similar experiences can help dismantle these internalized barriers. Campus staff can collaborate to design and build these spaces and events, share responsibility for marketing them, and attend campus activities and visit welcoming student spaces to support inclusion of Neurodivergent students. Universities should also simplify the process of requesting support by allowing students to access temporary accommodations without a formal diagnosis, particularly in cases where diagnostic pathways are delayed (Anderson et al., 2018). The current system often requires students to navigate extensive bureaucratic procedures before they can access even minor adjustments, reinforcing the idea that seeking support is burdensome. Streamlining these processes would ensure that students receive assistance when they need it, rather than after they have already struggled unnecessarily. Redesigning processes can also be a collaborative effort shared across university departments.

Mentorship programs also play a crucial role in fostering a more inclusive learning environment and can also benefit from collaborative endeavors. Pairing Neurodivergent students with upper year mentors who share similar experiences can help build confidence, improve self-advocacy skills, and combat feelings of isolation (Vincent & Ralston, 2024). Structured mentorship programs, in which mentors receive training on how to provide effective support, can empower students to take control of their academic experience. Additionally, social support groups can provide platforms for students to share experiences, discuss challenges, and develop coping strategies in a non-judgmental environment (Pellicano et al., 2014).

To ensure that all students receive appropriate support, universities must move beyond reactive accommodations toward a more inclusive model that does not rely on formal diagnosis. The widespread adoption of Universal Design for Learning (UDL) is essential in achieving this. UDL is an evidence-based framework that promotes accessible and flexible teaching practices, ensuring that course materials and assessments are designed to accommodate a wide range of learning styles (CAST, 2024). Many students struggle academically due to undiagnosed neurodivergence, and rather than forcing them to prove they qualify for accommodations, institutions should adopt a needs-based approach where support is provided based on challenges faced rather than diagnostic labels (Moriña, 2017).

One of the most effective ways to implement this shift is by embedding flexibility into course structures. Instead of limiting deadline extensions to students with official accommodations, universities can introduce policies that allow all students a limited number of flexible deadline requests per term (Seale, 2014). This removes the stigma of asking for help and ensures that those who need accommodations do not feel singled out. Similarly, providing assistive technology such as text-to-speech software, note-taking tools, and alternative exam formats should not be restricted to students with diagnosed disabilities (CAST, 2024). These tools benefit a wide range of learners, from those with executive functioning difficulties to international students who process written English more slowly.

Creating quiet study areas that are accessible to all students, rather than requiring a diagnosis to access a sensory-friendly environment, is another crucial step in ensuring an inclusive learning experience (Vincent & Fabri, 2020). Many Neurodivergent students struggle with sensory overload in traditional study spaces, yet they often avoid requesting accommodations due to fear of being perceived as a burden (Dean, 2019). If universities normalize the availability of these spaces, they can help dismantle the internalized stigma that prevents students from advocating for their needs. Similarly, providing anonymous access to mental health support can be beneficial for students who suspect they may be neurodiverse but lack a formal diagnosis (Irvine & MacLeod, 2022). The pressure to "prove" one's struggles to access help can deter many students from seeking support, particularly those who have spent years masking their difficulties (Cage & Troxell-Whitman, 2019; Raymaker et al., 2020).

By embedding UDL principles into course design, universities can create environments where all students—regardless of disability status—can thrive. The goal should not be to accommodate Neurodivergent students after they encounter barriers but to design learning environments that prevent those barriers from arising in the first place (Meyer et al., 2014). For too long, the responsibility has been placed on students to navigate inaccessible systems, reinforcing cycles of learned helplessness and self-doubt. By shifting to a model where accessibility is the default, rather than an exception, institutions can share the responsibility for student learning and ensure that every student can succeed without feeling like they must fight for the right to be included.

RECOMMENDATIONS FOR FUTURE RESEARCH

While this chapter highlights key barriers faced by Neurodivergent students in higher education, further research is necessary to develop and refine evidence-based interventions. The following areas warrant additional investigation.

Employment Outcomes and Workplace Inclusion

Research should explore how alternative hiring practices, structured interviews, and workplace mentorship programs impact employment outcomes for Neurodivergent graduates. Studies such as Austin & Pisano (2017) have demonstrated that structured hiring initiatives improve autistic employment rates, but further research is needed on how universities can support the transition from higher education to employment.

Impact of Universal Design for Learning (UDL)

While UDL has been identified as a promising framework for inclusive teaching (CAST, 2024; Moriña, 2017), more empirical studies are required to measure its impact on student success in UK higher education. Research should evaluate whether integrating flexible assessments, multiple forms of participation, and assistive technology improves academic engagement and retention rates for Neurodivergent students.

Barriers to Diagnosis

Cultural stigma and gender biases in autism diagnosis remain underexplored. Research should examine how universities across the globe can create more inclusive diagnostic pathways, ensuring that international students and women can access accommodations even in the absence of a formal diagnosis.

Long-term Psychological Impact of Masking

Camouflaging behaviors among autistic individuals are associated with anxiety, burnout, and mental health deterioration (Cage & Troxell-Whitman, 2019; Hull et al., 2017). Future research should investigate the long-term effects of masking on student well-being, academic performance, and professional development, as well as strategies to reduce the necessity of masking in educational settings.

RECOMMENDATIONS FOR SYSTEMIC CHANGE

To address persistent barriers, higher education institutions must adopt structural reforms that prioritize accessibility, inclusivity, and proactive support. The following recommendations are grounded in empirical research and best practices.

Shift from a Reactive to a Proactive Support Model

Universities should eliminate the requirement for a formal diagnosis as a prerequisite for accessing accommodations. Instead, institutions should implement needs-based support models that allow students to access adjustments based on reported challenges rather than diagnostic labels.

Operationalization

- Implement self-referral pathways for accommodations, where students can discuss support needs without requiring medical documentation (Anderson et al., 2018).
- Conduct early intervention outreach before students arrive on campus, providing workshops on self-advocacy, neurodivergence, and available services (Gurbuz et al., 2019).
- Train faculty and disability support staff in neurodiversity-affirming practices to ensure that students receive effective support without undue bureaucracy (Irvine & MacLeod, 2022).

Supporting Evidence

Research on self-advocacy interventions (Gibson, 2012) indicated that students who are proactively informed about support services are more likely to seek accommodations, leading to improved academic outcomes. Institutions may encounter resistance due to concerns about managing resources without formal diagnoses.

However, framing this as a pedagogical improvement rather than exclusively disability support can consolidate efforts, benefiting students experiencing various disadvantages, such as international students, those facing socioeconomic barriers, and disabled students, under a single comprehensive system, potentially resulting in overall cost efficiencies.

Adopt UDL Principles

UDL provides a flexible framework for designing accessible curricula that accommodate diverse learning styles, reducing the need for individual accommodations (CAST, 2024; Moriña, 2017).

Operationalization

- Incorporate multiple assessment formats (e.g., written reports, recorded presentations, and visual mind maps) to accommodate different cognitive strengths (Seale, 2014).
- Ensure lecture recordings and transcripts are available for all students to support varied processing speeds and sensory needs (CAST, 2024).
- Design courses with built-in flexibility for participation, allowing written and asynchronous contributions alongside verbal participation (Burgstahler, 2015).

Supporting Evidence

Studies on UDL implementation (Moriña, 2017) have shown that flexible assessment methods improve engagement among Neurodivergent students and contribute to overall student success.

Improve Career Support

Universities must bridge the gap between higher education and employment by collaborating with employers to develop neurodiversity-friendly hiring practices.

Operationalization

- Establish specialized career services for Neurodivergent students, offering mentorship programs and workshops on workplace self-advocacy (Vincent & Ralston, 2024).

- Develop alternative hiring pathways, such as work trials or task-based assessments, to reduce bias in traditional competency interviews (Austin & Pisano, 2017).
- Provide employer training on neurodivergent inclusion, emphasizing reasonable adjustments and bias reduction (McDowall et al., 2023).

Supporting Evidence

Data from the Autism@Work initiative (Austin & Pisano, 2017) demonstrated that structured hiring processes significantly increase employment rates for Autistic graduates.

Increase Institutional Accountability

Universities must legally ensure that accommodations are consistently implemented and accessible without excessive administrative barriers.

Operationalization

- Conduct annual audits of disability support services to evaluate the effectiveness and accessibility of accommodations (Pellicano et al., 2021).
- Establish an independent ombudsman for Neurodivergent students to address cases where universities fail to implement reasonable adjustments (Anderson et al., 2018).
- Provide faculty training on accommodations, ensuring that academic staff understand how to implement adjustments effectively (Irvine & MacLeod, 2022).

Supporting Evidence

Whilst there are financial costs to such accommodations, studies on higher education accessibility (Brown & Leigh, 2020) highlight that universities with formalized oversight mechanisms demonstrate better student satisfaction and retention rates. Improved retention rates equate to cost savings.

Culturally Responsive and Gender-Sensitive Support

To better support international and female Neurodivergent students, institutions must adopt culturally competent and gender-informed approaches to disability services.

Operationalization

- Develop culturally responsive disability services that consider international students' unique barriers to diagnosis and disclosure.
- Offer anonymous support pathways for students hesitant to disclose neurodivergence due to cultural stigma.
- Provide gender-sensitive autism screening and support programs, addressing the specific challenges of underdiagnosed female students (Hull et al., 2017).

Supporting Evidence

Research on gender disparities in autism diagnosis (Dean, 2019) and cultural barriers to disclosure (Rowan, 2024) highlighted the need for tailored interventions to support these populations effectively. To better support international and female Neurodivergent students, institutions must adopt culturally competent and gender-informed approaches to disability services.

CONCLUSION

This chapter highlights the systemic barriers that Neurodivergent students face in higher education within the UK. The findings reveal that, despite legal frameworks such as the Equality Act 2010 and the availability of funding schemes like the Disabled Students' Allowance, Neurodivergent students continue to encounter significant obstacles in accessing appropriate support. The rigid and bureaucratic nature of these systems often places undue burden on students to advocate for themselves, leading to stress, anxiety, and learned helplessness. These issues are further compounded for international students and female students, who face additional cultural and diagnostic challenges.

One of the most pressing concerns identified is the disparity in employment outcomes for Neurodivergent graduates. Despite achieving equivalent academic qualifications to their neuromajority peers, Autistic graduates face disproportionately high unemployment and underemployment rates due to biases in recruitment processes, lack of workplace accommodations, and limited career support during university. Similarly, the widespread underdiagnosis and misdiagnosis of autism in women result in delayed or inaccessible support, forcing many female students to rely on self-management strategies that contribute to long-term exhaustion and burnout.

The journey from secondary education to higher education and eventually to employment presents unique challenges for Autistic individuals and other Neurodivergent students, many of which build upon one another. In secondary education, Autistic students often encounter a structured environment with clear routines and additional support through special educational needs provisions. However, many secondary schools do not adequately prepare students for the self-advocacy and independence required at the university level. Misdiagnosis and diagnostic overshadowing in adolescence can also delay critical interventions, leaving students unaware of their needs until they face significant struggles in postsecondary education.

Upon transitioning to higher education, students must suddenly adapt to a more autonomous learning environment, often with fewer structured support systems. They may struggle with unstructured learning formats, large lecture halls, and a greater reliance on self-advocacy. The disconnect between secondary and postsecondary education means that students who received structured support in school often find themselves without equivalent accommodations in university.

As students move into employment, they encounter additional barriers, particularly in recruitment and workplace accommodations. Many hiring processes emphasize social competency, networking, and ambiguous interview questions that disadvantage autistic candidates. Employers may also engage in diagnostic overshadowing, attributing difficulties in communication or executive functioning to personality traits rather than considering neurodiverse needs. Furthermore, stigma around autism in professional settings often discourages disclosure, leaving Neurodivergent employees without the accommodations necessary to thrive in their roles.

To address these challenges, educational institutions must ensure a smoother transition between these stages by creating clearer pathways for support, fostering self-advocacy skills early, and increasing awareness among educators and employers about the cumulative impact of these barriers.

CASE STUDIES AND DISCUSSION QUESTIONS

Case Study 1: Jiahao's Story

Jiahao, a 24-year-old international student, arrived in the UK to pursue a one-year master's degree in finance. Coming from a highly structured academic environment in China, where rote learning and high parental expectations were the norm, Jiahao faced significant cultural adjustments upon entering the British higher education system. Unlike his UK peers, who were accustomed to interactive learning and self-advocacy, Jiahao struggled with seminar discussions, group work, and networking opportunities.

From the outset, Jiahao found it difficult to integrate with UK students due to cultural and linguistic barriers. His tendency to avoid eye contact and his difficulty in interpreting indirect communication led to misunderstandings with both peers and professors. In group assignments, he found it challenging to assert his opinions, often deferring to others, which resulted in his contributions being overlooked. One incident stood out during a finance group project, where his groupmates assumed his silence meant disengagement rather than difficulty in formulating responses in a second language. As a result, they distributed tasks among themselves without consulting him, reinforcing his sense of exclusion.

Social isolation compounded Jiahao's difficulties. While other international students formed social circles based on shared cultural backgrounds, Jiahao struggled to connect even with fellow Chinese students, who often prioritized social harmony over directly confronting personal challenges. A particularly disheartening moment occurred during a networking event where he attempted to engage in small talk with classmates but was repeatedly interrupted or ignored. This led him to withdraw further, avoiding similar events in the future despite their importance for career progression.

Jiahao had long suspected he was autistic but had never pursued a diagnosis due to the stigma surrounding autism in China. His parents discouraged him from seeking formal assessment, fearing that a label might harm his future employment prospects. Upon arriving in the UK, he considered seeking a diagnosis to access university accommodations, but the bureaucratic and time-consuming process deterred him. Additionally, he was unaware of how to navigate the UK healthcare system, which required a general practitioner (GP) referral to access autism assessment services. By the time he understood the process, he realized that the waiting list for an adult autism diagnosis meant it would not be done before his degree was finished.

Even without a formal diagnosis, Jiahao considered disclosing his suspected autism to university disability services, as they could have provided informal support. However, he hesitated, fearing discrimination from both professors and classmates. In Chinese culture, academic and professional success is closely tied to family honor, and he worried that acknowledging his difficulties might be seen as a personal failing. His experiences with previous teachers in China had reinforced the idea that accommodations were a sign of weakness rather than a tool for equity. During a feedback session, one of his professors expressed concerns about his lack of engagement in discussions, unknowingly exacerbating his anxiety rather than offering alternative participation methods.

Although UK universities offer various disability accommodations, Jiahao found the system confusing and difficult to navigate. He had been told that additional support, such as extended deadlines and mentoring, was available for Autistic students, yet he lacked the documentation required to access these adjustments. A university-appointed peer mentor was assigned to help him transition into the academic environment. However, the mentor, a former undergraduate student, frequently forgot to meet him and provided little meaningful guidance when they did meet.

Jiahao, rather than expressing frustration, responded with gratitude for the attempt, reflecting a broader trend among international students who have low expectations for institutional support and may not feel entitled to demand better accommodations.

Jiahao's struggles led to increasing stress and self-doubt. His academic performance suffered as he spent excessive time trying to mask his difficulties rather than seeking help. He frequently experienced sensory overload in large lecture halls, particularly when seated in the middle of a crowded room with overlapping conversations and shifting noise levels. On one occasion, after an especially overwhelming seminar, he left abruptly and skipped the rest of the day's classes, feeling drained and disoriented. The lack of structured support, combined with cultural stigma around mental health, meant that he did not seek counselling services, despite experiencing symptoms of anxiety and burnout.

Questions

1. What are some of the key barriers that prevented Jiahao from accessing an autism diagnosis and accommodations in the UK? How might these barriers disproportionately affect international students?
2. How can UK universities create clearer pathways for international students to seek disability support, particularly for those without a prior diagnosis?
3. In what ways can universities improve cultural competency among faculty and staff to better support neurodivergent international students?
4. What role can peer mentoring programs play in reducing feelings of isolation for autistic international students like Jiahao?
5. How can universities encourage international students to disclose suspected autism without fear of stigma or discrimination?
6. How can universities employ collaboration between faculty, staff, and administration to address the barriers to success for international Neurodivergent students?

Case Study 2: Lucy's Story

Lucy, an undergraduate maths student, had received her autism diagnosis only since leaving formal education, in the summer of her eighteenth birthday. As a previously undiagnosed autistic woman, she had spent years assuming that she simply needed to work harder to keep up with her peers. By the time she received formal recognition of neurodivergence, she had internalized the belief that support was an exception rather than a right. When she was finally offered adjustments, she was relieved, not because they fundamentally changed her experience, but because for the first time, her difficulties were being acknowledged.

One such adjustment intended to support her in navigating the academic environment meant she did not have to stay in a crowded, overstimulating lecture theatre but could work on her calculations with a PhD student who would check in with her in a designated quiet room and offer additional help if she needed it. However, this adjustment was not consistently implemented. “They’re supposed to have it so that one of the PhD students come up to one of the rooms I’m in and ask if I need any extra help, but that didn’t happen the last few times, so I’m going to have to kind of ask why and try and get it sorted.” Even as she described a failure of service that had persisted for weeks, Lucy’s focus was not on the lack of follow-through but on the intent behind the accommodation. She did not express anger or frustration that the support had not materialized; rather, she accepted the situation as an unfortunate but unsurprising reality. Her reaction demonstrated the extent to which she had been conditioned to expect little in terms of support and to see even a poorly executed attempt at accommodation as something for which she should be grateful.

Instead of dwelling on the disappointment of not receiving the promised assistance, Lucy praised the university for attempting to implement changes at all. “I really appreciate that they’re even trying. It’s more than I ever expected. The fact that they put something in place means they actually care, even if it’s not always working.” Her words revealed an ingrained sense of low expectations; so accustomed to being overlooked, she saw any effort, however ineffective, as a significant gesture of goodwill. This response exemplifies the paradox many autistic women face; they learn to navigate a world where accommodations are rare, and as a result, they find validation not in the actual support they receive but in the mere acknowledgment that their struggles exist.

Lucy’s case is not an isolated one. Many autistic women who have spent their lives masking their difficulties develop an overwhelming sense of relief when accommodations are even suggested, regardless of whether they are properly implemented. For these women, recognition itself becomes a source of comfort, even if it does not translate into meaningful change. While the failure of institutions to provide consistent support remains a critical issue, Lucy’s case highlights the deep emotional impact of being seen, even imperfectly. Her story underscores the necessity of ensuring that adjustments are not just proposed but actively maintained and upheld, not only for their practical benefits but for the psychological well-being of Neurodivergent individuals who have learned to expect little from the systems meant to support them.

Questions

1. What institutional factors contributed to Lucy's low expectations for support? How could these be changed to create a more inclusive environment?
2. What role does masking play in autistic women's experiences in higher education, and how does it influence their willingness to seek accommodations?
3. How can universities improve the consistency and reliability of adjustments to prevent students like Lucy from experiencing inconsistent support?
4. What strategies can be used to empower autistic female students to advocate for their needs without reinforcing the burden of self-advocacy?
5. How do these issues compound socialization and learned helplessness?
6. How can faculty, staff, and administrators come together to address the support needs of students like Lucy?

Case Study 3: Universal Design in an Undergraduate Module

Hannah, a second-year business studies student, had struggled with university teaching formats since her first year. Diagnosed as autistic in her late teens, she found traditional lecture-heavy modules overwhelming, with large, noisy lecture halls triggering sensory overload. Group discussions felt impossible; by the time she had processed a question and formulated a response, the conversation had already moved on. Although she had access to some accommodations, she hesitated to use them, feeling as though she was "making a fuss" by asking for adjustments.

When Hannah enrolled in a redesigned module that followed Universal Design for Learning (UDL) principles, she immediately noticed a difference. Instead of requiring in-person attendance at large lectures, pre-recorded lectures were made available in advance. This allowed her to engage with the material at her own pace, pausing or replaying sections when needed. Live sessions were still offered, but rather than being lecture-based, they focused on open discussions and Q&A, allowing students to participate in ways that suited them.

Group work had also changed. Previously, discussions were limited to in-person debates where quick thinking and verbal participation were expected. Now, students could engage in online forums throughout the week, where they had time to process and respond thoughtfully. Hannah, who had previously stayed silent in class, found herself contributing regularly to discussions online.

The most significant change, however, came with assessments. The module had moved away from rigid, high-stakes exams and essays, instead allowing students to demonstrate their understanding in different ways. Students could choose between written reports, recorded presentations, or visual mind maps. For the first time,

Hannah felt she was being assessed on what she knew, rather than how well she could perform under pressure in neuromajority learning environments.

Throughout the module, students were also encouraged to practice self-advocacy in a structured, low-pressure way. In the first week, they were asked to complete an anonymous survey about their preferred learning styles and any barriers they faced. Later in the term, they had an optional exercise in drafting an email requesting an adjustment, a small step toward normalizing self-advocacy. Hannah had never asked a lecturer for an adjustment before, but after completing the exercise, she felt more comfortable reaching out when she needed support.

By the end of the semester, Hannah's confidence in her abilities had grown. She no longer felt that success required masking or forcing herself to fit into a system that wasn't designed for her. The module had not only improved her academic experience but also showed her that learning could be flexible, inclusive, and accessible without requiring students to fight for accommodations.

Questions

1. How did the implementation of Universal Design for Learning (UDL) help break the cycle of learned helplessness for Hannah?
2. Why is it important to normalize different learning styles rather than framing them as "special accommodations"?
3. What were the most impactful changes in the module, and how did they benefit all students, not just neurodivergent ones?
4. How can faculty be encouraged to adopt UDL principles in their teaching, particularly in institutions resistant to change?
5. What challenges might arise in implementing UDL on a larger scale, and how can they be addressed?
6. What kind of collaboration across campus would be needed to effectively implement UDL in teaching and learning?

REFERENCES

Adams, M., & Brown, S. (Eds.). (2006). *Towards inclusive learning in higher education: Developing curricula for disabled students*. Routledge. DOI: 10.4324/9780203088623

Anderson, A. H., Carter, M., & Stephenson, J. (2018). Perspectives of university students with Autism Spectrum Disorder. *Journal of Autism and Developmental Disorders*, *50*(3), 935–946. DOI: 10.1007/s10803-017-3257-3 PMID: 28756552

Anderson, A. H., Stephenson, J., Carter, M., & Carlon, S. (2019). A systematic literature review of empirical research on postsecondary students with Autism Spectrum Disorder. *Journal of Autism and Developmental Disorders*, *49*(4), 1531–1558. DOI: 10.1007/s10803-018-3840-2 PMID: 30536219

Association on Higher Education And Disability. (2021). *AHEAD annual report 2021*. AHEAD. https://www.ahead.ie/userfiles/files/AHEAD_Report_2021_digital.pdf

Attwood, T. (2006). *The complete guide to Asperger's syndrome*. Jessica Kingsley Publishers.

Attwood, T. (2007). *Autism and girls*. Future Horizons.

Austin, R. D., & Pisano, G. P. (2017). Neurodiversity as a competitive advantage. *Harvard Business Review*, *95*(3), 96–103. https://celebratingneurodiversity365.com/wp-content/uploads/2019/08/Neurodiversity-Is-a-Competitive-Advantage-article-in-Harvard-Biz-Review.pdf

Baio, J., Wiggins, L., Christensen, D. L., Maenner, M. J., Daniels, J., Warren, Z., Kurzius-Spencer, M., Zahorodny, W., Robinson, C., Rosenberg, , White, T., Durkin, M. S., Imm, P., Nikolaou, L., Yeargin-Allsopp, M., Lee, L.-C., Harrington, R., Lopez, M., Fitzgerald, R. T., & Dowling, N. F. (2018). Prevalence of Autism Spectrum Disorder among children aged 8 years—Autism and developmental disabilities monitoring network, 11 sites, United States, 2014. *MMWR. Surveillance Summaries*, *67*(6), 1–23. DOI: 10.15585/mmwr.ss6706a1 PMID: 29701730

Bandura, A. (1977). *Social learning theory*. Prentice Hall.

Bandura, A. (1986). *Social foundations of thought and action: A social cognitive theory*. Prentice Hall.

Bargiela, S., Steward, R., & Mandy, W. (2016). The experiences of late-diagnosed women with autism spectrum conditions: An investigation of the female autism phenotype. *Journal of Autism and Developmental Disorders, 46*(10), 3281–3294. DOI: 10.1007/s10803-016-2872-8 PMID: 27457364

Bashe, P. R., & Kirby, B. L. (2005). *The OASIS guide to Asperger syndrome: Advice, support, insight, and inspiration*. Crown Publishing.

Bathmaker, A.-M. (2015). Thinking with Bourdieu: Thinking after Bourdieu. Using 'field' to consider in/equalities in the changing field of English higher education. *Cambridge Journal of Education, 45*(1), 61–80. DOI: 10.1080/0305764X.2014.988683

Begeer, S., Mandell, D., Wijnker-Holmes, B., Venderbosch, S., Rem, D., Stekelenburg, F., & Koot, H. M. (2013). Sex differences in the timing of identification among children and adults with Autism Spectrum Disorders. *Journal of Autism and Developmental Disorders, 43*(5), 1151–1156. DOI: 10.1007/s10803-012-1656-z PMID: 23001766

Bishop-Fitzpatrick, L., Minshew, N. J., & Eack, S. M. (2013). A systematic review of psychosocial interventions for adults with Autism Spectrum Disorders. *Journal of Autism and Developmental Disorders, 47*(3), 1953–1967. DOI: 10.1007/s10803-012-1615-8 PMID: 22825929

Bolton, P. (2023). *Tuition fee statistics* (CBP-917). House of Commons Library. https://commonslibrary.parliament.uk/research-briefings/sn00917/

Botha, M., & Frost, D. M. (2020). Extending the minority stress model to understand mental health problems experienced by the autistic population. *Society and Mental Health, 10*(1), 20–34. DOI: 10.1177/2156869318804297

Brickhill, R., Atherton, G., Piovesan, A., & Cross, L. (2023). Autism, thy name is man: Exploring implicit and explicit gender bias in autism perceptions. *PLoS One, 18*(8), e0284013. DOI: 10.1371/journal.pone.0284013 PMID: 37611041

Brown, N., & Leigh, J. (2020). *Ableism in academia: Theorising experiences of disabilities and chronic illnesses in higher education*. UCL Press. DOI: 10.2307/j.ctv13xprjr

Burgstahler, S. (2015). *Universal design in higher education: From principles to practice* (2nd ed.). Harvard Education Press.

Bury, S. M., Jellett, R., Spoor, J. R., & Hedley, D. (2020). "It defines who I am" or "It's something I have": What language do Autistic Australian adults on the autism spectrum prefer? *Disability & Society, 35*(9), 1514–1537. DOI: 10.1007/s10803-020-04425-3 PMID: 32112234

Cage, E., Monaco, J., & Newell, V. (2018). Experiences of autism acceptance and mental health in autistic adults. *Journal of Autism and Developmental Disorders*, *48*(2), 473–484. DOI: 10.1007/s10803-017-3342-7 PMID: 29071566

Cage, E., & Troxell-Whitman, Z. (2019). Understanding the reasons, contexts, and costs of camouflaging for autistic adults. *Journal of Autism and Developmental Disorders*, *49*(5), 1899–1911. DOI: 10.1007/s10803-018-03878-x PMID: 30627892

Cai, R. Y., & Richdale, A. L. (2016). Educational experiences and needs of higher education students with Autism Spectrum Disorder. *Journal of Autism and Developmental Disorders*, *46*(1), 31–41. DOI: 10.1007/s10803-015-2535-1 PMID: 26216381

Cassidy, S., Bradley, L., Shaw, R., & Baron-Cohen, S. (2018). Risk markers for suicidality in autistic adults. *Molecular Autism*, *9*(1), 42. DOI: 10.1186/s13229-018-0226-4 PMID: 30083306

CAST. (2024). *Universal design for learning guidelines version 3.0.* CAST. Retrieved from https://udlguidelines.cast.org

Chen, P., Chavez, O., Ong, D. C., & Gunderson, B. (2017). Strategic resource use for learning: A self-administered intervention that guides self-reflection on effective resource use enhances academic performance. *Psychological Science*, *28*(6), 774–785. DOI: 10.1177/0956797617696456 PMID: 28447894

Children and Families Act. 2014, c. 6. (UK). https://www.legislation.gov.uk/ukpga/2014/6/contents/enacted

Cumin, J.. (2021). Positive and differential diagnosis of autism in verbal women of typical intelligence: A Delphi study. *Autism. Online First*, (1). Advance online publication. DOI: 10.1177/13623613211042719 PMID: 34514874

Daley, T. C. (2004). From symptom recognition to diagnosis: Children with autism in urban India. *Social Science & Medicine*, *58*(7), 1323–1335. DOI: 10.1016/S0277-9536(03)00330-7 PMID: 14759679

Davies, J., Heasman, B., Livesey, A., Walker, A., Pellicano, E., & Remington, A. (2022). Autistic adults' views and experiences of requesting and receiving workplace adjustments in the UK. *PLoS One*, *17*(8), e0272420. DOI: 10.1371/journal.pone.0272420 PMID: 35930548

Day, M., Wood, C., Corker, E., & Freeth, M. (2024). Understanding the barriers to hiring autistic people as perceived by employers in the United Kingdom. *Autism*. Advance online publication. DOI: 10.1177/13623613241301493 PMID: 39629787

Dean, L. (2019). *Building employability: An exploratory study of the experiences and perceptions of autistic higher education students in preparing for graduate work* [Doctoral thesis, University of Sheffield]. White Rose eTheses Online. https://etheses.whiterose.ac.uk/id/eprint/27441/

Doyle, N. (2020). Neurodiversity at work: A biopsychosocial model and the impact on working adults. *British Medical Bulletin, 135*(1), 108–125. DOI: 10.1093/bmb/ldaa021 PMID: 32996572

Edgewick, P.. (2021). Gender differences in mental health prevalence in autism. *Advances in Autism, 7*(3), 17. DOI: 10.1108/AIA-01-2020-0007

Equality Act. 2010, c. 15. (UK). https://www.legislation.gov.uk/ukpga/2010/15/contents

Gelbar, N. W., Smith, I., & Reichow, B. (2014). Systematic review of articles describing experience and supports of individuals with autism enrolled in college and university programs. *Journal of Autism and Developmental Disorders, 44*(10), 2593–2601. DOI: 10.1007/s10803-014-2135-5 PMID: 24816943

Giarelli, E., Wiggins, L. D., Rice, C. E., Levy, S. E., Kirby, R. S., Pinto-Martin, J., & Mandell, D. (2010). Sex differences in the evaluation and diagnosis of Autism Spectrum Disorders among children. *Journal of the American Academy of Child and Adolescent Psychiatry, 49*(8), 789–800. DOI: 10.1016/j.dhjo.2009.07.001 PMID: 21122776

Gibson, S. (2012). Narrative accounts of university education: Sociocultural perspectives on the learning experiences of students with disabilities. *Disability & Society, 27*(3), 353–369. DOI: 10.1080/09687599.2012.654987

Gobbo, K., & Shmulsky, S. (2012). Classroom needs of community college students with Asperger's disorder and Autism Spectrum Disorders. *Community College Journal of Research and Practice, 37*(1), 40–51. DOI: 10.1080/10668920903381813

Gould, J., & Ashton-Smith, J. (2011). Missed diagnosis or misdiagnosis? Girls and women on the autism spectrum. [GAP]. *Good Autism Practice, 12*(1), 34–41.

Gu, Q., & Schweisfurth, M. (2015). Transnational connections, competences, and identities: Experiences of Chinese international students after their return "home.". *British Educational Research Journal, 41*(6), 947–970. DOI: 10.1002/berj.3175

Gurbuz, E., Hanley, M., & Riby, D. M. (2019). University students with autism: The social and academic experiences of university in the UK. *Journal of Autism and Developmental Disorders, 49*(2), 617–631. DOI: 10.1007/s10803-018-3741-4 PMID: 30173311

Higher Education Statistics Agency (HESA). (2022). *Where do HE students come from?* https://www.hesa.ac.uk/data-and-analysis/students/where-from

Hirota, T., Cheon, K.-A., & Lai, M.-C. (2024). Neurodiversity paradigms and their development across cultures: Some reflections in East Asian contexts. *Autism, 28*(11), 2685–2689. DOI: 10.1177/13623613241285678 PMID: 39370696

Hull, L., Levy, L., Lai, M.-C., Petrides, K. V., Baron-Cohen, S., Allison, C., Smith, P., & Mandy, W. (2020). Is social camouflaging associated with anxiety and depression in autistic adults? *Molecular Autism, 12*(1), 13. Advance online publication. DOI: 10.1186/s13229-021-00421-1 PMID: 33593423

Hull, L., Petrides, K. V., Allison, C., Smith, P., Baron-Cohen, S., Lai, M.-C., & Mandy, W. (2017). 'Putting on my best normal': Social camouflaging in adults with autism spectrum conditions. *Journal of Autism and Developmental Disorders, 47*(8), 2519–2534. DOI: 10.1007/s10803-017-3166-5 PMID: 28527095

Hull, L., Petrides, K. V., & Mandy, W. (2020). The female autism phenotype and camouflaging: A narrative review. *Review Journal of Autism and Developmental Disorders, 7*(4), 306–317. DOI: 10.1007/s40489-020-00197-9

Irvine, B., & MacLeod, A. (2022). What are the challenges and successes reported by autistic students at university?: A literature review. *Good Autism Practice., 23*(1), 49–59.

Jackson, S. L. J., Hart, L., Brown, J. T., & Volkmar, F. R. (2018). Brief report: Self-reported academic, social, and mental health experiences of post-secondary students with Autism Spectrum Disorder. *Journal of Autism and Developmental Disorders, 48*(2), 643–650. DOI: 10.1007/s10803-017-3315-x PMID: 29022149

Kelly, E. (2021). *Higher education funding in England* (CBP-7973). House of Commons Library. https://commonslibrary.parliament.uk/research-briefings/cbp-7973/

Kentrou, V., Livingston, L. A., Grove, R., Hoekstra, R. A., & Begeer, S. (2024). Perceived misdiagnosis of psychiatric conditions in autistic adults. *EClinicalMedicine, 71*, 102586. DOI: 10.1016/j.eclinm.2024.102586 PMID: 38596613

Kopp, S., & Gillberg, C. (1997). Selective mutism: A population-based study: A research note. *Journal of Child Psychology and Psychiatry, and Allied Disciplines, 38*(2), 257–262. DOI: 10.1111/j.1469-7610.1997.tb01859.x PMID: 9232472

Kopp, S., Kelly, K. B., & Gillberg, C. (2009). Girls with social and/or attention deficits: A descriptive study of 100 clinic attenders. *Journal of Attention Disorders, 14*(2), 167–181. DOI: 10.1177/1087054709332458 PMID: 19541882

Lai, M.-C., Lombardo, M. V., Ruigrok, A. N., Chakrabarti, B., Auyeung, B., Szatmari, P., Happé, F., & Baron-Cohen, S.MRC AIMS Consortium. (2015). Quantifying and exploring camouflaging in men and women with autism. *Autism, 21*(6), 690–702. DOI: 10.1177/1362361316671012 PMID: 27899710

Leedham, A., Thompson, A. R., Smith, R., & Freeth, M. (2019). 'I was exhausted trying to figure it out': The experiences of females receiving an autism diagnosis in middle to late adulthood. *Autism, 24*(1), 135–146. DOI: 10.1177/1362361319853442 PMID: 31144507

Leng, L. L., Zhu, Y. W., & Zhou, L. G. (2023). Explaining differences in autism detection timing: Age of diagnosis and associated individual and socio-familial factors in Chinese children. *Autism, 28*(4), 896–907. DOI: 10.1177/13623613231187184 PMID: 37491952

Lin, X. (2024). Chinese teachers' perspective on integrating autistic children in mainstream primary school classes. *SHS Web of Conferences*, 187, 03006. DOI: 10.1051/shsconf/202418703006

Loomes, R., Hull, L., & Mandy, W. P. L. (2017). What is the male-to-female ratio in Autism Spectrum Disorder? A systematic review and meta-analysis. *Journal of the American Academy of Child and Adolescent Psychiatry, 56*(6), 466–474. DOI: 10.1016/j.jaac.2017.03.013 PMID: 28545751

Lorenz, T., & Heinitz, K. (2014). Aspergers – different, not less: Occupational strengths and job interests of individuals with Asperger's syndrome. *PLoS One, 9*(6), e100358. DOI: 10.1371/journal.pone.0100358 PMID: 24950060

Ma, Y., Siu, A., & Tse, W. S. (2018). The role of high parental expectations in adolescents' academic performance and depression in Hong Kong. *Journal of Family Issues, 39*(9), 2505–2522. DOI: 10.1177/0192513X18755194

Mandy, W. (2019). Social camouflaging in autism: Is it time to lose the mask? *Autism, 23*(8), 1879–1881. DOI: 10.1177/1362361319878559 PMID: 31552745

Marginson, S. (2019). Higher education in the global knowledge economy. *Procedia: Social and Behavioral Sciences, 2*(5), 6962–6980. DOI: 10.1016/j.sbspro.2010.05.049

Mattila, M. L., Kielinen, M., Jussila, K., Linna, S. L., Bloigu, R., Ebeling, H., & Moilanen, I. (2007). An epidemiological and diagnostic study of Asperger syndrome according to four sets of diagnostic criteria. *Journal of the American Academy of Child and Adolescent Psychiatry, 46*(5), 636–646. DOI: 10.1097/chi.0b013e318033ff42 PMID: 17450055

McDowall, A., Doyle, N., & Kisleva, M. (2023). *Neurodiversity at work: A supply and demand gap analysis*. Neurodiversity in Business. https://neurodiversityinbusiness.org/research/neurodiversity-in-business-research-report-2023/

Meyer, A., Rose, D. H., & Gordon, D. (2014). *Universal Design for Learning: Theory and practice*. CAST Professional Publishing. https://www.cast.org/books-media/universal-design-for-learning-meyer-rose-gordon

Milner, V., McIntosh, H., Colvert, E., & Happé, F. (2019). A qualitative exploration of the female experience of Autism Spectrum Disorder (ASD). *Journal of Autism and Developmental Disorders*, *49*(6), 2389–2402. DOI: 10.1007/s10803-019-03906-4 PMID: 30790191

Milton, D. (2014). Autistic expertise: A critical reflection on the production of knowledge in autism studies. *Autism*, *18*(7), 794–802. DOI: 10.1177/1362361314525281 PMID: 24637428

Moriña, A. (2017). Inclusive education in higher education: Challenges and opportunities. *European Journal of Special Needs Education*, *32*(1), 3–17. DOI: 10.1080/08856257.2016.1254964

National Autistic Society. (2022). Now I Know Campaign. https://www.autism.org.uk/what-we-do/acceptance-and-awareness/now-i-know-campaign

National Autistic Society. (2023). Autism facts and history. https://www.autism.org.uk/advice-and-guidance/what-is-autism/autism-facts-and-history

National Autistic Society (NAS). (2021). *Left waiting: The crisis in autism diagnosis and employment outcomes*. https://www.autism.org.uk

National Institute for Health and Care Excellence (NICE). (2016). *Autism Spectrum Disorder in adults: Diagnosis and management*. https://www.nice.org.uk/guidance/cg142

Ng, C. S. M., & Ng, S. S. L. (2022). A qualitative study on the experience of stigma for Chinese parents of children with Autism Spectrum Disorder. *Scientific Reports*, *12*(1), 19885. Advance online publication. DOI: 10.1038/s41598-022-23978-0 PMID: 36379973

Office for Students. (2022). *Funding for higher education providers*. https://www.officeforstudents.org.uk/advice-and-guidance/funding-for-providers/

Pellicano, E., Dinsmore, A., & Charman, T. (2021). What should autism research focus upon? Community views and priorities. *Autism*, *25*(3), 756–770. DOI: 10.1177/1362361314529627 PMID: 24789871

Peterson, C., Maier, S. F., & Seligman, M. E. P. (1993). *Learned helplessness: A theory for the age of personal control.* Oxford University Press. DOI: 10.1093/oso/9780195044669.001.0001

Price, D. (2022). *Unmasking autism: Discovering the new faces of neurodiversity.* Harmony Books.

Raymaker, D. M., Teo, A. R., Steckler, N. A., Lentz, B., Scharer, M., Delos Santos, A., Kapp, S. K., Hunter, M., Joyce, A., & Nicolaidis, C. (2020). "Having all of your internal resources exhausted beyond measure and being left with no clean-up crew": Defining autistic burnout. *Autism in Adulthood: Challenges and Management, 2*(2), 132–143. DOI: 10.1089/aut.2019.0079 PMID: 32851204

Reiss, S., & Szyszko, J. (1983). Diagnostic overshadowing and professional experience with mentally retarded persons. *American Journal of Mental Deficiency, 87*(4), 396–402. https://europepmc.org/article/med/6829617 PMID: 6829617

Rowan, A. (2024). Beyond 'reasonable': Experiences of disabled international students in UK higher education. *Journal of Inclusive Practice in Further and Higher Education, 16*(1). https://nadp-uk.org/wp-content/uploads/2024/06/5.-A-Rowan-Beyond-Reasonable-Experiences-of-disabled-international-students-in-UK-Higher-Education.docx.pdf

Russell, G., Stapley, S., Newlove-Delgado, T., Salmon, A., White, R., Warren, F., & Ford, T. (2020). Time trends in autism diagnosis in the UK: Evidence from primary care records. *Journal of Autism and Developmental Disorders, 50*(12), 4358–4372. DOI: 10.1111/jcpp.13505 PMID: 34414570

Scott, M., Jacob, A., Hendrie, D., Parsons, R., Girdler, S., Falkmer, T., & Falkmer, M. (2017). Employers' perception of the costs and the benefits of hiring individuals with Autism Spectrum Disorder in open employment in Australia. *PLoS One, 12*(5), e0177607. DOI: 10.1371/journal.pone.0177607 PMID: 28542465

Seale, J. (2014). *E-learning and disability in higher education: Accessibility research and practice*. Routledge.

Seligman, M. (1975). *Helplessness: On depression, development, and death.* W. H. Freeman.

Shattuck, P. T., Durkin, M., Maenner, M., Newschaffer, C., Mandell, D. S., Wiggins, L., & Yeargin-Allsopp, M. (2009). Timing of identification among children with an Autism Spectrum Disorder: Findings from a population-based surveillance study. *Journal of the American Academy of Child and Adolescent Psychiatry, 48*(5), 474–483. DOI: 10.1097/CHI.0b013e31819b3848 PMID: 19318992

Shefcyk, A. (2015). Count us in: Addressing gender disparities in autism research. *Autism, 19*(2), 131–132. DOI: 10.1177/1362361314566585 PMID: 25789398

Solomon, M., Miller, M., Taylor, S. L., Hinshaw, S. P., & Carter, C. S. (2012). Autism symptoms and internalizing psychopathology in girls and boys with Autism Spectrum Disorders. *Journal of Autism and Developmental Disorders, 42*(1), 48–59. DOI: 10.1007/s10803-011-1215-z PMID: 21442362

The Buckland Review of Autism Employment. (2023). *Report and recommendations*. GOV.UK. https://www.gov.uk/government/publications/the-buckland-review-of-autism-employment-report-and-recommendations/the-buckland-review-of-autism-employment-report-and-recommendations

Ting, J. Y., & Hwang, W. C. (2009). Cultural influences on help-seeking attitudes in Asian American students. *The American Journal of Orthopsychiatry, 79*(1), 125–132. DOI: 10.1037/a0015394 PMID: 19290732

United Kingdom Council for International Student Affairs. (2023). *Annual Policy Review 2022–23*. UKCISA. https://www.ukcisa.org.uk/Research--Policy/Resource-bank/resources/250/Annual-policy-review-2022-23

Van Hees, V., Moyson, T., & Roeyers, H. (2015). Higher education experiences of students with Autism Spectrum Disorder: Challenges, benefits, and needs. *Journal of Autism and Developmental Disorders, 45*(6), 1673–1688. DOI: 10.1007/s10803-014-2324-2 PMID: 25448918

Van Wijngaarden-Cremers, P. J. M., van Eeten, E., Groen, W. B., Van Deurzen, P. A., Oosterling, I. J., & Van der Gaag, R. J. (2014). Gender and age differences in the core triad of impairments in Autism Spectrum Disorders: A systematic review and meta-analysis. *Journal of Autism and Developmental Disorders, 44*(3), 627–635. DOI: 10.1007/s10803-013-1913-9 PMID: 23989936

Vincent, J., & Fabri, M. (2020). The ecosystem of competitive employment for university graduates with autism. *International Journal of Disability Development and Education, 69*(6), 705–722. DOI: 10.1080/1034912X.2019.1626488

Vincent, J., & Ralston, K. (2024). Uncovering employment outcomes for autistic university graduates in the United Kingdom: An analysis of population data. *Autism, 28*(3), 732–743. DOI: 10.1177/13623613231182756 PMID: 37353923

Vygotsky, L. S. (1978). *Mind in society: The development of higher psychological processes*. Harvard University Press.

Wassell, C., & Burke, E. (2022). *Autism, girls, & keeping it all inside*. Autistic Girls Network. https://autisticgirlsnetwork.org/wp-content/uploads/2022/03/AGN-Report-Autism-Girls-Keeping-It-All-Inside.pdf

Yu, L., Stronach, S., & Harrison, A. J. (2020). Public knowledge and stigma of Autism Spectrum Disorder: Comparing China with the United States. *Autism*, *24*(6), 1531–1545. DOI: 10.1177/1362361319900839 PMID: 32338539

ADDITIONAL READING

Cage, E., & Troxell-Whitman, Z. (2019). Understanding the reasons, contexts, and costs of camouflaging for Autistic adults. *Journal of Autism and Developmental Disorders*, *49*(5), 1899–1911. DOI: 10.1007/s10803-018-03878-x PMID: 30627892

Hull, L., Petrides, K. V., Allison, C., Smith, P., Baron-Cohen, S., Lai, M.-C., & Mandy, W. (2017). 'Putting on my best normal': Social camouflaging in adults with autism spectrum conditions. *Journal of Autism and Developmental Disorders*, *47*(8), 2519–2534. DOI: 10.1007/s10803-017-3166-5 PMID: 28527095

Pellicano, E., Dinsmore, A., & Charman, T. (2014). What should autism research focus upon? Community views and priorities from the United Kingdom. *Autism*, *18*(7), 756–770. DOI: 10.1177/1362361314529627 PMID: 24789871

Vincent, J., & Ralston, K. (2024). Uncovering employment outcomes for Autistic university graduates in the United Kingdom: An analysis of population data. *Autism*, *28*(3), 732–743. DOI: 10.1177/13623613231182756 PMID: 37353923

Chapter 7
Empowering College Students With Intellectual Disability:
The Role of Self-Advocacy and Self-Determination

Jessie C. Green
https://orcid.org/0000-0002-7155-2457
The Ohio State University, USA

Andrew Buck
https://orcid.org/0000-0003-3770-9286
The Ohio State University, USA

Margo Izzo
The Ohio State University, USA

Emily Van Gaasbeek
https://orcid.org/0000-0001-9409-8157
The Ohio State University, USA

ABSTRACT

Youth with disabilities do not obtain employment at the same rates as their peers without disabilities. Many people with intellectual disability are enrolling in higher education as a step on their path to employment. Several inclusive postsecondary education programs in Ohio used structured interviews with program students, alumni, and past students to seek information on how programs are implementing the Think College Standards for Inclusive Higher Education. Thematic analysis

DOI: 10.4018/979-8-3693-8920-1.ch007

revealed extensive use of self-advocacy skills by students across five areas: academics, employment, social, staff, and with family. This chapter shares the use of self-advocacy skills by students and graduates across all areas.

INTRODUCTION

Researchers have found that young people with disabilities may have more difficulty finding employment than their peers without disabilities; Autistic students and those with an intellectual disability (ID), or multiple disabilities are often unprepared for adult life (Buck, 2022; Grigal & Hart, 2010; Mazzotti & et al., 2021). The number of people represented by the term Neurodivergent dramatically varies based on which definition is used (Dwyer, 2022; Legault et al., 2021). At the heart of neurodiversity is the idea that there are a variety of brains which means there are a variety of ways of thinking, learning, and interacting. Intellectual disability reflects one brain type within neurodiversity (Masataka, 2017). This chapter provides a look into how students with intellectual disability use self-advocacy while attending Inclusive Postsecondary Education (IPSE) programs in Ohio and how collaborative practices on campus help students use natural brain variation to develop and build deeper advocacy skills.

Statistics from the United States Department of Labor (2024) reveal that youth with disabilities between the ages of 20 and 24 have a lower labor force participation rate compared to youth without disabilities (46.9% versus 73.1%) and are nearly twice as likely to be unemployed (13.3% versus 7.1%). Survey data (N=12,410) from the Ohio Longitudinal Transition Study (OLTS) (Unger et al., 2022) found discrepancies between the planned and actual postschool employment outcomes of high school graduates with disabilities between 2010-2020. While 41% planned to work full time, fewer (36%) were working 35 or more hours per week during the year since leaving high school. Similarly, 36% anticipated working 20-34 hours per week but fewer (25%) reported part-time employment within the year after exit.

Fewer Neurodivergent students transition to higher education or training programs than their peers without disabilities (Newman et al., 2011). Among the OLTS sample of 2010-2020 graduates, about 34% (n=4,197) enrolled in two- or four-year colleges, which is less than state (53%) and national (63%) enrollment averages for nondisabled students (Unger et al., 2022). As with employment data, the survey found inconsistent rates between students planned and actual rates of enrollment in four-year colleges (27% versus 15%) and other training programs (9% versus 5%) after leaving high school. Morgan's story above demonstrates the many benefits to postsecondary education, including gains in independence, lifelong friendship development, and higher self-esteem (Grigal et al., 2024). Despite knowing these benefits, students with ID enroll in postsecondary education at the lowest rates compared to their peers with and without disabilities (Lipscomb et al., 2017; Newman et al., 2011).

Self-determination within the intellectual disability field is defined by Wehmeyer (2001) as "acting as the primary causal agent in one's life and making choices and decisions regarding one's quality of life free from undue external influence or interference (p. 30)." Self-advocacy is a component of self-determination and is defined as "an individual's ability to effectively communicate, convey, negotiate or assert his or her own interests, desires, needs, and rights. It involves making informed decisions and taking responsibility for those decisions" (Van Reusen et al., 2002, p. 1). Both self-determination and self-advocacy are shown to be evidenced-based predictors of post-school outcomes for students with disabilities (Mazzotti et al., 2021).

Bridging the gap to meet and exceed students' aspirations is an educational and societal imperative. It requires effective policy and practice to fortify students with essential transition skills that predict positive outcomes (Shogren et al., 2021). Two such skills, self-advocacy and self-determination, have been identified by research to be positively correlated with engagement in postsecondary education and employment, and new evidence suggests that self-determination is a predictor of independent living (Mazzotti et al., 2021; Petcu et al., 2017; Shogren et al., 2017); Morgan is a prime example since as they built their skills, they gained the confidence to now live on their own.

Comprehensive Transition Postsecondary (CTP) programs allow eligible students with intellectual disability to apply for existing federal financial aid mechanisms (e.g., PELL grants) to assist with the costs of attending inclusive postsecondary education programs.

The Higher Education Opportunity Act (HEOA) (2008) defines a student with an intellectual disability as having a cognitive impairment, characterized by significant limitations in: (i) intellectual and cognitive functioning; and (ii) adaptive behavior as expressed in conceptual, social, and practical adaptive skills (Madaus et al., 2012). In addition, students are formally or currently eligible for a free appropriate public education under the Individuals with Disabilities Education Act, which includes transitioned aged youth with disabilities through 22 years of age. Additionally, the HEOA established model demonstration programs which focus on four areas: "academic enrichment; socialization; independent living skills, including self-advocacy; and integrated work experiences and career skills that lead to gainful employment" (Voelker, 2013, p. 33).

By nature of the disability, traditional college pathways have not been available for students with intellectual disability due to typical entrance requirements, including competitive grade point averages, standardized assessment results, and essays, as well as engagement in extracurricular activities (Grigal & Hart, 2010). Increasing the number of accredited CTP programs nationwide is imperative, so more students with ID can access federal financial aid to help fund their postsecondary education.

There are many benefits to postsecondary education including gains in independence, lifelong friendship development, and higher self-esteem (Grigal et al., 2024). Despite knowing these benefits, students with ID enroll in postsecondary education at the lowest rates compared to their peers with and without disabilities according to the National Longitudinal Transition Study – 2 (Newman et al., 2011). According to Ohio's Indicator 14 data 53.5% of students report they plan to enroll in postsecondary education, yet only 26.7% of those students actually do enroll (Unger et al., 2022, p. 19). This discrepancy in postsecondary intentions could be due to a lack of strong self-determination skills.

Collectively, the Americans with Disabilities Act (ADA), HEOA, and Workforce Innovation Opportunity Act (WIOA) create a framework from which students with intellectual disability can be supported to successful. Self-advocacy is a learnable behavior by which an individual assertively and willfully represents their own interests and conveys personal preferences to others (Schmidt et al., 2020). Test et al. (2005) argued that an individual's ability to effectively utilize self-advocacy is crucial to actualizing self-determination. Furthermore, key components of self-determination, including goal setting, decision-making, self-realization (i.e., understanding one's strengths and support needs), and psychological empowerment (i.e., a belief in the relationship between one's actions and outcomes), have also been found to be independent predictors of postschool success (Mazzotti et al., 2021).

Developing self-advocacy and self-determination skills through collaborative direct instruction and multiple, varied opportunities for practice is a fundamental strategy for advancing equitable educational and employment outcomes for students with intellectual disability (Shogren et al., 2021; Wehmeyer, 2020). In this chapter, we will: (i) provide background information by describing a pivotal policy that aims to advance higher education opportunities for this population; (ii) discuss results from research interviews conducted with students enrolled in Inclusive Postsecondary Education (IPSE) programs; and (iii) explore case studies that emphasize the importance of self-advocacy and self-determination in promoting student success.

Numerous barriers to individuals with disabilities becoming strong self-advocates and self-determined individuals exist. Petri et al. (2021) used a qualitative analysis to highlight the economic barriers of becoming professional advocates, as many disability supporting organizations do not promote the self-advocate voice in meaningful ways. Self-advocates have described disclosing as a barrier to self-advocacy because disclosing can lead to continued stigmatization of individuals (Karpicz, 2020). Finally, themes emerging from Vaucher et al.'s 2020 study found environmental (e.g., institutional constraints, limited choices), personal (e.g., fear, communication), and relational (e.g., staff, family) barriers to being a more self-determined individual.

SELF-ADVOCACY AND SELF-DETERMINATION AS EVIDENCED-BASED PREDICTORS

Wehmeyer (2005, p.117) defined self-determined behavior as "volitional actions that enable one to act as the primary causal agent in one's life and to maintain or improve one's quality of life." Essential characteristics of self-determination include: autonomy, self-regulation, psychological empowerment, and self-realization (Buck, 2022; Shogren et al., 2007; Wehmeyer, 2005; Wehmeyer & Palmer, 2003). More recently, Rowe et al. (2015) combined self-determination and self-advocacy into the following definition: "the ability to make choices, solve problems, set goals, evaluate options, take initiative to reach one's goals, and accept consequences of one's actions."

Scholars (Buck, 2022; Test et al., 2009; Mazzotti et al., 2016; Mazzotti et al., 2021) have suggested elements that predict success in postsecondary outcomes in education, employment, and independent living for students with disabilities. These predictors include: goal setting, psychological empowerment, self-determination/self-advocacy, self-realization, and youth autonomy/decision making.

Federal Policy

Under the Americans with Disabilities Act (ADA), individuals with disabilities cannot be discriminated on based upon their disability across "major life areas" including in employment and educational settings. The ADA ensures reasonable accommodations such as physical access to public spaces, plain or clear language availability, workplace accommodations, accessible communication, and a process by which to report barriers to access. In 2014, the Workforce Innovation Opportunity Act (WIOA) was passed, providing resources to individuals with disabilities to find "meaningful competitive integrated employment" (Thelin & Grigal, 2019). Higher education is supported and even emphasized by WIOA as a path to competitive integrated employment.

The final federal policy impacting self-determination is the Higher Education Opportunity Act (HEOA; 2008) which reauthorized the Higher Education Act, adding two key provisions for students with intellectual disability in college settings. First, it established grants to develop model Transition and Postsecondary Programs for Students with Intellectual Disabilities (TPSID), which facilitate inclusive college classes, work experiences, social activities, and instruction in independent living skills, including self-advocacy and self-determination. These TPSID programs are part of a larger network of Inclusive Postsecondary Education (IPSE) programs across the nation. Second, HEOA established a national coordinating center, known as Think College, which is housed in the Institute for Community Inclusion at the

University of Massachusetts Boston. The act also provides a regulatory definition of a Comprehensive Transition and Postsecondary (CTP) program and mandated that the national coordinating center determine a formal program accreditation process.

Think College Standards and Accreditation Process

The HEOA of 2008 mandated the National Coordinating Center, Think College, to work toward a national accreditation process for IPSE programs (National Coordinating Center Accreditation Workgroup and Inclusive Higher Education Accreditation Council, 2024). In the first five years, the workgroup, made up of a variety of stakeholders, researched the field of accreditation and established the Think College Standards for Inclusive Higher Education (TCSIHE) for use by programs to develop and enhance high-quality IPSE programs (Green et al., 2024). During the second five years, the work group field tested the standards with programs, sought feedback from a variety of stakeholders, and engaged existing accrediting bodies to determine an accreditor (Think College National Coordinating Center Accreditation Workgroup, 2021). Finally, the current work group, established in 2020, created a non-profit, the Inclusive Higher Education Accreditation Council (IHEAC) and accredited the first three programs, with two additional under review (National Coordinating Center Accreditation Workgroup and Inclusive Education Accreditation Council, 2024). The group and IHEAC are working to determine the roll-out of the open accreditation process to the field of more than 350 programs (Think College, 2020).

The 2011 version of the Think College Standards for Inclusive Higher Education included eight standards, with 18 indicators with dozens more benchmarks (Grigal et al., 2011). These standards were refined into the new accreditation standards over time resulting in 10 standards with 38 sub-standards (Think College, 2020). These standards work to establish a program built on collaboration across campus and the university community.

Self-determination, including self-advocacy, is intertwined within both the former standards and the new accreditation standards. The development of self-determination and self-advocacy skills is an essential element of higher education programs for students with ID as it is specifically called out in the HEOA (2008) definitions. The fifth standard of the Think College Standards for Inclusive Higher Education outlines eight elements that address quality indicators of inclusive postsecondary education programs. The fifth standard, self-determination, includes the following essential practices: (1) student-directed process, or person-centered plans, to tailor individualized programming; (2) opportunities to practice and improve self-determination skills in academic, employment, and social settings; and (3) parent or family engagement that respects student autonomy. Self-determination and self-advocacy skills are evidence-based predictors of positive transition outcomes for students with disabilities, including enrolling in postsecondary education or training programs and gaining employment, and a promising practice for independent living (Mazzotti et al., 2021; Petcu et al., 2017; Shogren et al., 2017).

STUDENT VOICE

Students gain new knowledge that can encourage them to positively direct their own lives when their perspectives are shared more widely (Garratt et al., 2022). Student voice also leads to authentic higher education experiences for students "rather than tokenistic" practices (Kubiak, 2017) opportunities. Student voice is imperative to collect and for programs to respond to. Gaining insights into what individuals who have experienced inclusive postsecondary education (current or previous) helps to support practices that increase self-determination of students (Morningstar & Clavenna-Deane, 2018; Haber et al., 2016) and improve programs to better meet the needs of today's student with an intellectual disability. Thus, the Ohio Statewide Consortium set out to evaluate practices of inclusive postsecondary education programs from the student perspective.

The Approach to Gaining Student Voice

Our research team developed and conducted a qualitative research study using a case study evaluation approach. Data collection occurred in a multi-modal manner. We first created a structured interview to survey current and former program participants through an online meeting. The questions asked of research participants were aligned to the Think Colleges Standard for Inclusive Higher Education (Think College, 2020) as the new accreditation standards had not been released yet. Questions included dichotomous (i.e., yes, no), multiple-choice, and open-ended responses to gauge programs' adherence to quality indicators and gain deeper insights about students' experiences. For Standard 5 (i.e., Self-Determination), as an example, we asked students: (1) Do you have planning meetings with program staff? If they indicated 'yes,' we followed-up by asking: (a) Do you think your ideas and voice are heard during your planning meetings?; (b) Do you think your preferences and interests are included in your program plan?; and (c) Do you lead your planning meetings or co-lead your planning meetings with support from program staff? In addition, we asked students if they learned self-advocacy skills in their program, and how they used self-advocacy skills in academic, employment, and social settings.

The structured interview survey was chosen as the method for this study for several reasons. First, we aimed to increase accessibility to participate in the research. We believe simply sending out a survey to research participants would not have yielded the response rate that it did. While limited to Zoom videoconference for these interviews, the research team likely would still have chosen this method to enable access to the participants located off-site and to be able to present the questions in multiple ways, meeting the needs of how different brains acquire and use information and allowing for a larger pool of students to share and have their voice amplified. Presenting the questions on the shared screen and reading the questions aloud enabled participants to utilize a method of learning and understanding best for them (Hollomotz, 2018). The research team was also trying to increase the reliability of responses from the participants. Questions were written more simply to aid in the understanding of the question by each of the research participants. Some questions had support prompts available to aid the researcher if there was a limited understanding of the question. The research team also tried to elicit deeper, contextual responses from the individuals participating in the research study. By having a researcher present, built-in support prompts could be utilized to gain deeper and richer responses.

Participants

There were three groups of participants identified for this study: students currently participating in an inclusive postsecondary program, graduates of inclusive postsecondary programs, and students who began, but did not complete an inclusive higher education program (who will be referred to as non-completers from this point forward). Research participants were identified in five of Ohio's inclusive postsecondary programs. These schools, identified as Columbus State Community College, Marietta College, The Ohio State University, University of Cincinnati, and Youngstown State University, were the schools of selection because they had received funding from the 2015-2020 grant cycle of federal Transition Programs for Students with Intellectual Disability (TPSID) funding held by The Ohio State University.

The research team emailed the program directors of the five programs and requested they forward a recruitment email, which included an embedded video link describing the study, to the three groups of participants sought for the study. Emails were sent at the beginning of the week, with reminder emails sent at the end of the week. Participants were given multiple methods to respond to the research team with interest or to find out more information.

Ultimately, 19 participants were recruited from three of the five identified schools, including two four-year institutions and one community college. Eleven were current students, seven were graduates, and one was a non-completer. In addition, 10 students were male, eight were female, and one did not disclose their sex. A majority (n = 13) reported their race as white, two as African American/Black, one as Asian, and one participant did not disclose their race. Twelve students reported they lived at home with family and three students mentioned they lived in the dorms during the academic year. An additional four resided on campus, and two did not live at home with family or on campus. Finally, participants shared their disability diagnosis as three being autistic, three having cerebral palsy, five had an intellectual disability (e.g. Down's syndrome, William's syndrome), one had a specific learning disability and one reported having autism and a specific learning disability as their diagnoses.

Data Collection

Participants were interviewed via Zoom videoconference using a survey-based structured interview. The research team member opened a Qualtrics survey while in Zoom to gain consent and/or assent from the study participant and continue with the survey questions. Many of the questions were dichotomous, yes/no response questions. These questions were often followed by an open-ended question or "check all that apply" question related to the previous question. An example of this questioning series from the survey is as follows in Table 1.

Table 1. Example of Survey Question Series

TCSIHE Standard	Interview Survey Question with follow-up question based on first response	Response options
4.1C: The program disseminates data and evaluation findings to key stakeholders.	Have you received any information from your staff about program outcomes or achievements, or overall student results? *Support prompt: Overall student results may include how many students have enrolled or graduated, how many students got a job after graduation, or other program outcome information.	Yes, No, I Don't Know
	If yes, what information did your program send to you or did you learn about your program's outcomes or student results?	Open-ended, I Don't Know
	If no, what information would you like to learn about your program's outcomes or student results?	Open-ended, I Don't Know

During the structured interview, which was shared on the screen with participants, interviewers selected or typed participants' responses to the questions. Interviewers were trained to capture quotes verbatim, if feasible, or to paraphrase responses.

Analysis of Student Voice

Responses from the structured interview were later reviewed for accuracy by checking the recorded meeting's transcript. The research team downloaded a raw data file from Qualtrics as an Excel spreadsheet to extract all responses and tabulate results, including conversion into charts and graphs to visualize the data. Dichotomous results were calculated as a percentage of affirmative and negative responses, and percentages were also used to measure the selection of different multiple-choice options. The research team employed thematic analysis to code, group, and summarize open-ended responses while highlighting quotes to emphasize key findings and unique insights. This study was not a mixed methods study because the research team did not have two separate arms of the study which were to be combined at the end. While results from the study yielded both quantitative and qualitative results, these were done in tandem to best support the research participant, not for the purpose of developing meta-inferences.

Researcher Positionality

The authors of this chapter have varied individual backgrounds, experiences, and roles within the project. This may have influenced our perspectives and contributions to the work. Three of us were heavily involved in the design, implementation, and analysis of the project, bringing our expertise to the process. The fourth author was a student at the time of the research, contributing her expertise to a portion of the project. Additionally, at the time of this research, two of the authors were involved directly with one of the inclusive programs as faculty director and manager which may have influenced this project to some extent. Conversely, being connected to the programs helped the researchers to design the study to be more accessible and to make sense of the text. We acknowledge our understanding and representation of the findings are shaped by our collective positionalities, including our professional roles, institutional affiliations, and personal experiences. We aimed to approach this work with reflexivity, ensuring that diverse perspectives are considered and that our interpretations remain grounded in the voices and experiences central to the students with whom we work.

SELF-DETERMINATION AND SELF-ADVOCACY WITHIN ACADEMICS

Academic opportunities are included within the accreditation standards in several ways, including using student learning outcomes tied to meeting Satisfactory Academic Progress, access to a wide variety of inclusive university courses, and review of progress toward program completion with advising based upon a person-centered plan (NCCW & IHEA, 2024). A key mechanism IPSE programs use to document individualization of student goals and steps to achieve those goals is a person-centered plan which by design is an interdisciplinary process. Most students (n=14) thought their ideas and voices were heard during meetings and they thought their preferences and interests were included in their plan. These students also indicated that they lead or co-lead their planning meetings with support from program staff.

Nearly all students (n=18) agreed that they learned self-advocacy skills in their program. Students described self-advocacy within academic settings as asking for help to understand course material or complete homework. They requested this assistance from program staff and their professors. One student noted that they discuss academic progress with program staff "every other week, or call them if I have any problems," and another student said, "on Tuesdays and Thursdays, we work on our homework during Academic Support first." Students described asking to use accommodations as well as for support in meeting university health requirements. Self-advocacy was shown through choosing classes and by emailing professors to request meetings. Students mentioned, "[I] told [staff name] what classes I wanted" and I had a "meeting with a professor during office hours about an issue I had." A student described how self-advocacy can look: "if we don't know something, we raise our hands or wait until they are done, and they ask if we have any questions or comments on the situation and then we would answer it." An additional description of a successful use of self-advocacy skills was when a student was reflecting on using their advocacy skills in class related to health protocol saying, "I spoke in [staff name] class. They make us do a health check every time we do. I spoke up to see if they needed my green health screen to show that I took my temperature."

One student spoke of how self-advocacy skills allowed them to be more included in their course stating, "it helped me to listen more; the classes were bigger, and I could learn with my friends their opinions and what the teacher's opinions are," and another student shared that course content built their self-advocacy skills saying, "I learned how to speak with my hands and how to speak using eye contact; how to speak more clearly and loudly." One student shared their goal was "to be independent and self-advocate," while another student described how they built leadership skills "sharing duties with the teachers in my class." Another student provided an example of how they leverage their own skills to serve as a peer mentor:

> *I use them by helping the other students learn what they need to do. Like, with a resume, for example. They didn't know how to make a resume, but I already had mine done, so I could help them. I am also an ambassador to help the new students when they come to college.*

Importantly, all but one student was able to describe a personal and specific use of self-advocacy skills in an academic setting, which underscored an understanding of individual needs, knowledge of who and how to ask for help, and use for greater independence and leadership.

Over half of the students (n=10) selected "get the support that I needed to do well in classes (e.g., accommodations, tutoring)" as the most helpful thing that program staff did to support them with college classes. Moreover, all students indicated satisfaction with the meetings and communication that they had with program staff, and many (n=7) specifically mentioned their appreciation for school-related support. One student reminisced, "I was taking a class, and it was a really hard class, but then I talked to my [staff support], and she helped me understand that I was auditing the class and didn't need to take the exam." Often, auditing students must seek permission of the course instructor for enrollment. Programs can collaborate with departments to help streamline this process for students when the department faculty are aware of the program and provide supports for both student and faculty. This awareness helps to speed up the timeline of seeking the appropriate approvals, particularly in cases where the course instructor has not been assigned. The student also added that the staff member helped them with homework and understanding content.

Most students (n=16) agreed that they had access to the school's disability services office or accessibility resources office staff, but two students said that they did not. One student did not know if they had access to the disability services office. Of those that had access to disability services, most (n=12) indicated that they met with the school's disability services or accessibility resources staff to request academic accommodations. Two students indicated that they did not meet with disability services staff to request accommodations, and two students did not know. One student said that they had peer tutors, and the other student said that they had someone in class to help with notetaking to support their academic success. Students who were seeking to use their accommodations through the disability services office were voicing their needs, a prime example of self-advocacy in action.

Programs can collaborate with their disability service offices or campus offices dedicated to improving the teaching practices of faculty on initiatives focused on Universal Design for Learning (UDL) or neurodiversity awareness. Students can practice disclosing their disability when seeking supports from disability services for the first time. UDL practices can support faculty in adding variety to the ways they share knowledge and assess for knowledge gain (Tarconish et al., 2023). Neurodiversity awareness helps faculty to understand and accept why a Neurodivergent student may engage in a way that is not typical of most college students. Self-advocacy skills, on the other hand, empower students to express their needs and make informed decisions about disclosing their disability to access academic accommodations that support their academic success (Smith & Mueller, 2022). Communicating with educators equips them with knowledge to adapt their practice, address unique learning needs, and enhance education through accessible teaching strategies.

SELF-DETERMINATION AND SELF-ADVOCACY WITHIN VOCATIONAL ACTIVITIES

The HEOA (2008) states gainful employment is a goal of inclusive postsecondary education programs. Therefore, there are several accreditation standards tied to employment, including individualized employment outcomes established through a person-centered planning process, ongoing progress monitoring of employment goals, and participation in career development activities. Person-centered planning is at the heart of IPSE programs (NCCW & IHEA, 2024). The person-centered planning process intentionally brings together a team of people, including family members, Vocational Rehabilitation (VR) and Developmental Disability (DD) agency staff, program staff, and university personnel to help engage the student in setting and achieving their employment goals.

Employment-related assistance was one of the most helpful supports that program staff provided students, such as "going to class, then going to my practicum. Sometimes [they] would come to my practicum to see what we do and how we interact and meet after to see what we did good and what we need to work on." In this case, program staff members were integral in providing feedback that the student used to monitor and improve their work skills. Another student said they get, "job supervision and feedback on my performance," elaborating that "feedback is helpful to understand how well I'm doing on the job." These quotes illustrate examples of how program staff can collaborate with internship and worksites for the betterment of the student by strengthening a student's skills in the form of job coaching. Furthermore, students listed their DD Service Support Administrator, VR counselor, and managers as people who supported them to reach their vocational goals. These are people who students went to "ask for help and show me how to do something." Students noted that these team members were "respectful of how hard I work and take my job." DD and VR staff should be working through person-centered planning with the program to determine who will be providing specific services and supports to a student, including job coaching, transportation, or paying for a course leading to an industry recognized credential.

About 84% of the students (n=16) indicated that they participated in work-based learning related to their career interests. Workplace readiness skills learned through program participation included time management and communication skills. A student explained that on the job they need to "speak clearly, focus, and pay attention" while another shared how staff "helped me learn what to do and what not to do during an important time during work hours (you don't talk to the people, but after work hours, you can talk to your coworkers)." When asked about what they are required to do to graduate from their program, one student mentioned, "I have to go to my job on time and go to meetings on time, as well."

Many students mentioned that they use self-advocacy skills in employment settings to ask for help, when needed, and request accommodations on-the-job. "One of the things I needed at [my place of employment] was to ask for a to-do list to help me know what to do," stated one student. This is an opportunity for employers, VR, and job developers and coaches to work together to meet student vocational needs. One participant indicated, "I tell [my supervisor and co-workers] I need help." In recalling an example, another student said, "I was working with someone, and I got some help to do some of the same parts at work." A different student shared, "If I don't know, I ask one of my managers who knows more, and I can go to them and ask them. If there is something that I am doing that I am not positive how to do, I will ask for help." An additional anecdote included, "I was cleaning a bunch of rec center equipment, and I had trouble with the high bars on the pull up machine, and I asked [my supervisor] for help." Importantly, one student shared how their self-advocacy supported their career advancement: "I did ticket taking and ushering, but then I sent my boss an email that I wanted to do more, and I got my paid job at the [employer] because of that." These examples demonstrate how program participation prepares students with job readiness skills, promotes the ability to request reasonable job accommodations, and builds confidence to communicate career ambitions with an employer.

SELF-DETERMINATION AND SELF-ADVOCACY WITHIN SOCIAL EXPERIENCES

Like academic and vocational areas, students show self-advocacy skills in a variety of ways that also connect to the accreditation standards. For instance, students should have the same opportunities and access as all other students enrolled at the institution to activities and facilities (NCCW & IHEA, 2024). A prime example is how Ohio State University's program designed and implemented an alternative spring break trip appropriate in tasks and staffing for the students in its program by collaborating with the BuckiServ office, which coordinates service and civic engagement experiences for students during semester breaks. There is always a university staff member on the trip. This role was filled by program staff with two students serving as leaders to plan outings and other activities. Two peer mentors with the program also volunteered to be trip leaders. The remaining spots in the group were filled by program students and other students from the university. This partnership has continued with a total of four trips completed, each looking a little different and meeting the needs of all stakeholders. In one case, there was a student who wanted to go on a different trip because they preferred the service component. He advocated his desires and successfully attended the trip as a valued member of that team.

In addition, programs created policies for evaluating student learning outcomes related to social skills and community engagement which are developed through the person-centered planning process (NCCW & IHEA, 2024). About 70% of the students (n=13) indicated that they made many friends during their program experience, and about a quarter (n=5) said that they made a few friends. One student reported not making any friends from their classes. Another student said, "Mainly, I just like how [program staff] can help me learn about how friendships work and how to make a good friendship," which exemplifies the crucial role program staff play in supporting social integration and skill development.

Most students (n=17) made a choice to join or participate in a student organization, club, or other type of school program, and two students did not. Clubs and organizations are an inclusive space for students to engage with other students, different from themselves, around a common interest. Some students may need support from peer mentors while others attend these meetings and events independently. Students have shown great success in their independence, even traveling out of town for special functions. Over half of the students who engaged in a campus program (n=9) agreed that they needed support from program staff to join or participate in the program, although eight students said that they did not need support. Regardless, inclusion in university-sanctioned extracurricular organizations provides opportunities for different student populations to interact and collaborate, which promotes a culture of belongingness (Van Gaasbeek & Tassè, 2024).

Belongingness

While belongingness has long been studied among marginalized college students, it is a relatively new topic among adults with ID (Raines et al., 2023). Belongingness is a fundamental human need and motivational construct that enables individuals to create and maintain reciprocal social relationships characterized by attachment, companionship, and support (Baumeister & Leary, 1995). In school settings, belonging is "the extent to which students feel personally accepted, respected, included, and supported by others in the school" and involves an "individual's cognitive evaluation of his or her role in relation to the group" (Goodenow, 1993, p. 80; Hurtado & Carter, 1997, p. 328). In other words, a sense of belonging in college relies both on the experience of having satisfying, meaningful relationships, but also one's perception of social fit within a given context.

Belongingness is associated with many positive outcomes at school, including academic achievement, motivation, and school completion (Connell et al., 1995; Croninger & Lee, 2001; Gillen-O'Neel & Fuligni, 2013; Rumberger & Rotermund, 2012; Sánchez et al., 2005). Belongingness also has a negative relationship with mental health symptoms, particularly depressive symptoms, and can act as a protective factor for stress and loneliness (Çivitci, 2015; Dutcher et al., 2022; Zhou et al., 2023). A recent study found there was a negative relationship between a sense of belonging and mental health symptoms (i.e., anxiety and depression) in college students with ID (Van Gaasbeek, 2024). Understanding the relationship between belongingness and mental health may be particularly important for adults with ID, as they are at an increased risk of psychopathology compared to neuromajority peers (Cooper et al., 2015).

In the current study, college students were asked questions about their experiences of belonging within their IPSE programs (see Figure 1). In terms of classroom experiences, while most students (n=13) reported they always feel comfortable sharing their ideas with other students in their classes, some students (n=7) reported they sometimes or always are afraid to ask questions in front of other students.

In terms of social relationships, most students (n=17) reported that they sometimes or always are invited to do things socially by other students from their classes. Students (n=18) also overwhelmingly reported that students from their classes are friendly to them outside of class. However, some students (n=4) reported feeling left out among other students in their classes.

This pattern of results aligns with past research on belongingness among college students with ID. A study of 129 college students with ID from 21 IPSE programs found that most students with ID (54.3%) reported students in their classes were friendly to them (Van Gaasbeek, 2024). Many students with ID also reported feeling comfortable at school (59.7%) and that they felt like part of the school community (54.3%). However, within the classroom, some students (13.2%) reported that they felt other students did not take their opinions seriously. These results, much like those in the current study, suggest that students in IPSE programs generally feel welcomed by their college peers, yet still feel marginalized within classroom settings (i.e., other students do not take their opinions seriously, students with ID are afraid to ask questions in front of other students). The discrepancy between belongingness experiences in and out of the classroom is perhaps unsurprising given the focus on intellectual ability in college classrooms, but also the fact that a sense of belonging can fluctuate across settings (Ruedas-Gracia et al., 2023). Further research is required to examine how a sense of belonging can vary across contexts for students in IPSE programs, such as in segregated (i.e., with peers from their IPSE program) and inclusive (i.e., with neuromajority peers) settings.

Figure 1. Results of Student Belongingness Reporting

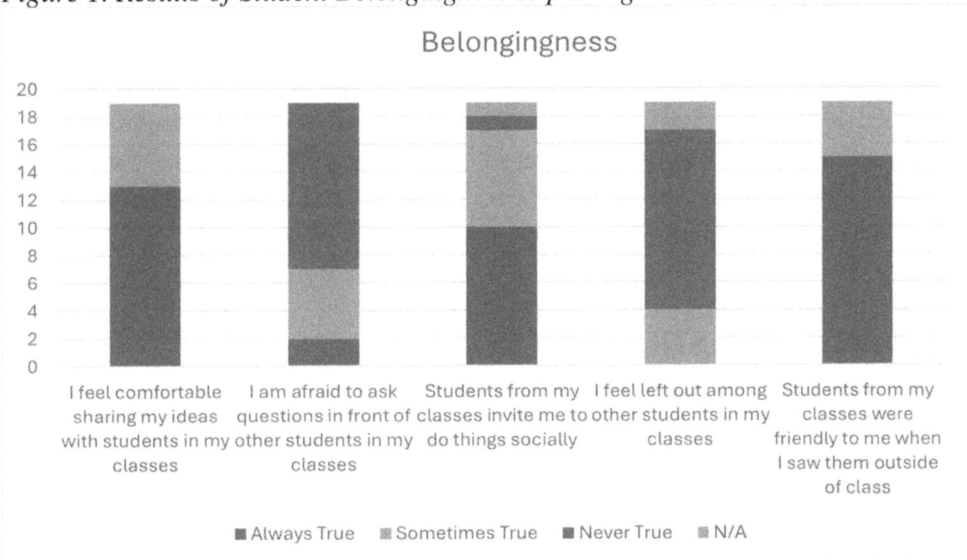

SELF-DETERMINATION AND SELF-ADVOCACY WITH IPSE PROGRAM STAFF AND SUPPORTS

Program staff should be retained within the program using adequate job descriptions with regular evaluation and ongoing professional development as outlined in the accreditation standards (NCCW & IHEA, 2024). Training should be delivered not only to staff, but also peer mentors, faculty, and university partners and staff. Because these roles are vital to student success, one program's peer mentors and program staff worked together to present at a professional conference on how to develop peer mentoring programs at other institutions. Peer mentors serve in a variety of roles and can be paid employees, earn course credit, or be volunteers. At a school where peer mentors receive credit, the program works with another department to get the practicum courses set up in the university system, meet syllabi requirements, and determine how to collectively recruit mentors for the program.

Ten students indicated that they met with or communicated with program staff weekly, and four students met daily. Two students met monthly, and two students met with staff each grading period. One student met every other week with staff but made contact in between if they had any questions or needs. All students were happy with meetings and communications they had with program staff evidenced by the statements: "They help me a lot and are really understanding if we need them or have something going on, you can always go to them and talk to them," or "They listen to me."

Finally, most students (n=18) indicated that program staff helped them learn how to use the technology well (e.g., access class materials, do schoolwork, turn work into teachers and staff), but one student disagreed. A student shared, "They're nice; they know how to help me if I get stuck with something. If there is something I don't understand, they can help me." One student shared how they problem solved with staff and "made phone calls when staff didn't show up."

SELF-DETERMINATION AND SELF-ADVOCACY WITH FAMILY SUPPORT

While each inclusive postsecondary education program wants to build the independence of their students, family involvement is a predictor of post-school success (Test et al., 2009). Programs should be seeking input from families but also engaging and communicating with families (NCCW & IHEA, 2024). This often looks like participation in person-centered planning meetings, program newsletters trainings, social media groups, or family member liaisons. Families have also been heavily involved in advocating at the state and federal level for IPSE programs (Grigal & Hart, 2010).

Most students (n=17) agreed that they had an involved or helpful family member or guardian during their program experience. A student said, "[They] come to meetings with program staff and myself." Only ten of these students (59%) indicated that they decided how much the family member or guardian would be involved or when they would help. This is an area for students and programs to better communicate on how much involvement is desired from the family. This could be as simple as a program staff saying to a student, "I am going to email you the notes from this meeting today, would you like me to copy your family on the email?" This gives the student the opportunity to control how much and when information gets passed onto families. This could also be a more significant factor in team meetings in which a student needs more direct support. Sometimes program staff will need to explain to students why involving their family may be in their best interest but ultimately they must leave the decision-making up to the student. This enhances students' dignity and risk management which sometimes programs and families fond uncomfortable for different reasons. These reasons include fear of mistreatment, risk of failure, and concerns of negative consequences (Bumble et al., 2021). Most students (n=16) agreed that program staff asked them for consent or permission before involving parents, family members, or guardians. One student said "If I have a meeting, my mom will take me. I will let my mom know if I have a meeting," and

My mom is going to help me move out of my house to Florida to my dream in Disneyworld for a job in Orlando, Florida. My mom is mainly a TAP ambassador, too, and she does special meetings they have, and she is on an Advisory Board for TAP.

Students shared how they have utilized their families to be more successful, including using technology independently as the main way to communicate with families. A student said, "I'm asked if I want to have text-based reminders." Additionally, "Mom helps with my paycheck and social security," and "They will take me to TAP events - help with transportation."

CONCLUSION

The mantra "nothing about us, without us" used by self-advocates with disabilities extends into the research space. IPSE programs and this research project allows "[students] to have a strong voice in their own education and can teach them a great deal about self-advocacy and self-determination," by empowering them to set and achieve their postsecondary education, employment and independent living goals (U.S. Department of Education, 2020). When multiple stakeholders come together to solve problems, build infrastructure, and believe that students with intellectual disability can successfully attend college, we create an opportunity to learn and grow from our different experiences.

Moving forward, other programs from across the nation need to add student voices to their evaluation process to further align with the inclusive higher education accreditation standards. Institutional leadership, not just programs, needs to articulate clearly that students with intellectual disability are integral to the fabric of their universities through inclusion in strategic plans, administrative leadership with the program, realignment of policies to include students with intellectual disability and representation in all facets of campus life including in student government, living in housing even if it is full, and as full alumni upon graduation from the institution. Additionally, further research is needed to operationalize youth autonomy/decision making and goal setting (Mazzotti et al., 2016) and to study the impact of these newly distinguished predictors on postsecondary outcomes.

Not only is self-advocacy paramount to increasing inclusion as laid out in HEOA, but it is clear that self-advocacy should be taught early (Palmer et al., 2017), as a part of the Individuals with Disabilities Education Act (IDEA) (2004), but it also continues after a student graduates from secondary and/or postsecondary education under the WIOA (2014). Using these three federal laws for guidance, university stakeholders need to work in conjunction with each other to ensure seamless support of an individual as they progress across their lifespan. Institutions prioritizing the use of the Inclusive Higher Education Accreditation standards will not only meet the floor of HEOA, IDEA, and WIOA, but far exceed the minimum standards.

CASE STUDIES AND DISCUSSION QUESTIONS

Case Study #1: Effective Self-Advocacy in Academic and Employment Settings

Alex, a 21-year-old, male diagnosed with William's Syndrome, enrolled in an IPSE program at a large public university in Ohio to improve independence, pursue academic goals, and build skills for future employment. The program provided Alex with direct instruction and coaching on self-advocacy skills to teach and reinforce strategies for expressing needs clearly, seeking assistance when necessary, and communicating effectively with authority figures, including professors and supervisors, as well as peers. Alex described himself as feeling comfortable sharing ideas with classmates and not being afraid to ask questions in front of them.

In the academic setting, Alex encountered initial challenges, particularly in understanding certain course materials and assignments. With the help of self-advocacy training, Alex learned to confidently approach professors and explain specific needs by expressing those needs, requesting accommodations and support, and building confidence and leadership skills. Initiating open and honest communication with faculty, especially to express confusion or concerns about understanding course content, is critical for helping teachers respond to students' unique learning needs. Employing multiple communication modalities, as well as providing additional, concrete, and practical examples or hands-on activities that demonstrate how to do something are effective strategies for supporting diverse learners.

In recognizing their need for extra time on assignments and assessments, Alex requested accommodations through the university's disability services office, which supported their planning and information processing needs to be a successful student. Self-advocacy is a fundamental aspect of becoming aware of personal needs, building a positive sense of identity, and being empowered to request support and access legal rights, such as academic accommodations for students with disabilities. While disability disclosure is a personal choice, Alex selected the choice of getting the support that he needed to do well in classes. When individuals are aware of their own needs and know how to ask for help, they can be better equipped to recognize the needs of others and provide specific assistance. Alex served as an ambassador to help new students and leveraged their career development knowledge and advocacy skills to provide peer mentorship.

Alex also used self-advocacy skills while engaged in work experiences arranged through the inclusive postsecondary education program. He worked on campus at a local theater, at one of the city's museums, and in grocery stores. These environments required similar forms of assertive communication. For tasks that were challenging, Alex would proactively ask for written guidance, which helped maintain productivity and avoid misunderstandings. Alex extended his self-advocacy skills to communicate his career goals with an employer, which resulted in a formal job offer. While internships provide formidable opportunities to learn basic employment knowledge and skills, they also offer job seekers with chances to demonstrate competence and character sought by employers, as well as valuable connections to resources, mentors, and references for future job applications. By expressing needs assertively and requesting support respectfully, Alex demonstrated self-awareness and elemental soft skills that elevated his confidence, competency, and career trajectory.

Questions

1. How can those supporting Alex help him use existing self-advocacy skills to interact with his family, whom he finds to be overbearing at times and not in agreement with his decisions?
2. What additional instruction could be put in place to increase Alex's independence (or interdependence) upon graduation as he transitions out of the program?
3. How can Alex utilize his self-advocacy skills to empower more novice students in the program to develop and use their self-advocacy skills?

Case Study #2: Advocacy and Autonomy in Community College

Casey, a 25-year-old non-binary student, diagnosed with Autism Spectrum Disorder and an undiagnosed intellectual disability, enrolled in an IPSE program at a community college to engage in academics and build skills for future employment. It should be noted that Casey moved to Ohio as an adult and was not connected to the Vocational Rehabilitation or Developmental Disability systems in their previous state or in Ohio. However, Casey was also PELL and Federal Work-Study eligible. The program provided Casey with direct instruction and coaching on self-advocacy skills to build confidence in articulating their needs, particularly to authority figures. Casey's team, including family members and program staff, recognized that stronger self-advocacy skills were needed to support how they manage mental health needs, design and implements goal setting strategies, and enact independent living skills. Casey was enrolled part time each semester to help them manage the many responsibilities they have while being successful with their studies at home and in the community.

Casey, very early on, identified a need for extended time on assignments, exams, and quizzes. Each semester, Casey sent an email to their course instructor to request extended time, which is identified as a necessary accommodation by the campus disability services office. They followed up in person to remind the instructor of this accommodation. Casey's program staff worked with them to develop a script and practice the conversation through role playing exercises, which prepared them to do this on their own. Now, Casey no longer needs to role play. They simply review the script before the first-class meeting, in which they request their accommodations with the instructor.

Additionally, Casey felt more time in the tutoring center would help provide the additional structure needed to focus on their assignments. Casey sought the support of program staff to assist them in building this regular time into their digital calendar, which provided reminders and notifications that supported them daily and weekly with time management. Casey also worked with staff to create a plan to help them chunk large readings and assignments into more manageable pieces.

Casey has struggled with anxiety for as long as they could remember. They routinely used self-advocacy skills to address their mental health needs. Casey was aware that they became more anxious when working with one staff member. Due to ongoing counseling, they recognized the need to address this challenge with support rather than avoid this staff person. Casey worked with the program director to learn how they could better engage with this staff member, understand their thinking, and find ways to build a better relationship. While uncomfortable, Casey scheduled an appointment with the staff member they struggled with to work explicitly on building a relationship. They requested they not have their traditional meeting, but rather, they have a walking meeting outside where they could chat about topics, such as pets, sports, or personal hobbies. In developing a personal connection through an informal conversation about individual preferences and interests, Casey became comfortable disclosing their mental health condition to the staff member to help each other become more aware of each other's preferences, interests, needs, and strengths (PINS). Casey showed an ability to understand academic accommodations needed to be successful in their courses through requesting support, as well as their knowledge of using technology to increase success. Furthermore, by recognizing the need to develop a relationship built on trust and transparency, Casey knew they could reduce the anxiety they had when meeting with the staff member.

Early in their time at the community college, Casey secured a volunteer position in the institution's food pantry and continued to spend time there throughout their schooling. Additionally, she was eligible for federal work-study and is currently seeking paid employment at her institution through this program. During the summer months when not enrolled in classes, Casey set a goal to volunteer 100 hours in the school's food pantry. They worked with program staff to identify a weekly schedule that allowed them time to focus on sleep, social activities with friends, and managing their home and necessary medical appointments. This schedule helped Casey feel in control of all aspects of their life, amassing more than double their initial volunteer hour goal.

Casey has grown into a leader in the school's food pantry, due in part to the longevity they have volunteered there, which includes periods of transitional leadership, administrative turnover, and supervisory changes. This has brought challenges and successes for Casey. They found challenges in the changes in new leadership. Casey was able to engage program staff to help them process the changes occurring and find support for their increased anxiety. In this way, Casey utilized her expertise to provide on-the-job training to her new supervisor(s).

Being a federal work-study eligible student, there is a specific way the institution would like them to review and apply for eligible jobs. However, the system would not allow them access. Program staff could not find them in the system. They worked with their career counselor to identify the issue. Together, they were not able to solve this problem. Casey knew another staff member had connections to others who might be able to help in this situation. Casey scheduled an appointment with that staff to discuss the problem. Casey leveraged her professional network to identify appropriate team members to help her overcome this barrier.

Casey was able to reach their goals and solve problems by communicating their needs and building an effective team indicating growth in their autonomy.

Questions

1. How can those supporting Casey help them to use existing self-advocacy skills to increase their paid employment opportunities?
2. What additional instruction could be put in place to increase Casey's independence (or interdependence) upon graduation from college?
3. How could Casey use their self-advocacy skills to connect with other community supports?

REFERENCES

Americans with Disabilities Act. (n.d.). *Introduction to the Americans with Disabilities Act.* https://www.ada.gov/topics/intro-to-ada/

Baumeister, R. F., & Leary, M. R. (1995). The need to belong: Desire for interpersonal attachments as a fundamental human motivation. *Psychological Bulletin, 117*(3), 497–529. DOI: 10.1037/0033-2909.117.3.497 PMID: 7777651

Buck, A. (2022). *Exploring the impact of EnvisionIT curriculum implementation on IEP transition goals and student participation in the transition planning process: A qualitative case study* (Order No. 29730322) [Doctoral dissertation, The Ohio State University]. ProQuest Dissertations & Theses Global. https://www.proquest.com/docview/2720903749

Bumble, J. L., Worth, C. R. J., Athamanah, L. S., Rooney-Kron, M., Regester, A., & Lidgus, J. (2021). "Messy inclusion": A call for dignity of risk in inclusive post-secondary education. *In Practice, 1*(2), 64–69. DOI: 10.1177/27324745211050023

Çivitci, A. (2015). Perceived stress and life satisfaction in college students: Belonging and extracurricular participation as moderators. *Procedia: Social and Behavioral Sciences, 205*, 271–281. DOI: 10.1016/j.sbspro.2015.09.077

Connell, J. P., Halpem-Felsher, B. L., Clifford, E., Crichlow, W., & Usinger, P. (1995). Hanging in there: Behavioral, psychological, and contextual factors affecting whether African American adolescents stay in high school. *Journal of Adolescent Research, 10*(1), 41–63. DOI: 10.1177/0743554895101004

Cooper, S. A., McLean, G., Guthrie, B., McConnachie, A., Mercer, S., Sullivan, F., & Morrison, J. (2015). Multiple physical and mental health comorbidity in adults with intellectual disabilities: Population-based cross-sectional analysis. *BMC Family Practice, 16*(1), 110. Advance online publication. DOI: 10.1186/s12875-015-0329-3 PMID: 26310664

Croninger, R., & Lee, V. (2001). Social capital and dropping out of high school: Benefits to at-risk students of teachers. *Teachers College Record, 103*(4), 548–581. DOI: 10.1111/0161-4681.00127

Dutcher, J. M., Lederman, J., Jain, M., Price, S., Kumar, A., Villalba, D. K., Tumminia, M. J., Doryab, A., Cresswell, K. G., Riskin, E., Sefdigar, Y., Seo, W., Mankoff, J., Cohen, S., Dey, A., & Creswell, J. D. (2022). Lack of belonging predicts depressive symptomatology in college students. *Psychological Science, 33*(7), 1048–1067. DOI: 10.1177/09567976211073135 PMID: 35735353

Dwyer, P. (2022). The neurodiversity approach (es): What are they and what do they mean for researchers? *Human Development*, *66*(2), 73–92. DOI: 10.1159/000523723 PMID: 36158596

Garratt, D., Johnson, K., Millear, A., Picken, S., Slattery, J., & Walmsley, J. (2022). Celebrating thirty years of inclusive research. *Social Sciences (Basel, Switzerland)*, *11*(9), 385. DOI: 10.3390/socsci11090385

Gillen-O'Neel, C., & Fuligni, A. (2013). A longitudinal study of school belonging and academic motivation across high school. *Child Development*, *84*(2), 678–692. DOI: 10.1111/j.1467-8624.2012.01862.x PMID: 23002809

Goodenow, C. (1993). Classroom belonging among early adolescent students: Relationships to motivation and achievement. *The Journal of Early Adolescence*, *13*(1), 21–43. DOI: 10.1177/0272431693013001002

Green, J. C., Buck, A., & Izzo, M. (2024). Evaluating Ohio's postsecondary programs for students with intellectual disability: A survey of program directors. *DADD Online Journal*, *11*(1), 114–130. https://daddcec.com/sites/default/files/2025-01/doj_2024_final.pdf

Grigal, M., & Hart, D. (2010). *Think College. Postsecondary education options for students with intellectual disabilities*. Brookes Publishing.

Grigal, M., Hart, D., & Weir, C. (2011). *Think college standards quality indicators, and benchmarks for inclusive higher education.* University of Massachusetts Boston, Institute for Community Inclusion. https://www.mass.edu/strategic/maicei/documents/think-college-standards.pdf

Grigal, M., Soldovieri, S. J., Myers, B., Papay, C., & Bukaty, C. A. (2024). Benefits of postsecondary education experiences for adults with intellectual and developmental disability. *International Review of Research in Developmental Disabilities*, *66*, 1–31. Advance online publication. DOI: 10.1016/bs.irrdd.2024.09.003

Haber, M. G., Mazzotti, V. L., Mustian, A. L., Rowe, D. A., Bartholomew, A. L., Test, D. W., & Fowler, C. H. (2016). What works, when, for whom, and with whom: A meta-analytic review of predictors of postsecondary success for students with disabilities. *Review of Educational Research*, *86*(1), 123–162. DOI: 10.3102/0034654315583135

Higher Education Opportunity Act. 20 U.S.C. §1140 (2008). https://www.govinfo.gov/content/pkg/PLAW-110publ315/pdf/PLAW-110publ315.pdf

Hollomotz, A. (2018). Successful interviews with people with intellectual disability. *Qualitative Research*, *18*(2), 153–170. DOI: 10.1177/1468794117713810

Hurtado, S., & Carter, D. F. (1997). Effects of college transition and perceptions of the campus racial climate on Latino college students' sense of belonging. *Sociology of Education*, *70*(4), 324–345. DOI: 10.2307/2673270

Individuals with Disabilities Education Act, 20 U.S.C. § 1400 et seq. (2004). https://sites.ed.gov/idea/statute-chapter-33/subchapter-i/1400

Karpicz, J. R. (2020). Just my being here is self-advocacy. *Journal Committed to Social Change on Race and Ethnicity*, *6*(1), 138–163. https://www.jstor.org/stable/48644514

Kubiak, J. (2017). Using 'voice' to understand what college students with intellectual disabilities say about the teaching and learning process. *Journal of Research in Special Educational Needs*, *17*(1), 41–48. DOI: 10.1111/1471-3802.12098

Legault, M., Bourdon, J. N., & Poirier, P. (2021). From neurodiversity to neurodivergence: The role of epistemic and cognitive marginalization. *Synthese*, *199*(5-6), 12843–12868. DOI: 10.1007/s11229-021-03356-5

Lipscomb, S., Haimson, J., Liu, A. Y., Burghardt, J., Johnson, D. R., & Thurlow, M. L. (2017). *Preparing for life after high school: The characteristics and experiences of youth in special education. Findings from the National Longitudinal Transition Study 2012*; *Comparisons across disability groups: Full report (NCEE 2017–4018).* Department of Education, Institute of Education Sciences, National Center for Education Evaluation and Regional Assistance: Volume 2. https://ies.ed.gov/ncee/projects/evaluation/disabilities_nlts2012.asp

Madaus, J. W., Kowitt, J. S., & Lalor, A. R. (2012). The higher education opportunity act: Impact on students with disabilities. *Rehabilitation Research, Policy, and Education*, *26*(1), 33–41. DOI: 10.1891/216866512805000893

Masataka, N. (2017). Implications of the idea of neurodiversity for understanding the origins of developmental disorders. *Physics of Life Reviews*, *20*, 85–108. DOI: 10.1016/j.plrev.2016.11.002 PMID: 27876343

Mazzotti, V. L., Rowe, D. A., Kwiatek, S., Voggt, A., Chang, W.-H., Fowler, C. H., Poppen, M., Sinclair, J., & Test, D. W. (2021). Secondary transition predictors of postschool success: An update to the research base. *Career Development and Transition for Exceptional Individuals*, *44*(1), 47–64. DOI: 10.1177/2165143420959793

Mazzotti, V. L., Rowe, D. A., Sinclair, J., Poppen, M., Woods, W. E., & Shearer, M. L. (2016). Predictors of post-school success: A systematic review of NLTS2 secondary analyses. *Career Development and Transition for Exceptional Individuals, 39*(4), 196–215. https://psycnet.apa.org/doi/10.1177/2165143415588047. DOI: 10.1177/2165143415588047

Morningstar. M., & Clavenna-Deane, B. (2018). *Your complete guide to transition planning and services.* Brookes Publishing.

National Coordinating Center Accreditation Workgroup and Inclusive Higher Education Accreditation Council. (2024). The 2024 guide to accreditation for higher education programs for students with intellectual disability. University of Massachusetts Boston, Institute for Community Inclusion. https://thinkcollege.net/sites/default/files/files/resources/PDF%202024%20accreditation%20guide%20.pdf

Newman, L., Wagner, M., Knokey, A.-M., Marder, C., Nagle, K., Shaver, D., Wei, X., Cameto, R., Contreras, E., Ferguson, K., Greene, S., & Schwarting, M. (2011). *The post-high school outcomes of young adults with disabilities up to 8 years after high school: A report from the National Longitudinal Transition Study-2 (NLTS2) (NCSER 2011-3005).* SRI International.

Palmer, S. B., Wehmeyer, M. L., & Shogren, K. A. (2017). The development of self-determination during childhood. In Wehmeyer, M., Shogren, K., Little, T., & Lopez, S. (Eds.), *Development of Self-Determination Through the Life-Course* (pp. 71–88). Springer., DOI: 10.1007/978-94-024-1042-6_6

Petcu, S. D., Van Horn, M. L., & Shogren, K. A. (2017). Self-determination and the enrollment in and completion of postsecondary education for students with disabilities. *Career Development and Transition for Exceptional Individuals, 40*(4), 225–234. DOI: 10.1177/2165143416670135

Petri, G., Beadle-Brown, J., & Bradshaw, J. (2021). 'Even a self-advocate needs to buy milk': Economic barriers to self-advocacy in the autism and intellectual disability movement. *Scandinavian Journal of Disability Research, 23*(1), 180–191. DOI: 10.16993/sjdr.738

Raines, A. R., Francis, G. L., Fujita, M., & Macedonia, A. (2023). Belonging from the perspectives of individuals with disabilities: A scoping review. *Psychology in the Schools, 60*(6), 2112–2127. DOI: 10.1002/pits.22864

Rowe, D. A., Alverson, C. Y., Unruh, D. K., Fowler, C. H., Kellems, R., & Test, D. W. (2015). A Delphi study to operationalize evidence-based predictors in secondary transition. *Career Development and Transition for Exceptional Individuals, 38*(2), 113–126. DOI: 10.1177/2165143414526429

Ruedas-Gracia, N., Jiang, G., & Maghsoodi, A. H. (2023). Is belonging stable over time?: A four-year longitudinal examination of university belonging differences among students. *Emerging Adulthood*, *11*(4), 1022–1038. DOI: 10.1177/21676968231181720

Rumberger, R. W., & Rotermund, S. (2012). The relationship between engagement and high school dropout. In S. L. Christenson, A. L. Reschly, & C. Wylie (Eds.), *Handbook of Research on Student Engagement* (pp. 491–513). Springer Science + Business Media. DOI: 10.1007/978-1-4614-2018-7_24

Sánchez, B., Colón, Y., & Esparza, P. (2005). The role of sense of school belonging and gender in the academic adjustment of Latino adolescents. *Journal of Youth and Adolescence*, *34*(6), 619–628. DOI: 10.1007/s10964-005-8950-4

Schmidt, E. K., Faieta, J., & Tanner, K. (2020). Scoping review of self-advocacy education interventions to improve care. *The Occupational Therapy Journal of Research*, *40*(1), 50–56. DOI: 10.1177/1539449219860583 PMID: 31342850

Shogren, K. A., Garnier Villarreal, M., Lang, K., & Seo, H. (2017). Mediating role of self-determination constructs in explaining the relationship between school factors and postschool outcomes. *Exceptional Children*, *83*(2), 165–180. DOI: 10.1177/0014402916660089

Shogren, K. A., Luckasson, R., & Schalock, R. L. (2021). Leveraging the power of context in disability policy development, implementation, and evaluation: Multiple applications to enhance personal outcomes. *Journal of Disability Policy Studies*, *31*(4), 230–243. DOI: 10.1177/1044207320923656

Shogren, K. A., Wehmeyer, M. L., Palmer, S. B., Soukup, J. H., Little, T. D., Garner, N., & Lawrence, M. (2007). Examining individual and ecological predictors of the self-determination of students with disabilities. *Exceptional Children*, *73*(4), 488–510. DOI: 10.1177/001440290707300406

Smith, I., & Mueller, C. O. (2022). The importance of disability identity, self-advocacy, and disability activism. *In Practice*, *1*(2), 47–54. DOI: 10.1177/27324745211057155

Tarconish, E., Lombardi, A., & Taconet, A. (2023). Disability awareness & inclusive teaching online training videos for college instructors featuring students with disabilities. *Journal of Postsecondary Education and Disability*, *35*(4), 339–353.

Test, D. W., Fowler, C. H., Wood, W. M., Brewer, D. M., & Eddy, S. (2005). A conceptual framework of self-advocacy for students with disabilities. *Remedial and Special Education*, *20*(1), 45–54. DOI: 10.1177/07419325050260010601

Test, D. W., Mazzotti, V. L., Mustian, A. L., Fowler, C. H., Kortering, L., & Kohler, P. (2009). Evidence-based secondary transition predictors for improving postschool outcomes for students with disabilities. *Career Development for Exceptional Individuals*, *32*(3), 160–181. https://psycnet.apa.org/doi/10.1177/0885728809346960. DOI: 10.1177/0885728809346960

Thelin, R., & Grigal, M. (2019). *Meeting the new requirements of WIOA through partnerships with institutions of higher education enrolling students with intellectual and developmental disabilities*. VR and Youth Rehabilitation Research and Training Center Practice Brief, Issue No. 02. TransCen, Inc.

Think College. (2020). *Think college standards for inclusive higher education.* (Rev. ed.). University of Massachusetts Boston, Institute for Community Inclusion. https://thinkcollege.net/sites/default/files/files/tc_standards%2Bchecklists_draftFeb2020_0.pdf

Think College National Coordinating Center Accreditation Workgroup. (2021). Report on model accreditation standards for higher education programs for students with intellectual disability: Progress on the path to education, employment, and community living. University of Massachusetts Boston, Institute for Community Inclusion. https://thinkcollege.net/sites/default/files/files/resources/TCreport_Accred_full_F3.pdf

U. S. Department of Labor. (2024). *Disability Employment Statistics*. https://www.dol.gov/agencies/odep/research-evaluation/statistics

Unger, D. D., Li, J., Shreffler, A., Puleo, M., & Wyant, S. (2022). *The Ohio longitudinal transition study: Indicator 14 data collection and reporting*. Kent State University. https://www-s3-live.kent.edu/s3fs-root/s3fs-public/file/2022%20OLTS%20Annual%20State%20Report_0.pdf?VersionId=HfN1s3tL04m8UftIsGFUuXG_uN6AVNp7

U.S. Department of Education. (2020). *A transition guide to postsecondary education and employment for students and youth with disabilities.* Washington, D.C., Office of Special Education and Rehabilitative Services. https://www.ed.gov/sites/ed/files/about/offices/list/osers/transition/products/postsecondary-transition-guide-08-2020.pdf

Van Gaasbeek, E. (2024). *Examining the predictors of life satisfaction in college students with intellectual disability* [Unpublished doctoral dissertation]. The Ohio State University.

Van Gaasbeek, E. K., & Tassé, M. J. (2024). Constructing a preliminary model of school belonging for students with intellectual disability. *Journal of Intellectual Disabilities, 28*(3), 591–614. DOI: 10.1177/17446295231164438 PMID: 37060351

Van Reusen, A. K., Bos, C. S., Schumaker, J. B., & Deshler, D. D. (2002). *The self-advocacy strategy for enhancing student motivation and self-determination: An education and transition planning process*. Edge Enterprises.

Vaucher, C., Cudré-Mauroux, A., & Piérart, G. (2020). Environmental, personal, and relational barriers and facilitators to self-determination among adults with intellectual disabilities. *Scandinavian Journal of Disability Research, 22*(1), 97–107. DOI: 10.16993/sjdr.624

Voelker, D. M. (2013). Evidence of academic access in higher education: College programs that include students with intellectual disabilities [Doctoral dissertation, University of Florida]. https://www.proquest.com/openview/a7c7ad9b0b7a9f314824ab755167f47a/1?pq-origsite=gscholar&cbl=18750 [proquest.com]

Wehmeyer, M. L. (2001). Self-determination and mental retardation. *International Review of Research in Mental Retardation, 24*, 1–48. DOI: 10.1016/S0074-7750(01)80004-5

Wehmeyer, M. L. (2005). Self-determination and individuals with severe disabilities: Re-examining meanings and misinterpretations. *Research and Practice for Persons with Severe Disabilities : the Journal of TASH, 30*(3), 113–120. DOI: 10.2511/rpsd.30.3.113

Wehmeyer, M. L. (2020). The importance of self-determination to the quality of life of people with intellectual disability: A perspective. *International Journal of Environmental Research and Public Health, 17*(19), 7121. DOI: 10.3390/ijerph17197121 PMID: 33003321

Wehmeyer, M. L., & Palmer, S. B. (2003). Adult outcomes for students with cognitive disabilities three-years after high school: The impact of self-determination. *Education and Training in Developmental Disabilities, 38*(2), 131–144. https://www.jstor.org/stable/23879591

Workforce Innovation & Opportunity Act 29 U.S.C. § 3101 et seq. (2014). https://www.govinfo.gov/app/details/USCODE-2023-title29/USCODE-2023-title29-chap32-sec3101

Zhou, C., Gao, M., Shi, X., & Zhang, Z. (2023). Suicidal behavior, depression and loneliness among college students: The role of school belonging. *Psychology Health and Medicine*, *28*(6), 1520–1526. DOI: 10.1080/13548506.2022.2113105 PMID: 35980293

ADDITIONAL READING

Blackburn, N., Domin, D., & Hart, D. (2019). *College experiences foster student self-determination and VR support. VR and Youth Rehabilitation Research and Training Center Practice Brief, Issue No. 06*. TransCen, Inc.

Connections, T. A. S. H. (2017). Postsecondary education and self-advocacy. *42*(2). https://tash.org/wp-content/uploads/2018/01/TASHConnections_Vol42_Issue2

Izzo, M. V., & Horne, L. (2016). *Empowering students with hidden disabilities: A path to pride and success*. Brookes Publishing.

Shogren, K. A., Wehmeyer, M. L., Shaw, L. A., Grigal, M., Hart, D., Smith, F. A., & Khamsi, S. (2018). Predictors of self-determination in postsecondary education for students with intellectual and developmental disabilities. *Education and Training in Autism and Developmental Disabilities*, *53*(2), 146–159. https://www.jstor.org/stable/26495266

Supporting Teens and Young Adults on the Autism Spectrum: Setting and Pursuing Self-Determined Goals: https://thinkcollege.net/sites/default/files/files/resources/Vanderbilt-selfdetermination-toolkit.pdf

Chapter 8
Neurodiversity in Higher Education Institutions:
A Case Study From Pakistan

Steven Michael Granich
https://orcid.org/0000-0002-7947-422X
Commonwealth University of Pennsylvania, USA

Sonia Omer
https://orcid.org/0000-0003-0345-2208
University of the Punjab, Pakistan

Munawar Malik
https://orcid.org/0009-0007-3468-813X
University of the Punjab, Pakistan

ABSTRACT

The collective capacities and capabilities of individuals within a society, including those with disabilities and neurodivergence, play a crucial role in the socio-economic development of a nation. Pakistan exhibits poor socio-economic indicators when it comes to the overall wellbeing of its people, including Neurodivergent individuals whose presence and needs are not recognized in comparison to those with physical disabilities. Despite Pakistan's commitment to the rights of persons with disabilities, the country fails to address the challenges faced by Neurodivergent students in postsecondary education. This chapter focuses on the issues within Pakistani universities that limit the inclusion of Neurodivergent individuals. It explores the barriers that hinder the practical implementation of inclusive policies regarding educational provisions for Neurodivergent individuals. The person-in-environment and strength-based perspectives of social work are explored as options for intervention.

DOI: 10.4018/979-8-3693-8920-1.ch008

INTRODUCTION

The collective capabilities, potentials, skills, and knowledge of individuals are pivotal for the social and economic development of any country. Sharing knowledge and fostering collaboration among individuals is important in creating a culture of resilience, learning, and adaptability. Neurodivergent individuals and people with disabilities require an inclusive environment designed to support their diverse needs. The person-in-environment model from the field of social work practice emphasizes that the physical, emotional, and cognitive abilities of individuals need to be considered in relation to the available physical spaces, supportive social structures, and accessible features. Modifying the available environment and the functioning of social institutions, including the institutions of family, education, and economics, can help significantly improve the experience and quality of life for Neurodivergent individuals (Jurgens, 2020).

Neurodiversity refers to the differences of human brain functioning across individuals. Neurodivergent individuals include, but are not limited to, those with autism, Attention Deficit Hyperactivity Disorder (ADHD), Tourette syndrome and learning disabilities such as dyslexia and dyscalculia. Among these, learning disabilities are the most commonly reported challenges in any given population, indicating that a large proportion of the people is neurodiverse. As reported, the absence of a support system leads to disparities among neurodiverse communities (Roy & Jain 2021). Neurodivergent individuals can contribute more significantly to the wellbeing of any society if their unique cognitive traits are recognized and their abilities are nurtured (Szulc et al., 2021). Investment through education and skill training maximizes the potential of all members of society, including Neurodivergent individuals. Students with disabilities often achieve lower levels of success compared to their peers, as evident in the disparities in employment, secondary education and independent living (Neuman, 2011; Laxton et. al, 2024). Limitations in educational support are reflected in increased poverty, unemployment and limited access to healthcare services for Neurodivergent individuals and those with disabilities (Laxton, et al., 2024).

As recorded in the 2023 Population Census, Pakistan is a developing country with a population of around 241.49 million. According to the Pakistan Bureau of Statistics (2023), 9.64% of the population has disabilities, including sensory, physical, and intellectual challenges. Although the census acknowledges disabilities such as physical and mental impairments, it fails to quantify Neurodivergent individuals. The lack of research on Neurodivergent individuals results in poor identification of this population. Hence, these individuals are deprived of an inclusive environment. Additionally, the stigmatization and neglect of Neurodivergent individuals is deeply rooted in Pakistani culture, further creating hurdles in the way of equitable opportunities for them (Bashir & Khanum, 2024). Pakistan is a signatory of United

Nations Convention for the Rights of the Persons with Disabilities (UNCRPD). The country has pledged to provide legislative support ensuring the provision of inclusive quality education for persons with disabilities.

A focus on investing in vulnerable groups, including minorities and individuals with educational challenges, is critical to provide quality education (Rasheed et al., 2023). Being a global partner for the socio-economic well-being of persons with disabilities, Pakistan has ratified UNCRPD and is committed to the Sustainable Development Goals (SDG) in the 2030 agenda. It is important to mention that while describing the term disability in different documents in Pakistan, the term neurodiversity is neglected and completely absent in any significant document. Additionally, the Higher Education Commission (HEC), a statutory body established by Government of Pakistan, is mandated to fund, oversee, regulate and accredit Higher Education Institutions (HEI's) in the country. HEC identifies gaps between policy and practice regarding the needs of people with disabilities (Government of Pakistan, 2018). In particular, this includes Neurodivergent learners whose needs are highly neglected in the formulation and implementation of policies at the higher education level. While educational and support services for Neurodivergent learners are available to some extent in Pakistan at clinics and during early school years, their scarcity at secondary and postsecondary levels significantly affects the development of neurodiverse human capital.

Pakistan lacks evidence-based data on neurodiverse populations. Only a few local research studies can be found that discuss autism or ADHD, and they are limited to the early years of childhood (Aftab et al., 2023; Nazim & Khalid, 2019; Noor et al., 2023). Individual researchers and private organizations are striving to conduct research instead of relying on official government data. This chapter focuses on universities in Pakistan that limit the inclusion phase for Neurodivergent individuals (Rahbar et al., 2011). It explores the limitations and barriers that hinder the translation of inclusive policies on educational provisions for Neurodivergent individuals into practical terms. The person-in-environment and strength-based perspectives of social work have been explored as options for intervention, as environmental factors can significantly minimize hurdles and challenges while maximizing growth opportunities for Neurodivergent individuals in the society.

The purpose of this chapter is to explain the current situation for Neurodivergent people in Pakistan and the implications for universities, faculty, and students. There is a lack of research base for understanding neurodiversity in Pakistan, and neurodiversity is not well identified within university settings. There is a scarcity of services at the postsecondary level. There are barriers for Neurodivergent students at Pakistani universities. The chapter investigates the challenges and issues neurodivergent individuals face at the universities in Pakistan. It throws light on provision, support and access of neurodivergent students in university level education which remains largely restricted for them due to certain factors ranging from social and cultural elements, scarcity of medical facilities, neglect of the government towards wellbeing of neurodivergent individuals and absence of awareness needed to support the needs of these individuals. While using a qualitative approach with 15 university faculty and staff, findings of the study reveal significant disconnection between policy and practice for neurodivergent individuals while the stigmatization and social and cultural barriers restrict these individuals to become productive members of the society. The chapter, in the end, advocates for a more inclusive educational landscape that recognizes the potential of all students, irrespective of neurological differences.

This chapter will explain the international context of neurodiversity and then move to the example of Pakistan as a case study including discussion of disabilities in Pakistan, higher education policies, and provisions of higher education practice. Then there will be an explanation of the challenges faced by Neurodivergent students in higher education. It will explore the person-in-environment approach as a possible intervention. By doing a qualitative study of university staff and faculty, further information was obtained on the social reality of Neurodivergent students at Pakistani universities. There are concluding remarks and policy recommendations which call for a collaborative approach at the university level in Pakistan. Finally, there are two case studies working with Neurodivergent students with a series of questions asked. There are international commitments to neurodiversity which Pakistan is part of with influences on policy and inclusion of people with neurodiversity in Pakistan. In the next section we cover these international commitments.

INTERNATIONAL COMMITMENTS ON NEURODIVERSITY

Neurodiversity movements across the globe emphasize the concept of equal rights, an acknowledgment of varied cognitive behaviors, and an argument against exclusion (Lollini, 2021). Significant international commitments or promises have been drafted to benefit Neurodivergent individuals as they stand protected through laws, acts and bindings (agreements) (Baker, 2011; Lollini, 2021). The Americans with Disabilities Act protects the rights of disabled people in the U.S. (United States Department of Justice and Civil Rights Division, 2024). The Equality Act 2010 in the United Kingdom (UK), for instance, prevents disability discrimination in all forms, be it academic, social, functional, or psychological. The law has its own accommodation for the neurodiverse population as it recognizes that neurodivergence may count as a disability, even if the individual does not consider themselves to be disabled. The act provides protection and mandates for reasonable accommodations through access to ordinary life experiences on an equity basis. It shields the neurodivergent population in areas of employment, education and public service (Fraser Butlin, 2011).

A key support for Neurodivergent individuals is extended through the UNCRPD and stresses the right to education through its Article 24. It signifies the importance of education in systems on an all-inclusive basis through full participation with peers. The U.S., Germany and Japan are at the forefront of disability rights and policy (Heyer, 2015). An increased emphasis on disabilities through research and education is setting new standards, particularly in the realms of health, prevention, and rehabilitation. Additionally, with more reliance on technology, the dream of inclusivity is turning into a reality (Chadwick et al., 2022).

Above are the glimpses of certain international commitments and support mechanisms extended to Neurodivergent persons in developed countries. In comparison with international commitments and support, the authors strive now to highlight and overview the status of commitment and support available in Pakistan for persons with disabilities in general, and Neurodiversit individuals in particular. Pakistan is very connected to an international context, and it is important to examine neurodiversity in Pakistan as a case study. It represents some of the challenges faced in developing countries addressing needs of Neurodivergent children and adults.

A CASE STUDY OF PAKISTAN

In Pakistan, there is a need to devise a dedicated policy that will guard the right to education for ND students in higher education systems. **Table 1** is a segment of the table from the 2023 Pakistan Census that shows that around 17 million people (ages 15-49) are experiencing a disabling condition. The Census specified disabilities and the number of citizens in Pakistan in each category. However, that representation is not visible in higher education institutions. This calls for attention on urgent grounds. A discussion of the accommodations and provisions at Higher Education Institutions (HEI's), working under the umbrella of Higher Education Commission of Pakistan (HEC), is imperative. The objective of the qualitative study undertaken at a Pakistani university was to examine the resolve of HEIs towards fostering inclusion and support for students with disabilities, particularly for Neurodivergent students. The research literature supported the need for this endeavor.

Table 1. Disability and Functional Limitation for Special Age Group (15-49-Year-Old), Pakistan 2023 Census

Specific Disability	Number of Individuals
Population	114,971,808
Disability	1,899,756
Functional limitation	7,212,031
Seeing	1,426,133
Hearing	1,562,148
Walking/Climbing	2,355,871
Communication	853,421
Memorization/Focus	1,209,963
Self-Care Etc.	725,290

Note. The indicators in Table 1 refer to sensory and physical disabilities; significantly, there is no mention of neurodiversity.

Higher Education Commission (HEC) Policy for Students with Disabilities

Pakistan needed to devise a dedicated policy that could guard the right to education for Neurodivergent students and those with disabilities in higher education systems. In 2002, the Pakistan HEC was established to fund, oversee, regulate, and accredit higher education institutions in public and private sectors. Apart from its various other roles of significance, the offices are dedicated to establishing educational policies and quality assurance in order to ascertain and maintain standards, thus uplifting student performance. The educational policies regarding HEIs are reviewed regularly, adapted, and reinforced to assure standards at international levels. HEC, reflecting national policies, devised its own policy for postsecondary students with disabilities. Commonly known as the "Policy for Students with Disabilities," it ensures that such students have equal opportunities to access and attain an education of their choice. When defining the term "disability," the educational policy refers to "any long-term physical, mental, intellectual, or sensory impairments which may hinder a student's ability to actively participate at par with their peers" (Hussain et al., 2020).

With the international commitment to "education for all," the policy aims to provide equal opportunity for students with disabilities in HEIs. The objective is ensured by creating inclusive environments in all domains of education, i.e. curricular, co-curricular, and extracurricular activities. The policy vows to eliminate any obstacle, be it physical, organizational, academic, or social. The policy further warrants non-discriminatory accommodations and support on an equity basis for students with disabilities in HEIs. The specific provisions of the higher education policies are important to consider.

Provisions Offered in the Policy

The policy urges the formation of accessibility committees at every HEI to determine possible accommodations, provide counseling, offer psychological support, and provide access to faculty advice during admissions, exams, and the dissertation process. The accessibility committee is also responsible for fundraising, promoting awareness, conducting seminars, as well as communicating the roles of the disability coordinator in each program. The policy discusses in detail admissions related matters, starting with the application procedure and identifying possible accommodations that might be required. The provision of disability certificates has been discussed while ensuring the elements of secrecy, bias, and discrimination (Hussain et al., 2020). The provision of disability is a document issued by the Pakistan government describing the disability of a person and the diagnosis; it allows the person then to access services and resources. The policy discusses that the certificate of disability should be issued without any bias or discrimination and with ensured secrecy of the applicant.

The policy mandates reasonable accommodations in the case of an entrance exam. This may include modified exam material, special material or lip-reading test for challenges in hearing, extra time, supervised breaks, use of computers, readers, and separate supervision for exams for students with disabilities. Financial aid, dedicated quotas, and age relaxations are also recommended in individual cases. In terms of quotas, all public sector universities dedicate one seat for higher qualification like MS/MPhil and PhD programs for students with disability. The HEC policy regarding such students generously defines reasonable accommodations in health and psychological issues through infrastructural accommodations, transportation, and assistive technology. The policy describes accommodation in exams and assessment as a subject of mutual consultation between the faculty member, disability coordinator, and the student. Residential accommodation within the university premises, participation in higher education, and vocational education are all discussed in the respective sections. Finally, the HEC policy allows and encourages establishing a special fund to support students through a defined budget provision on an annual basis (HEC Policy for Students with Disabilities, 2021).

Although Higher Education policy in Pakistan addresses some aspects of Neurodivergent students, there are many challenges and gaps.

Challenges and Gaps in Support of Neurodivergent Postsecondary Students

A point worth noting is that the higher education policy for persons with disabilities does not address Neurodivergent students specifically. In developed countries, the past few decades have witnessed cultural and community developments that support neurodiversity. However, postsecondary administrations continue to maintain deficit philosophical models (Muneeb, 2024). The same holds true for Pakistan where the implementation of the social model of disabilities is still struggling to become widespread. Students with learning disabilities such as dyslexia, autism, and speech disorders are not explicitly mentioned in the policy. Even the disability certificates mandated by the policy as an essential document for university admissions do not cater to Neurodivergent students (Halder & Squires, 2023). There is an urgent need to include the neurodivergent population in any disability policy formulated in the country.

Recognizing neurodiversity in Pakistan will result in a better understanding of diverse student needs, promote inclusion, and eventually create a more equitable educational landscape in Pakistan (Amin et al., 2024). Studies reveal significant challenges and barriers contributing to the vulnerability of Neurodivergent students in Pakistan, despite certain provisions in policies devised for their wellbeing. The general population in Pakistan remains unaware of the term neurodivergent. These disabilities are viewed through the lens of shame, stigma, fear, and pity (Halder & Squires, 2023; Warraich et al., 2024). Stigmatization is particularly pronounced in rural areas, where Neurodivergent individuals are kept in isolation. Rural areas in Pakistan face significant challenges regarding access to health care, education, and employment opportunities. Limited awareness among rural populations, combined with social and cultural barriers acts as a hurdle in the inclusion and acceptance of any form of disability, including neurodiversity (Choudhry et al., 2023). Neurodivergent individuals are excluded from educational institutions and later from employment opportunities. This situation makes these individuals dependent on their families and exacerbates the challenges they face in society. (Nizamani & Nizamani, 2022).

On the other hand, urban cities in Pakistan have better infrastructure, facilities, and provisions in health and education. The rural-urban disparity is a significant issue in Pakistan, which is evident in income inequalities, disparities in medical and educational facilities, employment opportunities and infrastructure gaps. Various government agencies in Pakistan have failed to provide equal opportunities to rural and urban populations, resulting in a widening class divide in the country (Ejaz & Mallawaarachchi, 2023). With the availability of more facilities, education, and awareness in cities, some progress can be witnessed in urban Pakistan. Individuals from the upper class have access to facilities for Neurodivergent individuals, such as diagnostic services, testing, therapy centers, and inclusive educational institutions. However, the majority of the neurodiverse population faces a severe lack of facilities (Khalid & Anjum, 2019).

Facilities for Neurodivergent individuals, such as private clinics in urban cities, are not funded by the state of Pakistan. This leads to inadequate services and understaffed facilities (Furrukh & Anjum, 2020). Widening inequality in medical facilities between rural and urban Pakistan is a critical issue that affects inclusion. A significant portion of Pakistan's population resides in rural areas, where poor medical facilities lead to poor health outcomes, further adding to the vulnerabilities faced by rural communities. There is a need for a collaborative approach in order to address the critical issues of inclusion. In order to address these challenges a person-in-environment perspective may be helpful in moving Pakistan toward a more effective approach for working with Neurodivergent students.

PERSON-IN-ENVIRONMENT PERSPECTIVE AS POSSIBLE INTERVENTION

Person-in-environment (PIE) is used as a model to suggest an effective solution for addressing the challenges faced by Neurodivergent students at universities in Pakistan. The person-in-environment perspective sees the individual as interacting with their surrounding environment and recognizing this interaction with the environment as important in resolving problems.

The significant characteristics of the PIE model focus on the fact that individual behavior and the overall wellbeing of people in society are influenced by the interaction of existing social, cultural, environmental, and physical traits within the society. Applying the framework of PIE demands that practitioners not only focus on fixing the issues, but also provide an enabling environment where such a diverse population can thrive and prosper in society (Whelpley et al., 2023).

While stressing the significance of context, the personal strength of individuals, and the collaborative role of social workers striving for change, the PIE and strength-based perspective provide an important framework for addressing the challenges faced by Neurodivergent individuals in Pakistan. In the domain of higher education, social workers play a crucial role for change and progress based on their code of ethics and interventions. Based on the absence of an inclusive approach to higher education for the neurodiverse population, the PIE perspective can be a significant framework to understand the needs of Neurodivergent individuals (Muneeb, 2024).

The PIE framework is a key element in attaining a holistic view of individuals. This framework primarily focuses on understanding needs, requirements, strengths, and abilities of each individual. The inclusion of professionals from social work in the formulation and implementation of policies for education can help universities understand the emotional, social, and cognitive functioning of Neurodivergent students by establishing a cooperative framework for intervention for Neurodivergent students (Whelpley et al., 2023).

One of the significant fields of social work is school social work which is missing in Pakistan. Schools and higher education institutes do not offer services of professional social workers in their institutes, unlike developed countries. The absence of school social workers exacerbates the challenges and issues faced by students on campuses. Without school social workers, there is an inability to create a collaborative environment where Neurodivergent students can grow and flourish. This particularly affects those with educational challenges, such as individuals with physical disabilities or Neurodivergent students (Knox, 2024).

The role of social workers, whether in schools or other settings, is pivotal in facilitating and assessing the environment of Neurodivergent students, specifically in clinical settings and within the limited number of institutions catering to their needs. School social workers can provide a variety of interventions to assist Neurodivergent students. These efforts can later pave the way for other higher education institutions to adopt similar inclusive practices. The placement of social workers in such settings may further help to investigate accessibility issues faced by Neurodivergent students in higher educational institutes, potentially acting as the missing piece of the puzzle.

Apart from assessing family dynamics, community environment, and societal pressure, social workers can help the neurodiverse population achieve an increased access to inclusive education by working with various systems to be supportive of their educational and social experience (Doyle, 2020). The Pakistani society has limited information regarding people experiencing autism, ADHD, dyslexia, and other forms of neurodiversity. While the urban population may have some access to information and an understanding of these conditions among their children, the greater part of the rural population has little understanding and focus on neurodiversity. Consequently, many children from rural areas are excluded from education from an early age. In a country like Pakistan, where social and cultural approaches and attitudes toward disability can often be stigmatizing, the PIE model can be instrumental in understanding the manifold layers of obstacles faced by Neurodivergent individuals by providing a systemic understanding of the challenges faced by Neurodivergent students.

Similarly, when it comes to policy and structural changes, the PIE perspective can play a crucial role in advocating for structural changes at multiple levels. For instance, the framework may help devise a clear guideline on inclusive education that can mandate resources for Neurodivergent students. This calls for faculty training and focuses on inclusive syllabi. The PIE methodology advocates for a universal service approach to make the environment more accommodating to the needs and aspirations of Neurodivergent individuals, rather than expecting them to conform to an educational model that operates on a one-size-fits-all principle (Lai et al., 2020).

Adopting a PIE approach can help raise awareness among the general population about neurodiversity, connect social spaces for Neurodivergent individuals, and help change societal attitudes by raising the consciousness of the general population and university faculty, staff, and administrators. This is especially important in a context where factors of shame and embarrassment stigmatize Neurodivergent individuals (Hussein et al., 2020).

The framework of PIE calls for an interdisciplinary approach to cater to the needs of Neurodivergent people. It advocates for a collaboration among social workers, psychologists, special education experts, and counselors to better support this population (Boobis, 2016). Such a collaboration ensures that various aspects of their needs: emotional, social, economic, and educational, are addressed. A social worker can reach out to families and communities to make sure that Neurodivergent individuals' needs are fulfilled. Mental health professionals can assist counseling and interventions. Similarly, a special education expert can help provide tools designed to enhance the academic success of individuals. This kind of holistic association of experts can ensure that Neurodivergent individuals have the services of seasoned professionals (Harrison, et al., 2024)

Similarly, the various social institutions within society can help mobilize and raise awareness. Family, as a primary institution, is important in understanding and recognizing the needs of Neurodivergent learners. The family's ability to address the stigmatization and shame associated with neurodiversity is important for students' wellbeing. Support from families serves as the first and foremost step in the growth and development of Neurodivergent individuals (Sohn et al., 2024).

Medical provisions from the state are needed in all corners of the country. Disparities exist between rural and urban Pakistan in medical facilities, acting as a major obstacle in addressing the challenges faced by Neurodivergent individuals who need a diagnosis to receive support. Furthermore, the role of mass media and non-governmental organizations is pivotal in creating awareness about neurodiversity. Whether through social support system, family, diagnostic centers, teaching pedagogies, instructional technologies, curriculum designs, or the provision of quiet, sensory-friendly environments, the collaborative efforts of professionals within the framework of PIE can produce productive and more effective results in higher education institutions (Bowman et al., 2021).

METHODOLOGY OF THE RESEARCH STUDY

The purpose of the qualitative study and document analysis completed was to better understand the situation in universities with Neurodivergent students and the faculty working with them. The goal was to investigate the degree of awareness and understanding of neurodiversity, policy/resource/research gaps, professional training, the lack of accommodation and modification in the instructional process, social stigmatization, and cultural barriers.

The authors adopted a qualitative design, using in-depth interviews that were analyzed thematically. The study highlighted the policies and provisions available in higher education institutes for Neurodivergent students. The participants of the study included university heads of departments and members of university management, such as student advisors and chairpersons of admissions committees. The authors independently developed the interview guide, considering key questions on the knowledge of and perception of Neurodivergent students in universities, challenges and provisions in admissions in higher education institutes for Neurodivergent students, policy implementation gaps, available facilities and infrastructure in universities, social stigmatization, and socio-economic barriers faced by Neurodivergent students.

Fifteen (15) respondents from two public sector universities in Lahore, Pakistan were selected. The participants of the study were selected with the help of a purposive sampling method. The purpose of the study was to obtain information from administrative as well as departmental heads of the universities. Fifteen interviews were conducted with the prior permission of the respondents in the offices of the participants in the universities until the researchers obtained an adequate sample.

The list of the administrative staff and faculty members was obtained from registrar offices of both the public sector universities. As mentioned in the study, all public sector universities have a quota system for intake of physically disabled students. None of the public sector universities have any criteria to admit Neurodivergent students. So, participants were selected on the basis of their administrative role as well as teaching role to gather data on challenges, available facilities (if any Neurodivergent individuals get admissions in the universities) and overall absence of Neurodivergent individuals in higher education institutes.

Participants were contacted before the interviews and were informed about the study. Written consent to participate in the study was obtained. The interview locations were agreed upon in advance while the duration of the interviews lasted between 30 to 45 minutes. Participants were given an opportunity to ask any question about the study prior to the interviews. The participants were also informed about the confidentiality of their responses, and they were ensured that their identity would not be revealed at any stage of the research. The interviews were professionally transcribed by one of the researchers familiar with transcription, and another author checked them thoroughly to maintain accuracy.

Thematic analysis was conducted with the help of the six-step framework developed by Braun and Clarke (2006) to identify important patterns in the data (Byrne, 2022). At the first stage, the authors familiarized themselves with the data by reading and rereading it to obtain a deep understanding of the content. Codes were generated by labeling the significant features of the data. The next significant step was to combine similar codes together to form overarching themes that showcased the true essence of the data. Before finalizing the significant themes, the authors made sure that these themes had relevance to the aim and objective of the study. The last stage involved reporting of the findings by explaining the themes. Verbatim quotations were used which provided richness to data and ensured the findings are presented in participants' own voices which helped in understanding of experiences and perspectives of the participants.

An additional aspect of the study involved conducting a document analysis of national policies pertaining to students with educational challenges, particularly the policy formulated by Higher Education Commission (2021) of Pakistan for Neurodivergent students. The objective was to critically review the policy, identify provisions for Neurodivergent students, and recommend amendments and policy implications. The authors became familiar with the content of the document of policies and received additional depth and information on the policy designed for Neurodivergent students which helped in writing background and a literature review. In addition, it facilitated the design of the interview guide.

Table 2 describes the participants in the study which included heads of departments, university management, student advisors, and chairpersons of admissions committees. The table gives the years of experience and age of each participant and the breakdown of their departments.

Table 2. Respondents' Roles, Years of Experience, and Age (N = 15)

Participant	Years of Experience	Age
	Head of Department (n=7)	
Ali	15	45
Imran	1	35
Sadia	10	37
Zegum	18	50
Sohail	15	43
Zakir	5	39

continued on following page

Table 2. Continued

Participant	Years of Experience	Age
Zubair	14	46
	Student Advisor (n=3)	
Usama	10	37
Razaq	23	52
Sonia	11	39
	Admissions Committee (n=2)	
Imer	13	41
Sarah	16	49
	Hostel (n=2)	
Miriam	21	52
Muhammad	16	50
	Registrar (n=1)	
Moshin	12	43

Note. Participant names are pseudonyms to protect their anonymity. Hostel refers to the place where students stay at the university in Pakistan.

Thematic Analysis

The themes derived from the research conducted included awareness and understanding of neurodiversity in Pakistan, policy implication gaps, the role of the Ministry of Education in professional training to support Neurodivergent individuals, the lack of accommodation and modification in the instructional process, social stigmatization, and cultural barriers faced by Neurodivergent individuals. The themes also involved the shortage of available resources and research data to identify Neurodivergent individuals and develop policies for their inclusion in all aspects of society. Below is the detailed discussion of the themes identified.

Awareness and Understanding of Neurodiversity in Pakistan

Pakistan has a literacy rate of approximately 62.3%, with 60 million adults being able to read (Government of Pakistan, 2020). The per capita income for the fiscal year 2023-2024 is around $1680, with a cruising inflation rate of 11.1% as of May 2024. Participants in the study argued that, due to the socio-economic conditions of the country, a significant portion of the population, around 21.9% lives below the poverty line (Asian Development Bank, 2024) and is combating unemployment. The social and cultural practices prevalent in Pakistan, combined with poverty, create significant challenges for individuals with disabilities. These individuals face multiple social, economic, and cultural barriers which further exacerbate their vulnerability (Asian Development Bank, 2024).

The general public tends to focus on noticeably physical and visual disabilities due to that emphasis within Pakistan society. As a result, there is better understanding of physical and disabilities in the country. This awareness is also reflected in policies and planning for the inclusion of individuals with physical disabilities, particularly in education and employment (Batool et al., 2019; Rathore et al., 2011). However, sensory and invisible conditions remain unnoticed by the masses and are sometimes ignored (Batool et al.,2019). Major cities have more to offer students with disabilities in terms of medical services, educational facilities, and employment opportunities. Yet, the outcomes remain dismal. (Shukat, 2023).

The responses of the participants support these conclusions. Sarah commented, *"We encourage, and we try to facilitate people with physical disabilities in our societies. University held meetings regarding policies for such students are full of deliberation, but it just primarily revolves around needs for students with physical disabilities and none other. Reality, however, is otherwise. I must say, despite the policies, even these physical disabilities have few accommodations and support. My university has several departments with multistory structures without any lifts, where there are staircases and chains at the entrances and a physically handicapped cannot access the class."*

The challenges faced by persons with disabilities are exacerbated by the general public's unwelcoming behavior toward them (Rathore et al., 2011; Shukat, 2023). Ali shared, *"Honestly if you ask me, I have heard of this term rarely in life. This term and people with cognitive issues are neither recognized nor are accepted in our society. There is no mechanism to identify these people, nor do people make efforts to have their diagnosis done. There may be some schools in a few major cities who deal with people having issues of autism or ADHD, but just to the benefit of elites who can afford them. Such children from the middle or upper class never make it to schools even."*

In order to improve this situation mentioned by the study participants, it is important to have a collaborative relationship among universities and society in order to improve this situation and make it more welcoming for people with neurodiversity.

Policy Implementation Gaps

Many participants noted that the concepts of "inclusive education" or the agenda of "education for all" exist only in text and policies made by the education ministry. However, significant barriers hinder the implementation of these policies. The education system fails to provide equal opportunities to individuals with different abilities and talents (Hussain et al., 2020)

The situation becomes more complex for Neurodivergent students who receive minimal educational provisions. They remain almost invisible at universities. The lack of a dedicated policy addressing neurodiversity makes matters worse. This lack of focus on Neurodivergent individuals results in numerous obstacles, such as an absence of specific policies, inadequate resources and accommodations, a lack of comprehensive needs assessment, nonprofessional staff/teachers, limited access to assistive devices and technologies, and the unavailability of learning centers (Naz et al., 2024).

"We have limited admissions, understanding and needs of people with disabilities. To cater to the needs of the disabled population, there are departments of special education in most of the public sector universities. These special education departments have students with physical and sensory disabilities enrolled in different programs. I have never heard of any department taking admission and fulfilling the needs of a neurodiverse group of the population," stated Muhammad.

The participants of the study admitted that universities lack mechanisms for the formal identification of individuals with dyslexia, autism or other neurodifferences. In each class, teachers may attempt to assess and identify students with learning difficulties, reading challenges, and attention deficits which are quite common, but they are not knowledgeable. The participants were of the view that faculty development training and programs by the Higher Education Commission of Pakistan must add training, syllabi modification, and infrastructure designed to address the needs of Neurodivergent individuals and students with diverse needs.

Imran, a professor said, "I can assess and I can identify students who are different from other students. Such neurodiverse groups silently get admission in universities. They are ones who somehow complete their school education and a greater majority is from influential urban families. The teachers are not trained; neither is the syllabus designed in a manner that can facilitate these individuals. They are socially isolated and misfits. They end up securing low grades eventually. In my opinion, ignoring such individuals is a great loss to the nation and the situation reveals how the state is ignoring strengthening human capital in the country, regardless of their diverse needs and capacities."

To improve this situation, it would be helpful to adapt a person-in-environment perspective in order to engage in collaboration between different elements of society to facilitate a more inclusive perspective on working with Neurodivergent students.

Lack of Accommodations and Modifications in the Instructional Process

Participants noted the absence of standardized policies and accommodations necessary to engage Neurodivergent students. This lack of provisions significantly hinders the learning experience for Neurodivergent students at universities. In the absence of educational facilities designed to cater to their needs, Neurodivergent students have to make extra efforts to engage with the content and teaching methodology which can lead to frustration and anxiety. This issue is similarly faced by students identified with autism or dyslexia during childhood who manage to enroll in universities. Due to the lack of identification of these individuals during university admissions, along with the absence of assistive technologies, modification of syllabi and teaching methods, the potential and abilities of these students remain limited. Neither are teachers adequately trained, nor are syllabi designed to accommodate the needs of Neurodivergent students.

Special education training is rarely included in teacher education programs in Pakistan, except for those specifically pursuing special education. (Tarhirkeli, 2022). Participants also emphasized the lack of collaboration between primary and secondary schools that work with Neurodivergent students and higher education institutes. Collaborative efforts, such as sharing of data on Neurodivergent students, exchanging teaching methods, and assisting in the designing of syllabi could greatly facilitate the enrollment of Neurodivergent students at HEIs.

> *"If the data is received and shared from schools and universities announce a special quota for neurodivergent, there are bright chances where such individuals can make it up to higher education institutes. Only then universities can think of teacher training and recruitment of special staff in the universities. The required syllabus and teaching aids can only make sure that there are mandatory admissions of this group in our universities," said Sarah.*

The national syllabus is designed in a rigid manner and follows a 'one size fits all' approach (Ali & Baig, 2012; Pakistan Curriculum, 2025). While cities do have several centers catering to the educational needs of students with disabilities, the number of such institutions is insufficient when compared to the size of the disabled population. The rigid curriculum structure eventually results in struggles for both individuals with physical disabilities and Neurodivergent students. Participants in the study were of the view that policy making in education is usually questioned due to the absence of real stakeholders in the process of policy making and the haphazardness of the process. Moreover, political and economic instability results in the halting of many policies designed on the basis of inclusivity in education (Jamil, 2009; Inclusion, 2021),

Teacher training programs in Pakistan primarily focus on class management and emphasize traditional methods of instruction. There is a lack of on-the-job teacher training in the classroom, especially for teaching those with diverse abilities. This poses a serious threat to successful inclusion. Additionally, there is a dearth of professionals equipped with counseling skills, therapy models, and support for these students (Ahmad & Yousaf, 2011; Shukat, 2023).

In such circumstances, it is difficult to expect Neurodivergent students to enroll in higher education institutes. The lack of comprehensive training programs for teachers results in an absence of the expertise necessary to address the challenges of inclusive education. Students with different abilities face emotional, behavioral, and academic challenges. The limited number of Neurodivergent students who enroll in universities often end up leaving in the absence of a supportive environment.

> *According to Zubair, "I really think the higher education commission of Pakistan as a regulatory body needs to take some candid measures to include this group on a distinct basis. All universities are bound to follow higher education policies in the country, and hence policy implementation measures should be revisited to ensure transparency and avoid biases." Although there are policies to handle situations with disability, there is a need for a more collaborative approach to address the real needs of Neurodivergent students through a person-in-environment approach.*

Social Stigmatization

The word "normalcy" is deep-seated in Pakistani culture and social practices, particularly when measuring academic success and social behavior. Individuals who face challenges with reading, writing, communication, and socialization are excluded and stigmatized in society. Participants in the study expressed that, due to poverty and low literacy rates, stigmatization of Neurodivergent individuals has become a general attitude. The disabled population faces visible social, cultural, and systemic hurdles in their daily lives. They are generally excluded from mainstream societal activities and are viewed through the lens of shame and pity (Dixon, 2023).

The neurodiverse population, in general, is linked with insanity or mental illness, and is largely misunderstood. Cultural practices, particularly in rural Pakistan, tend to view Neurodivergent individuals as "possessed," and many seek help from spiritual healers instead of pursuing medical diagnoses and educational support (Ahmad et al., 2023). As a result, these individuals are often expelled from schools, putting an end to inclusion efforts. Due to certain cultural beliefs, Neurodivergent individuals are stigmatized and misjudged. Rural Pakistan presents a very dismal picture when it comes to medical facilities. The facilities provided by the state are inadequate and people, even if they wish, are reluctant to avail themselves of these medical facilities

(Razzak et al., 2008; Tariq, 2021). Additionally, people in rural areas are habitually seeking treatment from spiritual healers and people who falsely represent themselves as healers. These misconceptions are deeply rooted in cultural beliefs and create a situation where neurodivergence in rural areas is totally misunderstood (Veesar et al., 2023). In such circumstances, where general medical ailments are treated in this way, the recognition and support of Neurodivergent individuals are severely neglected. Neurodivergent individuals are often linked to madness.

Socio-Economic Barriers

Literature has highlighted the poor socio-economic conditions of a large segment of Pakistani population which adds to the vulnerabilities of individuals and groups in need. The country reports high infant and maternal mortality rates (Tharwani et al. 2023). Issues like polio remain a medical challenge for Pakistan, making it one of the few countries where polio still exists (Sultan et al., 2023). As per the UNICEF 2023 report, approximately 28 million children in Pakistan are out of school. Participants in the study believed that Pakistan, as a social welfare state, faces challenges in providing medical and educational facilities as per needs and requirements. The country lacks both modern medical facilities and an effective education system. The large population is a significant burden on the state machinery due to meagre resources (Akhtar et al., 2013) In such circumstances, disabilities of any kind, including neurodiversity, become a serious issue in Pakistan as such individuals require extra attention, caring support, and facilities. The complexity of neurodiversity is compounded by limited awareness, poverty, socio-cultural practices, and inequality in the country. There is a significant focus on physical health by the health department of the country. However, neurodiversity receives less attention and facilitates due to stigmatization and socio-cultural barriers. Furthermore, the cultural practices of stigmatization add to the increased vulnerabilities of Neurodivergent individuals (Taj, 2015).

Lack of Research and Data

One significant issue regarding the acceptance and awareness of Neurodivergent students in Pakistan is the lack of data on the number of Neurodivergent students. The population census conducted in the country does not specifically categorize people with autism, dyslexia or other cognitive differences. This omission eventually leads to lack of policies and limited implementations, hindering the betterment of this segment of the population.

Due to the cultural stigmatization, a lack of public knowledge, and insufficient awareness efforts through mass media and other channels, this issue is largely unaddressed (Najmi, 2021). The matter does not end here. There is also a notable scarcity of research on the needs and challenges faced by these individuals. This lack of research and awareness eventually results in an absence of advocacy and support of neurodiversity in the country. The situation demands immediate attention, with efforts to raise public awareness (Imran et al., 2011, Najmi, 2021). There is a visible lack of government support as the state fails to recognize the neurodiverse population and does not create a conducive environment where the issues can be addressed. The lack of infrastructure in different spheres of life excludes this group from mainstream societal activities (Taj, 2015).

Mohsin said, "The entire process through which the wellbeing of such individuals can be made sure is expensive. The country, with few psychiatrists, psychologists, less people in special education, scarcity of diagnosis and rehabilitation centers makes this issue unapproachable for the general population." Sadia supported this argument by saying, "There is a serious issue of lack of funding of the Neurodivergent group of the population. The situation may improve if there is a mechanism of diagnosis first and later incentives are announced for them. The quota system only for this group of the population may be made mandatory in all educational institutions to ensure their smooth educational journey." The person-in-environment perspective can play a crucial role in advocating for structural changes at multiple levels, increasing public consciousness, and improving collaboration between different disciplines and institutions.

POLICY RECOMMENDATIONS

To create an environment that is conducive and inclusive, the authors of this chapter propose a multi-faceted approach to ensure that the neurodiverse population has acceptance, access, and recognition at Higher Education Institutes (HEIs). One significant factor is the development of linkages between public sector universities and schools or centers where Neurodivergent learners are present. Private schools in Pakistan have reported the enrollment of Neurodivergent individuals. Through data sharing, Neurodivergent individuals can be engaged, and their families can be convinced to ensure that their children study further at universities. Seminars and talks at schools, funded and organized by universities, can help create awareness about Neurodivergent individuals.

The authors strongly suggest a pilot program at major public sector universities, such as The University of the Punjab in Lahore, Pakistan, which has robust departments of psychology, special education and social work. A team consisting of the faculty members of these departments can come forward to establish connections with parents and schools where Neurodivergent students are enrolled. Public sector universities can also allocate quotas to ensure the enrollment of Neurodivergent students in different departments of the university. Additionally, developing teacher training workshops in these universities, sponsored by the Higher Education Commission of Pakistan, is important for recognizing and supporting these individuals. Necessary modifications in syllabi and assistive teaching tools are important to facilitate Neurodivergent student success in higher education institutes in Pakistan. Designing flexible syllabi and evaluation systems for such populations based on alternative methods such as presentations, group projects, and verbal exams can accommodate the unique needs of Neurodivergent students.

Integrating assistive technologies and accessible platforms at HEIs is important and can be a great initiative. Computer science departments at public sector universities can assist in devising teaching tools to help this population. Moreover, establishing peer networks with the help of student councils is important to reduce stigmatization. Initiatives led by students for the acceptance and support for Neurodivergent students will reduce shaming and break cultural barriers. For a country like Pakistan, it is significant to examine case studies from developing regions where Neurodivergent individuals are recognized at HEIs. For instance, the University of the Punjab and most of the public sector universities have foreign connections offices managed by full-fledged directors. Faculty members may be sent to international universities for training. Contact between local and international universities can create new avenues to include Neurodivergent students in mainstream society, building a more inclusive, empathetic, and diverse world for this group.

CONCLUSION

Pakistan, with limited resources and multiple commitments, is struggling to provide provisions deemed necessary in the developed world. In this context, the role of universities is pivotal in addressing the social and economic problems of the country. Universities can foster critical thinking among youth through inclusive education, encouragement of research, and raising awareness about socioeconomic issues. Collaboration at different levels, whether between students, researchers, teachers, or public and private educational institutions, under the umbrella of the Ministry of Education, can help initiate steps towards sustainable solutions. These efforts will eventually benefit all members of society, including those with different abilities and challenges (Nisar et al., 2023).

Pakistan ranks low on the Human Development Index due to unsatisfactory indicators, primarily in health, education, income, and gender disparities (Khan et al., 2019). In such circumstances, individuals with disabilities are deprived of various facilities, infrastructure, medical care, educational provisions and employment opportunities. Socio-cultural factors and practices contribute deeply to the marginalization of people with disabilities (Hussain et al., 2023). With a low level of education, the majority in Pakistan lack awareness on this pressing issue. The implementation of inclusive education in its true spirit is critical. There is a dire need to address all sorts of disabilities in policy formulation. An emphasis is required to ensure educational provisions for Neurodivergent individuals in particular.

In public and legal documents, individuals with neurodiversity are categorized as part of the general disability group and are recognized as "other disabilities" (Azeem et al., 2021). Neurodiversity is neither addressed nor is any policy made to improve the overall welfare of these individuals. The elite urban population of Pakistan has access to the limited available diagnostic centers which ensure educational provisions for these individuals (Furrukh & Anjum, 2020). However, a large number of Neurodivergent individuals miss out on educational opportunities from the beginning. In general, parents keep them at home due to feelings of shame and embarrassment, creating greater obstacles in the socialization process of such individuals (Marwat, 2023). The few who receive admission to universities face numerous challenges in the absence of trained faculty, curriculum accommodation, and other tools designed to aid such individuals. They are often viewed as slow learners, and they tend to pass semesters with low grades.

No university in Pakistan has a special program, quota or admission policy exclusively for Neurodivergent people. In fact, the idea of inclusive education exists at a very rudimentary level in Pakistan (Imran et al., 2024). The teaching skills and respective motivation of a teacher is a strong predictor in student success, and needs to be invested in through training of teachers at universities. Teacher training programs have been reported to have a direct and enhanced impact on the quality of services offered by teachers (Ahmed et al., 2021). Furthermore, in the absence of reliable data and research on neurodivergence, the present and future of such individuals presents a dismal situation in the country.

A person-in-environment collaborative effort can create an inclusive educational environment where Neurodivergent people can receive appropriate accommodations and education through interdisciplinary work, raising of public awareness, formulating appropriate policies, and advocating for structural change.

CASE STUDIES AND DISCUSSION QUESTIONS

Case Study 1: Moni's Story

Moni is a typical South Asian university student pursuing creative arts. Her education journey began early at the age of six where she was soon recognized as having difficulty in learning. When she attended high school, she had difficulty in mathematics and language subjects. Being part of a family with meager resources and limited education, she could hardly manage the school fee. The teachers frequently reported her as inattentive, talkative, and restless in class. As the demands of language skills increased, her performance worsened and she was on the verge of being expelled. Teachers had no clue why she performed better in arts and extracurricular activities but did not manage to pass other subjects. Her writing had spelling errors and grammatical mistakes, and these bothered her throughout school.

It was by chance that her drawings caught the attention of a visitor who happened to be a psychologist. She recognized the talent immediately and looked for Moni's portfolio. The psychologist was impressed with her drawing skills, and her parents, teachers, and managers were counseled, and the subject contents were changed according to her abilities with some dedicated coaching in the arts. She received her formal diagnosis as dyslexic. She obtained assistance from a dedicated support teacher who worked on her reading and writing skills. Upon the psychologist's advice, she received accommodations both in her instructional and assessment engagements. Today Moni is doing exceptionally well at her university. Not only is she enjoying her talent in arts, but has also improved in writing. She has learned to manage her language challenges.

Questions

1. How might Moni have done better if she was assessed for her performance in language and mathematics at an early age?
2. How might the experience of repeated failure be avoided and how might that have changed her learning outcomes?
3. Moni's artistic talents, if unrecognized and undervalued, could have been easily wasted. If her teachers had known about the challenges confronted by students like her, how might have they supported Moni in achieving success?
4. How can parents and teachers be educated in ways to identify exceptional abilities and support Neurodivergent learners in capitalizing on these talents?

Case Study 2: Babar's Story

Babar, born in an educated family, was developing like any other child of his age. It was around his third birthday when his parents started to realize there was some decline in his social and communication behaviors. His verbal repertoire was deteriorating and so was his social play. His play behavior was evolving, and he started preferring to play on his own. Being from an elite family, an allied health professional team including psychologists, a speech language therapist, and a special education teacher were approached for consultation. The parents were told that Babar suffered a mild form of autism. Not being knowledgeable about autism, the parents utilized the advice of professionals.

Babar benefitted from earlier enrollment in an inclusive school as per recommendation, where he received regular speech, occupational, and psychological therapies. The school teachers were well trained and assisted Babar in succeeding to the best of his abilities. Although Babar had his own pace of learning, he could easily meet expectations at the school. The real challenge unfolded as Babar transitioned to college. The expectations of parents and teachers at college were higher as compared to his previous school. The new environment, expectations, and crowd took a toll on his spirits. There were no quiet spaces where he could gather himself. His peers mocked him, adding to his challenges. The teachers, on the other hand, had no clue how to handle his academic needs. In addition, the teachers considered extra time and any other form of accommodation unethical and biased. During his school years, teachers were well acquainted with his abilities and provided him with support during instruction and assessment which the college teachers did not accept. Babar did survive in the challenging situation for two semesters before he decided to quit. At present, he is living at home with his parents and gets anxious as he thinks about his time spent in college.

Questions

1. How had Babar managed to get along in school with his autism?
2. How could his dropping out have been prevented?
3. How might one plan to secure the future of many others like Babar at universities?
4. What could teachers have done to support and retain Babar?
5. How could awareness about autism on the college campus have made a difference in this case?

REFERENCES

Aftab, R., Pirani, S., Mansoor, M., & Nadeem, T. (2023). Caregiver strain and its associated factors in Autism Spectrum Disorder in Karachi, Pakistan. *Journal of the College of Physicians and Surgeons—Pakistan*, *33*(7), 784–788. DOI: 0.29271/jcpsp.2023.07.784 PMID: 37401221

Ahmad, S., & Yousaf, M. (2011). Special education in Pakistan: Perspectives of educational policies and plans. *Academic Research International*, *1*(2), 228. http://www.savap.org.pk/journals/ARInt./Vol.1(2)/2011(1.2-21a).pdf

Ahmad, Z., Sanauddin, N., & Nawab, H. (2023). From hostage to host: The spirit possession, mediumship, and gender relations in Chitral, Pakistan. *Journal of Humanities. Social and Management Sciences*, *4*(1), 28–40. DOI: 10.47264/idea.jhsms/4.1.3

Ahmed, N., Pasha, A. R., & Malik, M. (2021). The role of teacher training programs in optimizing teacher motivation and professional development skills. *Bulletin of Education and Research,43*(2), 17-37. ISSN- 0555-7747. https://eric.ed.gov/?id=EJ1338294

Akhtar, S., Ahmed, A., Ahmad, A., Ali, Z., Riaz, M., & Ismail, T. (2013). Iron status of the Pakistani population: Current issues and strategies. *Asia Pacific Journal of Clinical Nutrition*, *22*(3), 340–347. DOI: 10.6133/apjcn.2013.22.3.17 PMID: 23945403

Ali, S. K., & Baig, L. A. (2012). Problems and issues in implementing an innovative curriculum in developing countries: The Pakistani experience. *BMC Medical Education*, *12*(1), 1–8. DOI: 10.1186/1472-6920-12-31 PMID: 22591729

Amin, N., Tariq, M., Arshad, M., & Cheema, M. A. (2024). Frequency of visual impairment in autistic children at an autism school in Lahore, Pakistan. *British Journal of Visual Impairment*, *42*(2), 478–485. DOI: 10.1177/02646196221145367

Asian Development Bank. (2024). *Pakistan and ADB*. Asian Development Bank. https://www.adb.org/countries/pakistan/main

Azeem, M. W., Imran, N., & Nazeer, A. (2021). Pakistan and autism. In *Encyclopedia of Autism Spectrum Disorders* (pp. 3260–3262). Springer International Publishing. DOI: 10.1007/978-3-319-91280-6_102029

Baker, D. L. (2011). *The politics of neurodiversity: Why people policy matters*. Lynne Rienner Publishers. DOI: 10.1515/9781685851224

Bashir, N., & Khanum, H. (2024). Autism in Pakistan: Understanding the challenges and seeking solutions. *Educational Research and Innovation*, *4*(1), 96–104. DOI: 10.61866/eri.v4i1.65

Batool, H., Khan, A. M., & Khanum, S. (2019). Evaluation of quality of life of parents having children with sensory disabilities. *Pakistan Journal of Humanities & Social Sciences Research*, *2*(2), 33–44. DOI: 10.37605/pjhssr.2.2.4

Boobis, S. (2016). *Evaluation of a dialogical psychologically informed environment (PIE) pilot: Addressing homelessness, re-offending, substance abuse, and mental illness*. Fulfilling Lives-Newcastle & Gateshead.

Bowman, K. S., Suarez, V. D., & Weiss, M. J. (2021). Standards for interprofessional collaboration in the treatment of individuals with autism. *Behavior Analysis in Practice*, *14*(4), 1191–1208. DOI: 10.1007/s40617-021-00560-0 PMID: 34868822

Braun, V., & Clarke, V. (2006). Using thematic analysis in psychology. *Qualitative Research in Psychology*, *3*(2), 77–101. DOI: 10.1191/1478088706qp063oa

Byrne, D. (2022). A worked example of Braun and Clarke's approach to reflexive thematic analysis. *Quality & Quantity*, *56*(3), 1391–1412. DOI: 10.1007/s11135-021-01182-y

Chadwick, D., Ågren, K. A., Caton, S., Chiner, E., Danker, J., Gómez-Puerta, M., Heitplatz, V., Johansson, S., Normand, C. L., Murphy, E., Plichta, P., Strnadová, I., & Wallén, E. F. (2022). Digital inclusion and participation of people with intellectual disabilities during COVID-19: A rapid review and international bricolage. *Journal of Policy and Practice in Intellectual Disabilities*, *19*(3), 242–256. DOI: 10.1111/jppi.12410

Choudhry, F. R., Khan, N., & Munawar, K. (2023). Barriers and facilitators to mental health care: A systematic review in Pakistan. *International Journal of Mental Health*, *52*(2), 124–162. DOI: 10.1080/00207411.2021.1941563

Dixon, A. (2023). *"I want to say that disabled people also want to live as human beings": Stigma experiences of women with disabilities in Pakistan* (Doctoral dissertation, University College London). UCL Discovery. https://discovery.ucl.ac.uk/id/eprint/10177028/

Doyle, N. (2020). Neurodiversity at work: A biopsychosocial model and the impact on working adults. *British Medical Bulletin*, *135*(1), 108–125. DOI: 10.1093/bmb/ldaa021 PMID: 32996572

Ejaz, N., & Mallawaarachchi, T. (2023). Disparities in economic achievement across the rural–urban divide in Pakistan: Implications for development planning. *Economic Analysis and Policy*, *77*, 487–512. DOI: 10.1016/j.eap.2022.11.023

Fraser Butlin, S. (2011). The UN Convention on the Rights of Persons with Disabilities: Does the Equality Act 2010 measure up to UK international commitments? *Industrial Law Journal*, *40*(4), 428–438. DOI: 10.1093/indlaw/dwr015

Furrukh, J., & Anjum, G. (2020). Coping with Autism Spectrum Disorder (ASD) in Pakistan: A phenomenology of mothers who have children with ASD. *Cogent Psychology*, *7*(1), 1728108. DOI: 10.1080/23311908.2020.1728108

Government of Pakistan, Ministry of Federal Education and Professional Training. (2018). *National education policy for persons with disabilities*. Government of Pakistan.

Government of Pakistan, Ministry of Federal Education and Professional Training. (2020). *Achievements in adult literacy*. Government of Pakistan.

Halder, S., & Squires, G. (2023). *Inclusion and diversity: Communities and practices across the world*. Routledge. DOI: 10.4324/9781003379034

Harrison, M., Rowlings, J., & Aivaliotis-Martinez, D. (2024). Supporting neurodivergent players. In *Press B to Belong* (pp. 65–77). Emerald Publishing Limited. DOI: 10.1108/978-1-80455-926-020241005

Heyer, K. (2015). *Rights enabled: The Disability Revolution, from the US, to Germany and. Japan, to the United Nations*. University of Michigan Press.

Higher Education Commission. (2021). *HEC policy for students with disabilities at higher education institutions in Pakistan*. Higher Education Commission of Pakistan.

Higher Education Commission. (2021). *Policy for students with disabilities at higher education institutions in Pakistan*. Higher Education Commission of Pakistan. https://www.hec.gov.pk/english/services/universities/pages/policy.aspx

Hussain, S., Alam, A., & Ullah, S. (2023). Persons with disabilities and the profession of social work in Pakistan: A review of literature. *Pakistan Journal of Society, Education and Language (PJSEL)*, *10*(1), 282–290. https://pjsel.jehanf.com/index.php/journal/article/view/1304

Hussain, S., Munir, A., & Ibrar, M. (2020). Children with disability: Problems and challenges in Pakistan. *Journal of the Humanities and Social Sciences*, *28*(1), 87–99. http://ojs.uop.edu.pk/jhss/article/view/387

Hussain, S., Shahzadi, U., & Khan, I. (2020). Challenges to learners with disabilities in higher education institutions in Pakistan: A review. [RJSSER]. *Research Journal of Social Sciences and Economics Review*, *1*(3), 12–19. DOI: 10.36902/rjsser-vol1-iss3-2020(12-19)

Imran, M., Oad, L., Jat, Z. G., Hafeez, A., & Sultana, Z. (2024). Enhancing support for slow learners evaluating inclusive education models in contemporary classrooms. *Research Journal for Societal Issues*, *6*(3), 156–177. DOI: 10.56976/rjsi.v6i3.268

Imran, N., Chaudry, M. R., Azeem, M. W., Bhatti, M. R., Choudhary, Z. I., & Cheema, M. A. (2011). A survey of autism knowledge and attitudes among healthcare professionals in Lahore, Pakistan. *BMC Pediatrics*, *11*(1), 1–6. DOI: 10.1186/1471-2431-11-107 PMID: 22107951

Inclusion. (2021). UNESCO. https://education-profiles.org/central-and-southern-asia/pakistan/~inclusion

Jamil, B. R. (2009, August). Curriculum reforms in Pakistan: A glass half full or half empty. In *Seminar on School Curriculum Policies and Practices in South Asian Countries* (pp. 10–12). NCERT., https://itacec.org/document/nep09/NCERT%20Pakistan%20paper%20BRJ.pdf

Jurgens, A. (2020). Neurodiversity in a neurotypical world: An enactive framework for investigating autism and social institutions. In Vecchi, D. J. (Ed.), *Neurodiversity studies: A new critical paradigm* (pp. 73–88). Routledge. DOI: 10.4324/9780429322297-8

Khalid, M., & Anjum, G. (2019). Use of remedial teaching approaches for dyslexic students: Experiences of remedial teachers working in urban Pakistan. *Cogent Psychology*, *6*(1), 1580181. Advance online publication. DOI: 10.1080/23311908.2019.1580181

Khan, N. H., Ju, Y., & Hassan, S. T. (2019). Investigating the determinants of human development index in Pakistan: An empirical analysis. *Environmental Science and Pollution Research International*, *26*(19), 19294–19304. DOI: 10.1007/s11356-019-05271-2 PMID: 31073836

Knox, K. (2024). Meeting the need of students and families: Adapting service delivery of Special Education Social Workers during a pandemic. *Children & Schools*, *46*(2), 107–116. DOI: 10.1093/cs/cdae002

Lai, , Anagnostou, E., Wiznitzer, M., Allison, C., & Baron-Cohen, S. (2020). Lai, M. C., Anagnostou, E., Wiznitzer, M., Allison, C., & Baron-Cohen, S. (2020). Evidence-based support for autistic people across the lifespan: Maximising potential, minimising barriers, and optimising the person–environment fit. *Lancet Neurology*, *19*(5), 434–451. DOI: 10.1016/S1474-4422(20)30034-X PMID: 32142628

Laxton, S., Moriarty, C., Sapiets, S., Hastings, R., & Totsika, V. (2024). Neighbourhood deprivation and access to early intervention and support for families of children with intellectual and developmental disabilities. *Journal of Policy and Practice in Intellectual Disabilities*, *21*(1), 1–10. DOI: 10.1111/jppi.12486

Lollini, A. (2021). Brain Equality: Legal Implication of Neurodiversity in a Comparative Perspective. *New York University Journal of International Law & Politics. New York University. International Law Society*, *51*, 70–133. http://hdl.handle.net/11585/817387

Marwat, A. (2023). Studying dyslexia and cognitive deficits in a global context to investigate learning difficulties in primary school students. *Journal of International Relations and Social Dynamics*, *2*(1), 1–10.

Muneeb, S. (2024). *Establishing the design space for educational technologies to support autistic children in the context of Pakistan* (Doctoral dissertation, Queensland University of Technology). Queensland University of Technology.

Najmi, S. (2021). *A communicative assessment of mental health literacy in Pakistan* (Master's thesis, Texas Southern University). Texas Southern University.

Naz, S., Majeed, Z., & Sulman, N. (2024). The challenges of accessibility and equity for students with disabilities in higher education institutions with special reference to the University of Karachi, Pakistan. *Siazga Research Journal*, *3*(3), 313–322. DOI: 10.58341/srj.v3i3.97

Nazim, A., & Khalid, R. (2019). Assessment of temperament in children with autism spectrum disorder. *JPMA. The Journal of the Pakistan Medical Association*, *69*(10), 1437–1441. DOI: 10.5455/JPMA.290521 PMID: 31622293

Neuman, W. L. (2011). *Social research methods: Qualitative and quantitative approaches* (7th ed.). Pearson.

Nisar, A., Bashir, I., & Naseem, A. (2023). Special needs students' lived experiences of support practices in higher educational institutes in Pakistan. *Journal of Asian Development Studies*, *12*(3), 1487–1497.

Nizamani, M. K., & Nizamani, A. (2022). Dyslexia: Emotional and psychological effects in relation to the social behavior of caretakers in Sindh, Pakistan. [LASSIJ]. *Liberal Arts and Social Sciences International Journal*, *6*(2), 43–62. DOI: 10.47264/idea.lassij/6.2.3

Noor, H., Khan, I. N., & Humara, B. (2023). Effectiveness of self-regulation training plan for the treatment of adolescents with Attention Deficit Hyperactivity Disorder *Pakistan Journal of Social Sciences, 43*(2),177-189. https://pjss.bzu.edu.pk/index.php/pjss/article/view/1254

Pakistan Bureau of Statistics. (2023). *Announcement of results of 7th Population and Housing Census–2023.* Pakistan Bureau of Statistics. https://www.pbs.gov.pk

Pakistan Curriculum. (2025). Department of Education and Knowledge, https://www.adek.gov.ae/en/Education-System/Private-Schools/Curriculum/Pakistani-Curriculum

Rahbar, M. H., Ibrahim, K., & Assassi, P. (2011). Knowledge and attitude of general practitioners regarding autism in Karachi, Pakistan. *Journal of Autism and Developmental Disorders, 41*(4), 465–474. DOI: 10.1007/s10803-010-1068-x PMID: 20632204

Rasheed, H., Hashmi, N. U., Bhutta, M. H., & Chaudhry, A. G. (2023). Social inclusion of persons with disabilities: A right-based approach. *Pakistan Islamacus: An International Journal of Islamic & Social Sciences, 3*(2), 426–441. https://www.pakistanislamicus.com/index.php/home/article/view/74

Rathore, F. A., New, P. W., & Iftikhar, A. (2011). A report on disability and rehabilitation medicine in Pakistan: Past, present, and future directions. *Archives of Physical Medicine and Rehabilitation, 92*(1), 161–166. DOI: 10.1016/j.apmr.2010.10.004 PMID: 21187218

Razzak, J. A., Hyder, A. A., Akhtar, T., Khan, M., & Khan, U. R. (2008). Assessing emergency medical care in low-income countries: A pilot study from Pakistan. *BMC Emergency Medicine, 8*(1), 8. Advance online publication. DOI: 10.1186/1471-227X-8-8 PMID: 18598353

Roy, R., & Jain, S. (2021). Global neurodiverse support systems: Primary research findings on key challenges and optimized solutions in Mumbai, India. *The Physician, 6*(3), 1–22. DOI: 10.38192/1.6.3.9

Shukat, S. (2023). Challenges for education of children with disabilities *in Pakistan. Intervention in School and Clinic, 59*(1), 75–80. DOI: 10.1177/10534512221130082

Sohn, M. A., Zhao, L. M., & Tadros, E. (2024). Integrating structural and experiential family therapy in neurodivergent families: A case study. *Issues in Mental Health Nursing, 45*(5), 477–487. DOI: 10.1080/01612840.2024.2328260 PMID: 38593465

Sultan, M. A., Closser, S., Majidulla, A., Ahmed, S., Naz, F., Nayyab, S., & Sohail, A. (2023). How to eradicate polio in Pakistan: Insights from community health workers. *PLOS Global Public Health, 3*(8), e0002289. DOI: 10.1371/journal.pgph.0002289 PMID: 37643151

Szulc, J. M., Davies, J., Tomczak, M. T., & McGregor, F. L. (2021). AMO perspectives on the well-being of neurodivergent human capital. *Employee Relations, 43*(4), 858–872. DOI: 10.1108/ER-09-2020-0446

Taj, R. (2015). Mental health in Pakistan. In Bhurga, D., Tse, S., Ng, R., & Takei, N. (Eds.), *Routledge handbook of psychiatry in Asia* (pp. 101–114). Routledge.

Tarhirkeli, H. (2022). Special education in Pakistan: Hope for children with special needs. *socialprotection.org.* https://socialprotection.org/discover/blog/special-education-pakistan-hope-children-special-needs-0

Tariq, N. (2021). Health care challenges in Pakistan. *Journal of Islamabad Medical & Dental College., 10*(4), 190–191. DOI: 10.35787/jimdc.v10i4.826

Tharwani, Z. H., Bilal, W., Khan, H. A., Kumar, P., Butt, M. S., Hamdana, A. H., Essar, M. Y., Nashwan, A. J., Habib, Z., & Marzo, R. R. (2023). Infant & child mortality in Pakistan and its determinants: A review. *Inquiry : a Journal of Medical Care Organization, Provision and Financing, 60*, 00469580231167024. Advance online publication. DOI: 10.1177/00469580231167024 PMID: 37085986

United States Department of Justice and Civil Rights Division. The American with Disabilities Act (2024). https://www.ada.gov/

Veesar, G. Y., Akhlaq, A., & Siddiqi, A. Q. (2023). The faces of deceptive healers: A scoping review of titles and traits associated with quacks across regions. *National Journal of Health Sciences, 8*(4), 203–211. DOI: 10.21089/njhs.84.0203

Warraich, A., Rauf, N. K., Ingersoll, D. S. S. B., & Khan, M. (2024). Exploring maternal perspectives on autism spectrum disorder in Pakistan: Communication, stigma, and intervention. *Remittances Review, 9*(4), 924-950. https://remittancesreview.com/menu-script/index.php/remittances/article/view/2197

Whelpley, C. E., Holladay-Sandidge, H. D., Woznyj, H. M., & Banks, G. C. (2023). The biopsychosocial model and neurodiversity: A person-centered approach. *Industrial and Organizational Psychology: Perspectives on Science and Practice, 16*(1), 25–30. DOI: 10.1017/iop.2022.95

ADDITIONAL READING

Ahmad, S., & Yousaf, M. (2011). Special education in Pakistan: Perspectives of educational policies and plans. *Academic Research International*, *1*(2), 228. http://www.savap.org.pk/journals/ARInt./Vol.1(2)/2011(1.2-21a).pdf

Dixon, A. (2023). *"I want to say that disabled people also want to live as human beings": Stigma experiences of women with disabilities in Pakistan* (Doctoral dissertation, University College London). UCL Discovery. https://discovery.ucl.ac.uk/id/eprint/10177028/

Higher Education Commission. (2021). *HEC policy for students with disabilities at higher education institutions in Pakistan*. Higher Education Commission.

Hussain, S., Munir, A., & Ibrar, M. (2020). Children with disability: Problems and challenges in Pakistan. *Journal of the Humanities and Social Sciences*, *28*(1), 87–99. http://ojs.uop.edu.pk/jhss/article/view/387

Rasheed, H., Hashmi, N. U., Bhutta, M. H., & Chaudhry, A. G. (2023). Social inclusion of persons with disabilities: A right-based approach. *Pakistan Islamacus: An International Journal of Islamic & Social Sciences, 3*(2), 426–441. https://www.pakistanislamicus.com/index.php/home/article/view/74

Whelpley, C. E., Holladay-Sandidge, H. D., Woznyj, H. M., & Banks, G. C. (2023). The biopsychosocial model and neurodiversity: A person-centered approach. *Industrial and Organizational Psychology: Perspectives on Science and Practice*, *16*(1), 25–30. DOI: 10.1017/iop.2022.95

Chapter 9
Building Neuroinclusive Campuses:
The NICE Program's Approach to Faculty Training

Roxanne Ross
https://orcid.org/0000-0003-0511-2389
University of Calgary, Canada

Heather Thompson
University of Calgary, Canada

Carly McMorris
University of Calgary, Canada

ABSTRACT

In this chapter, the authors highlight their efforts to advance neuroinclusivity at their institution through the development of a faculty and staff training program created in partnership with Neurodivergent students. Authors share the details of their program's design and implementation, weaving into their discussion two key frameworks guiding their practice, Universal Design for Learning (UDL) and Students as Partners (SaP). After illustrating their approach to teaching UDL alongside Neurodivergent students' lived experiences, they provide their adaptation of SaP approaches to ensure a neuro-affirming workplace for student partners. The chapter concludes with recommendations for developing and sustaining neurodiversity campus-wide training for faculty and staff.

DOI: 10.4018/979-8-3693-8920-1.ch009

INTRODUCTION

In recent decades, innovations in assessment, diagnosis, and accessibility have led to a significant increase in the number of Neurodivergent individuals pursuing higher education. In 2024, 15% of graduating students surveyed across Canadian universities identified as Neurodivergent (Canadian University Survey Consortium, 2024). Although Neurodivergent individuals have the academic abilities to excel in postsecondary education, many face significant barriers and challenges that impact their success (Anderson et al., 2017). These challenges are not solely due to their neurodiversity, but rather to limited available programs or supports, restrictions with accessibility, stigma, and an environment that fails to meet the unique needs of Neurodivergent students (Cage et al., 2020). Recent literature highlights the need for a system-wide approach that promotes inclusion of Neurodivergent students, staff and faculty in higher education, and to do so, researchers have recommended campus-wide neurodiversity training, and the implementation of neuro-affirming supports and programs (Dwyer et al., 2023). Neurodiversity training has been shown to foster more inclusive attitudes toward Neurodivergent students and a unified understanding of neuro-affirming pedagogical and programming approaches (Waisman et al., 2023). Despite this, the adoption of neuro-affirming approaches in higher education has progressed slowly. In this chapter, we outline the theory, development and implementation of the Neurodiversity Inclusive Campus Experience (NICE) workshop series. We detail the program's development with Neurodivergent student partners and the role of integrated Universal Design for Learning (UDL) and Students as Partners' (SaP) approaches. We conclude with recommendations and case examples to illustrate the breadth and potential impact of a collaborative approach to campus-wide training.

NEURODIVERSITY AND HIGHER EDUCATION

While the number of Neurodivergent students pursuing postsecondary education is increasing, Neurodivergent students experience several disability and accommodation related challenges (Clouder et al., 2020). These include co-occurring challenges with mental health (anxiety and depression), sensory sensitivities, difficult social relationships, changes in environment, and executive functioning demands (e.g., time management, planning, flexibility), that can impede success in higher education (van Hees, et al., 2015; Waisman & Alba, 2022). These individual challenges can also be exacerbated by a lack of available supports/programs (Ames et al., 2022) coupled with complicated processes for accessing them. Stigma and prejudice of fellow students, staff and faculty (Dwyer et al., 2023) also play a role all while

Neurodivergent students try to navigate a significant transition into adulthood. As a result, Neurodivergent students often report feeling disconnected, socially excluded, and misunderstood in higher education (Cage et al., 2020), contributing to either the onset or worsening of mental health symptoms, academic difficulties, and ultimately failure to graduate.

To improve retention rates of Neurodivergent students in higher education, there has been an emphasis on enhancing supports to meet their academic and non-academic needs. While this approach is valuable and effective, recently researchers and advocates have emphasized the importance of enhancing the postsecondary environment to be more neuroinclusive. Indeed, Dwyer et al. (2023) recommended system-wide training for faculty, staff and students to increase the knowledge and improve attitudes toward Autistic students in higher education, ultimately reducing stigma toward Neurodivergent students. This training would aim to cultivate more inclusive attitudes toward neurodiversity on campuses, creating an environment where Neurodivergent students feel empowered and safe to seek support whenever needed. This is particularly important as emerging evidence highlights that many Neurodivergent students in higher education do not disclose their diagnosis due to fear of judgement and negative consequences following disclosure to staff or faculty (Frost et al., 2019). This poses a challenge, as most higher education support services require a formal diagnosis to be accessed.

To date, two studies exist that have examined the benefits of offering neurodiversity trainings to staff and students. Seminal work by Waisman et al. (2023) demonstrated the value of providing an online autism and universal design training for faculty. In this study, faculty's autism knowledge, stigma, and attitudes toward universal design improved and were maintained up to one month following the training. Gillespie-Lynch et al. (2015) demonstrated a similar change in knowledge and attitudes on autism of neuromajority postsecondary students. Despite these promising findings and the frequent calls for neuro-inclusive campuses, there has been a slow shift in higher education settings to incorporate neuro-inclusive policies and practices. This requires greater awareness of Neurodivergent learner differences and an understanding of ways to make learning environments and student services programs more neuro-affirming.

BUILDING A NEURO-AFFIRMING CAMPUS THROUGH PROFESSIONAL DEVELOPMENT

In response to calls for a university-wide approach to inclusive campuses informed by principles of Universal Design for Learning (UDL) and Students as Partners (SaP), we worked alongside Neurodivergent students to develop the Neurodivergent

Immersive Campus Experience (NICE) workshop series for postsecondary faculty and staff. The series aims to facilitate participants' learning about neurodiversity as well as provide practical Universal Design strategies that are supportive for *all* students. Below we provide a brief scholarly overview of our two guiding frameworks, UDL and SaP, followed by an outline of the workshop series. We then turn to a detailed discussion of our practice, illustrating our integration of UDL and SaP throughout the program's design and implementation.

Universal Design for Learning

In designing the workshop series, our approach was significantly guided by Universal Design for Learning (UDL) principles. Emerging from the introduction of Universal Design and the design of physical and digital spaces to universally meet the needs of as many users as possible (Story et al., 1998), UDL is a teaching and learning framework aimed at increasing access for *all* learners by designing learning environments that honor and anticipate learner variation (Cumming & Rose, 2022). Established by the Center for Applied Special Technology (CAST, n.d.), UDL is grounded in neuroscience and learning sciences research. The framework focuses on designing flexibility into educational environments to respond to various and naturally occurring differences in the ways learners understand and process information (representation), express knowledge and strategically plan learning activities (action and expression) and engage in learning (engagement) (CAST, n.d.).

The principle of *multiple means of representation* encourages educators to consider ways in which information is shared, ensuring learning materials are accessible in a variety of modalities (e.g., audiovisual and written). *Multiple means of engagement* practices emphasize supporting students in finding meaning in learning while also creating a welcoming and comfortable space to learn. Lastly, the UDL framework advocates for *multiple means of action and expression,* stressing the importance of providing learners with various opportunities to communicate and express their knowledge. In addition, promoting ways in which educators can scaffold how learners plan and break down learning tasks strategically is a key part of this principle.

The most recent update of UDL, *Universal Design for Learning Guidelines 3.0*, launched in fall 2024 has included an expanded research base "to address critical barriers rooted in biases and systems for exclusion for learners with or without disabilities" (CAST, n.d., para. 5). The renewed guidelines demonstrate an expanded focus on the importance of honoring identity and multiple ways of knowing and more overtly position UDL as a key tool in broadly enhancing equity in education across students' intersectional identities (CAST, 2024).

Although applications of UDL are not currently widespread in higher education, particularly when compared to K-12 education systems, UDL approaches are frequently recommended in current research related to enhancing both the inclusivity of postsecondary education (Tobin & Behling, 2018) as well as supporting student wellbeing (Lindsay et al., 2022; Fovet, 2020). Recent studies engaging Neurodivergent participants have highlighted the strong alignment of UDL's focus on flexibility and the honoring of learner variation with neurodiversity and neuro-affirming campus initiatives (Accardo et al., 2024; Waisman et al., 2023).

Research demonstrating that UDL approaches enhance learning outcomes within higher education is currently limited (Cumming & Rose, 2022). However, we align with Waisman and colleagues (2023) in their assessment that the need for more formal research does not discount UDL as a promising practice. Early research demonstrates high student satisfaction (Cumming & Rose, 2022) and increases in emotional and cognitive engagement (Durgungoz & Durgungoz, 2025) in response to UDL applications in higher education. This, combined with the way the framework has strongly resonated with our Neurodivergent student partners, has made UDL a powerful lens with which to talk about ways to create neuro-inclusive university environments.

Students as Partners and Co-Creators

In addition to UDL, the development and implementation of our workshop program is grounded in a Students as Partners (SaP) model (Healey et al., 2014). SaP approaches engage students to work alongside faculty/staff to support pedagogical enhancements in higher education (Mercer-Mapstone et al., 2017). Partnerships between students and staff aspire to engage members in "reciprocal learning" (Healey et al., 2014. p.15) whereby each party brings unique and "essential expertise" (Mercer-Mapstone et al., 2017, p. 14). In addition to *reciprocity*, SaP models emphasize *respect,* the valuing of all partners' perspectives and a shared *responsibility* for teaching and learning by introducing the notion that students take on "some of the responsibility for pedagogy" and "faculty share some responsibility for learning" (Cook-Sather et al., 2014, p.5).

Critiques of SaP approaches have queried the efficacy of creating truly equal partnerships in traditionally hierarchical education systems (Mercer-Mapstone et al., 2017). Other scholars have pointed out that as a novel and unfamiliar way of working in postsecondary education, co-creation can be challenging for both student and staff/faculty participants (Lubicz-Nawrocka & Bovil, 2023). However, Lubicz-Nawrocka and Bovil (2023) also found that in a "trusting environment" (p. 1752) students involved in co-creation projects engaged in risks leading to deeper engagement and reported experiencing greater connection to community through relational interactions with staff and peers. In addition, Cook-Sather (2018) found that SaP approaches were supportive in helping postsecondary equity-deserving students develop an increased sense of agency. Importantly, neurodiversity scholarship also places a heavy emphasis on the importance of partnership with Neurodivergent students (Durgungoz & Durgungoz, 2025; Waisman et al., 2023) in neurodiversity research and program development. Participatory co-creative processes have been demonstrated to be more effective in the development of professional development programs (Waisman et al., 2023) and essential to countering systemic ableism (Pena et al. 2020). Similarly, in the development and implementation of NICE, partnering with Neurodivergent students has been an essential value of the program. Prior to illustrating the ways in which UDL and SaP are embedded within our program implementation, we first turn to an overview of the NICE workshop series.

THE NICE WORKSHOP SERIES: A NEURODIVERGENT STUDENT PERSPECTIVE

The first iteration of the NICE workshop series was developed in 2022 by a collaborative team of student affairs professionals and Neurodivergent students who were employed as NICE mentors. Using a social-ecological lens (Chapman, 2021), the series is designed for educators (e.g., course instructors, teaching assistants) and university staff (e.g., student services, counselling and advising staff) and focuses on strategies to better support the diverse learning needs of *all* postsecondary students, including those who identify as Neurodivergent. By sharing the experiences of Neurodivergent students more directly, the workshops also aim to reduce negative assumptions that NICE mentors and the literature tell us can be experienced by Neurodivergent people due to lack of understanding (Butcher & Lane, 2024). The series, titled A Neurodivergent Student Perspective, includes three 60-minute workshops: Teaching and Advising, Creating a Sensory-Friendly Environment and Navigating the University. Beginning in January 2023, workshops have been regularly delivered in each fall and winter term in both online and in-person formats and promoted through our university event channels. To date, the program has delivered 63 workshops and hosted 387 participants from across our institution.

Developing the Workshops

The initial year of workshop development began as a collaboration between staff members from our university wellness and academic support services, each with long time experience working alongside Neurodivergent students. As a first step, staff collectively recruited and hired paid student staff as NICE mentors. Staff approached hiring with a shared understanding of the value of neurodivergence self-identification and were open to hiring students who were themselves Neurodivergent or who had some life experience interacting with Neurodivergent people. However, all three NICE mentors hired identified as Neurodivergent.

Over the next four months, staff and NICE mentors met together as a cohort and individually for the purposes of developing and refining the workshop series. As a lead into discussing neuro-affirming environments, staff initially supplied the group with information on neurodiversity and the UDL framework. Mentors were invited to share their thoughts on these approaches as well as their perspectives on barriers in the postsecondary environment for Neurodivergent students. Staff provided students with multiple opportunities and means to participate in group meetings to generate, categorize and share their thoughts. Through iterative discussions, NICE mentors led the way on generating key themes. Topics arose organically, emerging out of students' shared conversations and personal experiences.

In addition, both staff and mentors took part in locating resources to augment lived experience and support the development of workshop content. The resources considered ranged from recorded videos of lived experiences, grey literature on strategies for creating neuro-affirming environments and scholarly research. After determining workshop themes and related content, each NICE mentor took ownership over creating an initial draft of one workshop. Mentors chose workshop topics based on what they felt was closest to their own experience.

Workshop drafts were shared and edited through an iterative and collaborative process during group and individual meetings ensuring mentors had the benefit of receiving feedback from both peers and staff.

Hands-on, interactive activities were collectively generated and woven throughout sessions to support participant learning and application. As a final step in the creation of the three initial workshops, the academic support services staff member, as the NICE program coordinator, edited and collated all the slides and activities into accessible templates. After a series of practice presentation sessions, the NICE mentors presented the pilot series in the winter of 2023. During each presentation, NICE mentors were supported by a designated staff member, who helped with room set up and co-facilitation of workshop questions.

Following this first development phase, workshops have been updated and revised each semester. Both new and continuing NICE mentors are invited into a similar collaborative process to revise workshop content based on staff and existing mentors' reflections, participant feedback and the fresh perspectives of new mentors. Below, we briefly describe the components of the workshop series.

Session 1: Teaching and Advising: A Neurodivergent Student Perspective

The Teaching and Advising workshop focuses on the potential challenges that classroom and advising environments can pose for Neurodivergent students. Examples of possible barriers based on NICE mentors' collective experiences and scholarship are provided to participants via short scenarios. In particular, the session highlights various ways that learning environments can be taxing on those with executive function differences in the areas of working memory, focus, task organization, forecasting, and communication (Conference Board of Canada, 2024; Durgungoz & Durgungoz, 2025). Workshop facilitators encourage participants to reflect on the complexities of commonplace postsecondary activities such as interacting with course outlines, registering for academic courses or communicating in office hours in the context of these potential challenges. This is followed by specific strategies for creating inclusive learning environments such as strategies for delivering information in varied formats, building in information processing time during interactions, and helping learners break down tasks.

Session 2: Creating a Sensory-friendly Environment: A Neurodivergent Student Perspective

The Creating a Sensory-Friendly Environment workshop offers an overview of sensory processing and how students may manage and respond to sensory information in various ways in a university environment. Participants are presented with different scenarios to illustrate sensory challenges and are provided with options on how they might adjust various settings to respond to students' needs. These suggestions derive from NICE mentors' experiences and current research examining typical sensory conditions in postsecondary spaces. These include, where possible, providing flexible lighting, adjustable volume levels and seating options as well as supporting students with advanced information on what they can expect from various environments across campus (Osifo & Terashima, 2024). Participants are also provided an opportunity to engage with video activities that share lived experiences of sensory overload, along with key neuro-affirming strategies for supporting students in these moments.

Session 3: Navigating the University: A Neurodivergent Student Perspective

This session offers insight more broadly into Neurodivergent students' experiences navigating the university environment by exploring common situations that students encounter such as finding classrooms, connecting with resources, managing university processes, asking questions in class, and getting to know their professors. While admittedly there is some overlap within this session with workshops 1 and 2, the focus of this workshop is on the various unique and collective impacts that navigating university may have on Neurodivergent students' wellbeing and success with the aim of challenging higher education's assumption that one size fits all. As with all workshops, recommendations from a UDL lens are provided to attendees, such as strategies for helping students locate and access information and learn what to expect prior to engaging in different university settings.

Theory to Practice: Applications of UDL and SaP

The NICE program provides a contextualized example of the ways in which UDL and SaP can be meaningfully applied to the development and implementation of a faculty and staff training program designed to support neuro-inclusion. Below, we share our practical applications of these frameworks embedded with the workshops and overall program.

Integrating UDL Principles within the Workshops

One of the realities of many postsecondary environments, including our current context, is that faculty familiarity with UDL principles remains limited (Cumming & Rose, 2022; Hills et al., 2022). Given that estimates of UDL faculty adoption in higher education is less than 10% (Tobin & Behling, 2018), it is highly likely that many of us have also not experienced UDL as learners. Therefore, one important learning outcome of the workshop series is to provide participants a UDL learning experience. Studies with higher education faculty have also illuminated issues related to the amount of time UDL takes to implement (Hills et al., 2022). Modelling UDL practices within each workshop also helps to demystify the time and energy used to implement UDL principles. To shed light on how we embed UDL throughout the workshop series, we share a few examples of the strategies we use for providing workshop attendees with multiple means of engagement, representation and expression. One caveat is that we truly adopt UDL as a "mindset" (Tobin & Behling, 2018, p.48), and therefore, our approach to UDL in our facilitation practices continues to be iterative, as we grow our shared understanding of the diversity of student learning experiences and the varied participants from across campus that attend the workshop program.

Multiple Means of Engagement: Supporting a Variety of Ways to Connect with Learners. Considering multiple means of engagement, we have focused our efforts on creating a welcoming and neuro-affirming environment that aims to provide participants with flexibility in how they engage in activities. To reduce potential anxiousness and create predictability, we send registrants a warm email the day prior to each workshop, sharing the location of the session and an introduction to the presenter(s) and the topics that will be covered along with the types of interactions and activities that will be included. In-person workshop spaces are arranged with soft lighting and sensory tools are available on each table for participants to use if they choose.

To provide attendees with a chance to connect with material more personally, we have aimed to develop content in relatable ways (e.g., student stories). Time for reflection and application to one's own context is built in throughout the session. Space to reflect is also critical in each session as we recognize that for some who are new to conversations of neurodiversity, workshop content has the potential to challenge deeply held beliefs about ways of learning and being in higher education. To facilitate participants' comfort and reduce fears of being asked to participate without preparation, we include and normalize explicit options for ways to engage throughout the session (e.g., reflect on your own or with someone beside you). While opportunities for sharing and group conversation are provided and encouraged in each session, we let participants know at the onset of each workshop that we will be present afterwards for anyone who would like to share their thoughts or ask questions individually.

Multiple Means of Representation: Sharing Information in Varied Ways. As mentioned above, workshop content is presented in a variety of modalities including story, images and captioned video. Where captions are not included for externally produced videos, transcripts are provided to participants in advance of the session. Beyond incorporating multiple presentations of information, guided by the revised UDL 3.0 guidelines (CAST, 2024), we also aim to include images and student profiles that honor diverse identities representative of our student population.

As clarifying vocabulary is another essential feature of knowledge representation in the UDL framework (CAST, 2024), we spend time at the onset of each workshop defining neurodiversity and various related terms. While these definitions are core to the content learning goals of each session, we strive to go beyond merely stating definitions. We create space for participants to first connect new terminology to any prior understandings they may have and invite discussion. This is then followed by defining terms through multiple presentations. For example, when presenting the term neurodiversity, we may begin with a video and reflection question (e.g., what surprised you if anything?). Participants are then engaged in a short optional discussion followed by a summary definition along with a visual representation.

Multiple Means of Action and Expression: Providing Varied Opportunities to Structure Tasks and Share Knowledge. As multiple means of action and expression encourages us as practitioners to "vary and honour the methods of response, navigation and movement" (CAST, 2024, para. 7), we have been intentional in embedding a variety of participation and response options throughout the workshop series. For instance, sessions are offered in both online and in-person modalities and participants can opt to take sessions in any order. Overlapping with engagement, we are also intentional about letting participants know that various forms of participation are valid and welcome (e.g., reflective listening, working alone or individually or sharing verbally with the group or privately with the facilitator after the session).

To scaffold the strategic learning component within the action and expression principle, we share our learning goals at the beginning of each session and design activities that engage participants in applications of content to real-life scenarios. This might include generating the steps in a common student process such as registering for courses or reviewing a sample course outline through a neuro-affirming lens with the goal of pointing out strengths and potential areas for enhancements. Facilitating a UDL experience for participants in each workshop highlights tangible universal design features in ways that inspire reflection on UDL applications to their own teaching and learning contexts.

UDL from a Neurodivergent Student Perspective

One of the ways we have found to present UDL in a way that is relatable and true to our growing understanding of Neurodivergent student needs has been to intentionally connect student stories of learning to UDL strategies. Beginning first by engaging with authentic Neurodivergent student experiences, we as program staff and mentors used this as an entry point to developing our approach to presenting UDL throughout the workshop series. Articulating focused challenges and strengths of Neurodivergent learners helped us to select UDL strategies that we collectively felt would be most impactful for supporting student learning and inclusion. The presentation of UDL within the workshop series mirrors this process by pairing specific UDL applications with examples of students' learning experiences. In Navigating the University Environment and Teaching and Advising Students, for instance, we present a number of student snapshots highlighting learning differences that may be experienced by a Neurodivergent learner. In essence, these snapshots represent composites of NICE mentors' personal experiences as well as program staff experiences working alongside Neurodivergent students within the NICE program. By providing relatable student snapshots, we aim to support participants' awareness of the variety of learners' challenges and strengths while at the same time set the context for the introduction of purposeful UDL approaches responsive to the needs of the learners in the snapshots.

For example, in our Teaching and Advising Students workshop session, we highlight a student who finds it challenging to identify the steps involved in an assignment that is presented in a paragraph description of big picture outcomes. We then offer a number of UDL-based strategies that might support this learner such as providing a breakdown of the steps involved in the assignment, a checklist detailing the tasks involved to complete the assignment or an optional templated version of the assignment to help students begin a draft. Not only has this approach enabled us to focus our workshop content on instructional strategies that NICE mentors attest are neuro-affirming, but we also find more personalized student snapshots have the added benefit of increasing participant interest and the relatability of UDL, which staff and faculty can find overwhelming in higher education settings (Cumming & Rose, 2022).

Although presenting UDL through the lens of students' experiences has been a helpful strategy, it is important to note that we approach the creation and presentation of student snapshots with great care. As with UDL's guiding philosophy, we have aimed to position student snapshots in ways that highlight the "barrier in the design, not the learner" (Sanjah et al., 2024, 9:34). In addition, we have been intentional about taking a strengths-based approach, referencing potentially unacknowledged strengths alongside felt barriers in neuromajority learning contexts. Lastly, care has been taken to respect NICE mentors' decisions on disclosure in the context of storytelling (Pena et al., 2020). Given that students are the primary presenters of each workshop, our strategy has been to create de-identified and composite student snapshots as well as incorporate video content. This has allowed us to honor a variety of Neurodivergent student experiences while also ensuring that presenters themselves do not feel obliged to share personal stories with audiences.

Being Explicit about Sensory Differences

Although research is limited surrounding the prevalence of sensory differences and their impact on Neurodivergent postsecondary students' experiences (Clince et al., 2016), more recent studies have demonstrated that postsecondary environments can pose a variety of sensory processing challenges (Dwyer et al., 2023; Nolan et al., 2023). Nolan et al. (2023) defined sensory processing as the way in which we "receive and interpret . . . information through our senses, which enables us to engage in our daily occupations such as eating, dressing, learning, working and socialising" (p. 367). Drawing on Dunn's (1997, as cited in Nolan et al., 2023) framework of sensory preferences which identified a range of sensory differences including high sensitivity and avoidance to low sensitivity registration and sensation seeking, Nolan et al. (2023) surveyed the sensory preferences of 150 students with disabilities. Results identified challenges that limited students' ability to learn and participate on campus ranging from harsh lighting and noise to crowded spaces and lack of clear wayfinding information. Likewise, we have been privileged to enhance our understanding of university environmental impacts on sensory processing differences from firsthand experiences shared by NICE Mentors.

While the UDL framework does not contain a detailed focus on the managing of sensory processing differences (Creaven, 2024), in the development of the workshop series, we consider this to be a critical component of engagement in terms of creating a welcoming space that seeks to minimize threats (CAST, 2024) within the learning environment. As such, raising awareness of the various ways that Neurodivergent students may be impacted by common sensory conditions found in postsecondary settings has played a significant role in the workshop series. In all workshops, we introduce terminology related to sensory-friendly environments, in addition to hosting a dedicated workshop on the topic.

Given that the inability to locate comfortable sensory spaces could impact students' opportunities to study and in extreme cases cause students to leave campus altogether (Nolan et al., 2023), building workshop participants' awareness of the varied ways that students can experience sensory input is critical to engaging in conversations about creating more flexible and inclusive sensory environments. In the sensory-friendly workshop in particular, we provide opportunities for participants to reflect on how they might introduce sensory-friendly options in their own settings such as the possibility of using adjustable or lower lighting, providing movement breaks or encouraging the use of sensory tools or offering access to breakout spaces for large events. Most importantly, this workshop has aimed to support participants to acknowledge sensory needs (both their own and those of learners) and to normalize options for meeting those needs. This is particularly important in spaces where we have less control over the sensory components of our environment such as a crowded lecture hall. For instance, acknowledging that lighting might not be ideal for everyone and normalizing the wearing of hats or sunglasses is one example. Additionally, we might provide clarity at the beginning of a longer class time, when breaks will occur. Openly encouraging students to reflect on and use aids to support them in learning during the session (e.g., doodling, using sensory tools, or noise mitigating earplugs) can help to foster a more inclusive space where sensory differences are acknowledged and explicitly considered.

Building Partnerships for a Neuro-Affirming Campus

Given the impacts of non-inclusive postsecondary environments on Neurodivergent students in relation to belonging, wellbeing and social engagement, building upon connections that are made with workshop participants from across campus has been key to growing UDL awareness as well as beginning to make tangible changes within our university context. In many ways, the workshop series has served as a catalyst to relationships and the development of shared goals. While the small group setting and relational approach to instruction that we have fostered aims to support the building of relationships, making time for individual conversations following sessions and broadening our content to be inclusive to a wide variety of staff and faculty audiences have also been important strategies. This has facilitated a broader reach of the program, sparking collaborative initiatives with colleagues across the university. These have included work to expand sensory-friendly options for our campus orientation programming, the introduction of Neurodivergent student support programming within faculties and dedicated training for faculty advising and student services offices.

As we begin to work with others in context, we have recognized the need for more iterative and nuanced conversations. This relational work requires a caring and attuned approach, developing an understanding of context and fostering conversations that facilitate shifts in "minds and practices" (Black & Fraser, 2019, p.248). In their work on establishing faculty partnerships in the context of UDL, Black and Fraser identify "five shifts in thinking" (2019, p. 249) several of which are helpful in the context of developing neuro-affirming initiatives more broadly across campus. They describe the process of "listening for shifts" in conversations as possible "entry point[s] to challenge thinking and offer a new way of looking at the situation" (p. 254).

In working with campus colleagues outside of faculty roles, two important shifts identified by Black and Fraser, shifts from "a medical to a social view of disability" (p. 249) and moving from "response to design" (p.249), have been most helpful in thinking about the ways in which we can create flexible engagement opportunities as part of the design process rather than providing accommodation responses once a program is launched. In the example of the orientation programming mentioned above, this has taken the form of building in a variety of sensory options for students to participate in programs ranging from providing ways to access content online, offering sunglasses and earplugs to students when attending a large-scale event and identifying sensory-friendly spaces where students can retreat during the day if feeling overloaded. This mindset acknowledged sensory variability at the design stage, rather than waiting for individual students to come forward to request accommodations or risk student pre-arrival anxiety about whether their needs can be met. In working with orientation student services partners, we were able to facilitate a sense of predictability and demonstrate care for Neurodivergent students during their initial engagement with the university.

Engaging Neurodivergent Students as Partners (SaP): Embedding SaP

A SaP approach has been instrumental to our development of the workshop series, in that each aspect of development has been co-created with NICE mentors. Partnership with NICE mentors ensures that workshop content honors the lived experience of Neurodivergent students and promotes change to university environments that are deemed meaningful by the people they are meant to support. As shared above, a SaP approach entails intention to actively create ways of working that are based on a trusting relationship. Although as student affairs staff, we had had experience co-creating with students on other projects, adapting this approach to ensure our ways of working with Neurodivergent students were also neuro-affirming was a critical part of our process. Below we describe how we blended SaP as a theory and practice with neuroinclusive ways of working in our partnership with NICE mentors.

Neuro-affirming Recruitment and Onboarding Practices

An important part of the NICE program is to ensure we have a welcoming, neuro-affirming, and accessible environment where NICE mentors feel they can be their true selves. Attention to this goal began with the recruitment and hiring process. We used plain language in preparing the job advertisement and encouraged students to talk with the NICE coordinator to learn more about the role prior to applying. The posting was included on our institution's central student job board and NICE staff also informed students engaged in our Neurodivergent student support programs about the opportunity. For those students who applied, we provided options for candidates to meet in a sensory-friendly environment or online and provided the interview questions in advance as well as a detailed description of what to expect in the interview.

Although we created a job profile indicating a number of job activities and designated hours, we let students know that these were flexible, and that we were interested in learning more about the ways they felt they could best contribute as a NICE mentor. Flexibility regarding the tasks NICE mentors might perform ranged from involvement in workshop development to co-presenting workshops with staff and/or other NICE mentors to taking on a role as a full facilitator. We also collaborated with each candidate to determine a comfortable number of weekly working hours ranging from three to ten. This approach proved to be important as some students initially interested in the role were tentative to apply, excited by the opportunity but unsure they could participate due to their own learning needs.

Building Relationships and Modeling Neuro-affirming Attitudes

To establish a trusting environment for co-creation, shift away from traditional staff/student hierarchies and support NICE mentors in doing their best work, we established several relational practices. The NICE coordinator hosted regular meetings with each NICE mentor to support mentors' sense of belonging and connection. In approaching relationship building within these meetings, we recognized that mentors, as Neurodivergent students, may have had less positive workplace and educational experiences or faced negative comparisons to their peers which might cause them to feel the need to hide or mask (Miller et al., 2021) their true selves. To support mentors in being their whole selves during these interactions, the NICE coordinator held explicit conversations about neurodiversity and shared the NICE program goals of learning from their expertise and working together to build more neuro-affirming spaces on campus. In addition, the NICE coordinator engaged mentors in conversations about workstyle and sensory preferences. Having discussions that foster ways to identify strengths and increase sense of self, while supporting NICE mentors' wellbeing, particularly with regards to experiences of shame or embarrassment, help to establish an environment that promotes the concept that it is okay to be who we are.

Establishing partnerships that reduce hierarchies and encourage co-creation also rely on adopting a position as learner in our professional roles, explicitly presenting ourselves as not always knowing the answers or being infallible of making mistakes. We adopted an open approach to program development and ways of working in which we were not imposing a predetermined notion of perfection. We also regularly invited feedback from mentors regarding what they felt was and wasn't working well. This aimed to create opportunities for us to collaboratively build options for NICE mentors to take on roles that they felt suited to, helping them build confidence and engage in decision-making. While these practices involved a significant time commitment, they were vital to building trusted, authentic partnerships and fostering reciprocal learning.

Fostering Community and Collaborative Ways of Working

Developing an engaged community has also been an essential part of our SaP approach within the NICE program. In addition to individual meetings with mentors, the NICE coordinator held working meetings that brought NICE mentors and professional staff together regularly. Working meetings were structured to explain the meeting outcome at the onset. This was followed by fifteen minutes of dedicated time for individuals to brainstorm verbally with a partner or on their own, engage in quiet reflection or craft mind maps or visuals. Mentors were then invited to come back together to share their insights and findings. Setting up the meetings in this way aimed to support mentors in understanding the meeting goals and provide individuals with dedicated time to gather and share their thoughts. We found that this method helped mentors to get to know each other's strengths and interests, gain familiarity with individual differences in approaches to work and ultimately enhance their skills of working together as a team while respecting and negotiating different workstyles.

It is in these meetings that mentors collectively determined the direction of the workshops as well as which workshop project they would each take responsibility for drafting. Engaging mentors fully and collectively in decision-making was intentional. Working meetings as a practice enabled us to weave an open, honest, and caring community, which we observed helped students to gain confidence in participating in a leadership role that they may not have even contemplated prior.

Providing Opportunities to Practice and Discuss

While our partnership model had mentors lead in many areas of workshop development, we also built in flexible supports throughout the process. This included creating spaces to process ideas and develop collaborative timelines. Creating collaborative timelines rather than imposing deadlines aimed to reduce challenges and time pressures for students while at the same time providing an agreed upon structure.

Having Neurodivergent mentors facilitate the workshops for faculty and staff is an incredibly powerful, yet potentially anxiety-inducing experience. As we moved closer to delivering the workshop series, we wanted to ensure mentors had a strong sense of support and grounding from staff partners. To achieve this, we held individual meetings with NICE mentors to generate approaches to facilitating their session. This was also a time to talk more privately about questions relating to disclosure and personal sharing in their mentor role as a presenter. We have continued to adopt the approach to disclosure advocated by Pena et al. (2020) in that we wanted to ensure "collaborators have control over their disclosure narratives" (p. 240). We talked with students about what they may or may not want to share and brainstormed ways to more confidentially share their own or fellow mentors' first-person Neurodivergent student experiences. In addition, meetings provided a tangible way to check in on project timelines and identify interim dates to ensure processes were moving forward.

Multiple opportunities to practice delivering sessions and receive feedback were also a key scaffold for mentors. Workshop simulations gave mentors a chance to present first one-on-one with the program staff, then with other mentors, and finally in a small group setting with workshop participants. In our experience, the one-on-one presentation opportunity was important in assisting students in gaining the confidence to present for a faculty and staff audience. The NICE coordinator modeled asking questions that may come up and talked through possible approaches for responding. Given that a program staff member attended every session, mentors also developed a private signal to allow staff to know that the student would like extra facilitation support at that point in the session. While all these activities required a large investment of time by the NICE coordinator, in our experience the result was that mentors demonstrated a tremendous amount of confidence and skill in co-creating and leading workshops, skills that will undoubtedly support them in future employment positions.

Program Outcomes

Although we have plans to conduct more formal evaluation of the NICE workshop series, up to this point we have engaged in an ongoing process of reflective practice, including regularly debriefing and adjusting workshop content and approaches. As staff members who are present at all workshops, we have the opportunity to witness firsthand how workshop attendees respond to session content. In this section, we highlight our general observations as practitioners.

Increased Awareness of Neurodiversity

One of the most frequent comments made by participants in sessions and included in our voluntary feedback form is that they experienced an increased understanding of neurodiversity as a concept. Attendees also provided feedback on the value of the contextualized, lived experiences that are included in the workshops, linking them directly to supporting their new or growing awareness of the obstacles that postsecondary settings can pose for Neurodivergent students. Occasionally, attendees demonstrated an increased self-awareness, articulating a new understanding of a barrier that they themselves had experienced in response to the workshop content. Although we have yet to formally measure the rate of increased awareness and its connection to participants' attitudes, within the conversations that arise in each workshop, there is often a shared recognition of new understanding and/or ways of thinking about neurodiversity and learner differences.

Bridging to Application

Even more promising is the way in which the questions asked by participants demonstrate real-time bridging work between workshop content and their professional contexts. The small group format is ideal for engaging in questions about how to apply new tools and strategies introduced in the workshop. Although we recognize that this represents a very early stage of change, we are encouraged to see so many participants demonstrate engagement at this level within the workshops.

Application: Changes to Practice

The most tangible impact of the workshop series that we have observed are the collaborations that they have generated which we referenced earlier. These include partnerships across the university that have resulted in documented changes to practice. These changes can occur on a smaller scale. For example, an advisor attends a workshop and reaches out to the program a week later for support with creating a neuro-affirming communication. Changes to practice have also been more significant in scale, such as the introduction of a tailored staff training program, which leads to a more substantial shift in the way services are offered. Although these shifts towards more neuro-affirming practices are not a direct result of only the learning provided in the workshop, it is the workshop series and the relational connections that are made within the session between attendees and NICE staff that build the initial inspiration for action.

RECOMMENDATIONS FOR FOSTERING A NEURO-AFFIRMING CAMPUS THROUGH TRAINING

As we consider our experiences implementing the NICE program and look to furthering our work, there are several considerations that we identify as important to future practice. These include finding ways to customize and continue workshop participants' learning, strategies for enlisting institutional support, and working to include research and evaluation.

A Campus Community Approach to Program Design and Implementation

As reflected in the literature (Waisman et al., 2023) and in our own experience, when designing a staff and faculty training program such as this, co-creation with Neurodivergent people is essential. In the postsecondary context, working with Neurodivergent students as partners presents the best opportunity to promote the types of shifts in perspective and changes to practice that will be most meaningful to Neurodivergent students. In addition, our program demonstrates the value that practitioners in student affairs' fields (e.g., learning support, accessibility services) bring to the development of campus-wide neuroinclusive initiatives.

In relation to postsecondary advancements in UDL, Black and Fraser (2019) have argued that accessibility services staff are "uniquely positioned…to bring clarity to the nuances of accommodations, accessibility, and UDL" (p.257), which in our perspective, is a critical step in creating more neuro-affirming campus environments. Similarly, learning support staff whose roles afford them the privilege of hearing a vast array of individual learning stories and the opportunity to work collaboratively with learners to support their success can offer unique insights, theory, and practice to conversations that have traditionally been housed in teaching and learning domains. Initiatives that include student affairs staff also present an opportunity to align staff and faculty training with concurrent student-facing programming. In our experience, engaging Neurodivergent students in university transition events and social programs offers the chance for professional and student staff to build their understanding of postsecondary student experiences in ways that authentically feed into faculty and staff workshop development and refinement.

However, the partnerships we continue to develop as the NICE program grows have also illuminated the benefit of engaging in this work within a multi-disciplinary community inclusive of researchers, faculty, teaching and learning and university administrators. This expanding community builds our capacity as program administrators and supports the development of more nuanced and contextualized programming. Partnering with experts in neurodiversity research also presents important opportunities to measure the impact of our program and contribute to the neurodiversity scholarship.

Opportunities for Customized, Ongoing Learning

As partnerships and relationships grow, it has become clear that workshop attendees frequently desire ongoing support with change implementation and further learning. This has been an extremely positive outcome of the workshop series and has allowed us to see firsthand the ways in which participants conceptualize and work to apply their learning to relevant contexts. Collaborating with others following workshops has also showcased for us the additional supports needed to bridge awareness of Neurodivergent student needs and inclusive teaching practices to particular contexts. As much as the sessions aim to provide participants with examples of application and "quick fix UDL solutions" (Hills et al., 2022, p.12), additional implementation support is often required. Rather than a limitation to the workshop series, we instead have begun to understand this extended collaborative support as a key part of an effective training program. This has challenged us to consider systematic ways to create ongoing engagement opportunities for workshop attendees within our existing resources. Following recommendations in the literature, next steps to develop sustainable learning communities may require working more directly with teaching and learning partners as well as faculty "early adopters" (Hills et al., 2022, p.13).

Engage Complementary Institutional Support

While we recognize the value of "bottom-up initiatives" (Hills et al., 2022, p.13) such as the one we describe here, we also support calls in the literature that advocate to include neurodiversity training initiatives in institutional approaches to equity (Dwyer et al., 2023). In relation to supporting more far-reaching implementations of UDL for instance, Hills et al. (2022) put forward several recommendations for concurrent "top-down approaches" (p. 13) that we feel also align with designing more neuroinclusive postsecondary environments. In addition to considering where UDL might be integrated into applicable institutional policies, they also suggest "reward[ing] UDL activities" and "invest[ing] in strategies that can mitigate barriers linked to faculty time and workload" (p. 13), such as introducing instructional resources. More visible institutional support would also help to align efforts across institutions, supporting connections and community-building that is essential to shifting postsecondary cultures.

Embedding Research and Evaluation into Initiatives

As the field moves to implement various initiatives aimed to foster a neuroinclusive postsecondary environment, engaging in research and evaluation alongside programming is necessary to determine how effective training is in changing faculty and staff's knowledge, attitudes and stigma related to neurodiversity. The inclusion of implementation science frameworks is key to identifying what strategies and determinants help or hinder the success of program implementation in postsecondary settings. This information can inform best approaches to scaling initiatives (e.g., within the faculties, or across universities), as well as demonstrating how to ensure training programs are sustained at the university. Future research is also needed to understand behavioral change following faculty trainings and/or policy changes at the faculty and university level. Only through concerted evaluation efforts, can we accurately demonstrate the impact of such initiatives for Neurodivergent postsecondary students.

CONCLUSION

Consistent with recommendations from advocates with lived experience, a shift in the focus of postsecondary supports for Neurodivergent learners is needed, that of ensuring adequate supports exist while *also* fostering an inclusive postsecondary environment. Grounded in a social-ecological lens and informed by the voices and experiences of Neurodivergent students, the NICE workshop series focuses on how learning and advising environments within higher education can better support the diverse learning needs of all students, including those who identify as Neurodivergent. Through the application of UDL and an adapted SaP model that is responsive to Neurodivergent students, the NICE workshop series has demonstrated that it is a feasible, cost-effective approach to improving faculty and staff's understanding of supporting Neurodivergent students. The series not only shows early evidence of improved faculty and staff knowledge/attitudes but offers leadership experiences for Neurodivergent mentors to facilitate the series, fostering confidence and a sense of accomplishment in these students. Further research is needed to understand the cascading impact of trainings and workshops, like NICE, to ensure that they are fostering a neuroinclusive environment for learners.

CASE STUDIES AND DISCUSSION QUESTIONS

Case Study 1: Supporting Sensory Differences in Advising

Julie is a graduate student advisor who is preparing to meet with Morgan, a Master of Science student in the last year of writing her thesis. She sees that in the appointment booking note that Morgan is having difficulties connecting with her supervisor and is feeling overwhelmed by how the interactions have gone lately. Julie greets Morgan in the waiting room and guides her back through a brightly lit hallway. She invites Morgan to take a seat in her office cubicle, which is situated among a number of additional cubicles where other advising appointments are occurring. Julie starts the conversation by sharing information on how to connect with a supervisor and Morgan nods her head in response, crosses her arms and looks down towards the floor. Julie begins to ask Morgan questions, but it seems as though Morgan is having trouble responding or interpreting the questions. Unsure how to proceed, Julie asks Morgan if the tips on meeting with her supervisor that she provided will be helpful. Morgan nods. Julie starts to wrap up the meeting notes and stands up saying, "It was nice meeting you Morgan," and Morgan heads back out towards the waiting room. As Julie reflects on the appointment, she is feeling unsure if the meeting was helpful and wonders in what other ways she might have approached the interaction.

Questions

1. What might be some causes of Morgan's lack of response to Julie's questions? What could be going on for Morgan during this interaction?
2. Using a UDL and sensory-friendly lens, what strategies might Julie employ to determine how and if she had met Morgan's advising needs?

Case Study 2: Supporting Neurodivergent Student Orientation

Cam is a staff member at the university and sits as a faculty representative on a committee that helps with student orientation for first-year students. Over 4000 students have registered this year to join in the activities. Cam oversees their faculty's welcome sessions which include leading students in a faculty cheer and providing them with an overview of their program. During the faculty cheer, Cam observes a few students covering their ears and moving to the sides of the room. During the faculty program overview, students are asked to find a friend to share more about themselves. Cam has a couple of students come up and ask if they have to participate in this activity and Cam encourages those students to pair up together. They then notice a few of those students leaving the room. During a break, an individual approaches Cam and introduces themselves as a parent of one of the attendees. The parent asks Cam if there are any reduced noise areas for their student. Cam lets the parent know that the only place that might be quiet could be the library, but even there, faculty tours going on that day could be noisy. The parent continues to ask if there are any options to participate in tours in smaller groups. Cam answers that as it is a large school and there are many students participating in this event, having a small group would not be possible. The parent thanks Cam for their time and Cam resumes the session. Cam later reflects on what ways the events of the day might not be supporting all students.

Questions

1. What challenges might be present in the event described above for Neurodivergent students?
2. How might you support Cam in identifying ways to adjust the event to be more neuroinclusive?

Case Study 3: Supporting Neurodivergent Student Staff as Partners

Ethan is an undergraduate student in their 3rd year of a Bachelor of Science degree in Biochemistry and is joining the Neurodivergent student staff team as a student partner. During the first meeting with the coordinator, Ethan expresses enthusiasm for the role, which will involve working with other student staff to develop and present workshops. As their rapport grows over the course of their individual meetings, Ethan shares that they have some concerns about how much collaborative work will be involved in the role. In the past, they have found working in groups challenging, particularly when others in the group seem to have different ways of approaching group tasks and the work includes a lot of impromptu brainstorming during group meetings. They also express that sometimes in conversation, especially if they are feeling anxious, it can take them time to process and respond to what others are saying. This can make it appear as if they don't have anything to contribute or that they are not being an active member of the group. Although they work better closer to a deadline, they have found this has also created tension in group projects. Ethan also shares that although they are looking forward to the presentation aspects of the role, they can get anxious presenting, to the point where they forget what they want to communicate. They have found this embarrassing and are worried about this happening while they are delivering workshops as part of their role. After the first meeting, the coordinator reflects on how to support Ethan in their role.

Questions

1. What strategies could the program coordinator employ to support Ethan to do their best work?
2. How could the program coordinator support Ethan's participation in collaborative group settings?
3. What strategies could Ethan and the coordinator employ to support Ethan while presenting workshops?

ACKNOWLEDGEMENTS

The NICE project was supported by a grant from the University of Calgary's Student Union Quality Money program.

REFERENCES

Accardo, A. L., Bomgardner, E. M., Rubinstein, M. B., & Woodruff, J. (2024). Valuing neurodiversity on campus: Perspectives and priorities of neurodivergent students, faculty, and professional staff. *Journal of Diversity in Higher Education*. Advance online publication. DOI: 10.1037/dhe0000571

Ames, M. E., Coombs, C. E. M., Duerksen, K., Vincent, J., & McMorris, C. A. (2022). Canadian mapping of autism-specific supports for postsecondary students. *Research in Autism Spectrum Disorders*, *90*, 101899. DOI: 10.1016/j.rasd.2021.101899

Anderson, A. H., Stephenson, J., & Carter, M. A. (2017). Systematic literature review of the experiences and supports of students with Autism Spectrum Disorder in postsecondary education. *Research in Autism Spectrum Disorders*, *39*, 33–53. DOI: 10.1016/j.rasd.2017.04.002

Black, J., & Fraser, R. (2019). Integration through collaboration: Building strategic faculty partnerships to shift minds and practices. In Bracken, S., & Novak, K. (Eds.), *Transforming higher education through universal design for learning: An international perspective* (pp. 244–257). Routledge. DOI: 10.4324/9781351132077-15

Butcher, L., & Lane, S. (2024). Neurodivergent (Autism and ADHD) student experiences of access and inclusion in higher education: An ecological systems theory perspective. *Higher Education*. Advance online publication. DOI: 10.1007/s10734-024-01319-6

Cage, E., De Andres, M., & Mahoney, P. (2020). Understanding the factors that affect university completion for autistic people. *Research in Autism Spectrum Disorders*, *72*, 101519. DOI: 10.1016/j.rasd.2020.101519

Canadian University Survey Consortium. (June, 2024). *2024 Graduating student survey master report*. https://cusc-ccreu.ca/wordpress/?lang=en&download=3708&tmstv=1742270935

CAST. (2024). *Universal Design for Learning Guidelines version 3.0* [graphic organizer]. https://udlguidelines.cast.org/static/udlg3-graphicorganizer-digital-numbers-a11y.pdf

CAST. (n.d.). The UDL guidelines. *UDL Guidelines*. https://udlguidelines.cast.org/

Chapman, R. (2021). Neurodiversity and the Social Ecology of Mental Functions. *Perspectives on Psychological Science*, *16*(6), 1360–1372. https://doiorg.ezproxy.lib.ucalgary.ca/10.1177/1745691620959833. DOI: 10.1177/1745691620959833 PMID: 33577400

Clince, M., Connolly, L., & Nolan, C. (2016). Comparing and exploring the sensory processing patterns of higher education students with attention deficit hyperactivity disorder and Autism Spectrum Disorder. *The American Journal of Occupational Therapy*, *70*(2), 1–9. DOI: 10.5014/ajot.2016.016816 PMID: 26943106

Clouder, L., Karakus, M., Cinotti, A., Ferreyra, M. V., Fierros, G. A., & Rojo, P. (2020). Neurodiversity in higher education: A narrative synthesis. *Higher Education*, *80*(4), 757–778. DOI: 10.1007/s10734-020-00513-6

Cook-Sather, A. (2018). Listening to equity-seeking perspectives: How students' experiences of pedagogical partnership can inform wider discussions of student success. *Higher Education Research & Development*, *37*(5), 923–936. DOI: 10.1080/07294360.2018.1457629

Cook-Sather, A., Bovill, C., & Felten, P. (2014). *Engaging students as partners in learning and teaching: A guide for faculty* (1st ed.). Wiley.

Creaven, A. (2024). Considering the sensory and social needs of disabled students in higher education: A call to return to the roots of universal design. *Policy Futures in Education*, *23*(1), 259–266. DOI: 10.1177/14782103241240808

Cumming, T. M., & Rose, M. C. (2022). Exploring Universal Design for Learning as an accessibility tool in higher education: A review of the current literature. *Australian Educational Researcher*, *49*(5), 1025–1043. https://link.springer.com/article/10.1007/s13384-021-00471-7. DOI: 10.1007/s13384-021-00471-7

Durgungoz, F. C., & Durgungoz, A. (2025). "Interactive lessons are great, but too much is too much": Hearing out neurodivergent students, Universal Design for Learning and the case for integrating more anonymous technology in higher education. *Higher Education*. Advance online publication. DOI: 10.1007/s10734-024-01389-6

Dwyer, P., Mineo, E., Mifsud, K., Lindholm, C., Gurba, A., & Waisman, T. C. (2023). Building neurodiversity-inclusive postsecondary campuses: Recommendations for leaders in higher education. *Autism in Adulthood: Challenges and Management*, *5*(1), 1–14. DOI: 10.1089/aut.2021.0042 PMID: 36941859

Fovet, F. (2020). *Exploring the potential of universal design for learning with regards to mental health issues in higher education*. [conference proceedings]. Pacific Rim International Conference on Disability and Diversity. University of Hawai'i at Mānoa, Honolulu, Hawai'i. http://hdl.handle.net/10125/69333

Frost, K. M., Bailey, K. M., & Ingersoll, B. R. (2019). "I just want them to see me as…me": Identity, community, and disclosure practices among college students on the autism spectrum. *Autism in Adulthood: Challenges and Management, 1*(14), 268–275. DOI: 10.1089/aut.2018.0057 PMID: 36601323

Gillespie-Lynch, K., Brooks, P. J., Someki, F., Obeid, R., Shane-Simpson, C., Kapp, S. K., Daou, N., & Smith, D. S. (2015). Changing college students' conceptions of autism: An online training to increase knowledge and decrease stigma. *Journal of Autism and Developmental Disorders, 45*(8), 2553–2566. DOI: 10.1007/s10803-015-2422-9 PMID: 25796194

Healey, M., Flint, A., & Harrington, K. (2014). *Engagement through partnership: Students as partners in learning and teaching in higher education*. Higher Education Academy. https://www.advance-he.ac.uk/knowledge-hub/engagement-through-partnership-students-partners-learning-and-teaching-higher

Hills, M., Overend, A., & Hildebrandt, S. (2022). Faculty perspectives on UDL: Exploring bridges and barriers for broader adoption in higher education. *The Canadian Journal for the Scholarship of Teaching and Learning, 13*(1), 1–18. DOI: 10.5206/cjsotlrcacea.2022.1.13588

Lindsay, B. L., Bernier, E., Bowman, J. & Boyce, M. (2022). Understanding the connection between student wellbeing and teaching and learning at a Canadian research university: A qualitative student perspective. *Pedagogy in Health Promotion: The Scholarship of Teaching and Learning,* 1-12. DOI: 10.1177/23733799221089578

Lubicz-Nawrocka, T., & Bovill, C. (2023). Do students experience transformation through co-creating curriculum in higher education? *Teaching in Higher Education, 28*(7), 17441760. DOI: 10.1080/13562517.2021.1928060

Mercer-Mapstone, L., Dvorakova, S. L., Matthews, K. E., Abbot, S., Cheng, B., Felten, P., Knorr, K., Marquis, E., Shammas, R., & Swaim, K. (2017). A systematic literature review of students as partners in higher education. *International Journal for Students as Partners, 1*(1), 15–37. DOI: 10.15173/ijsap.v1i1.3119

Miller, D., Rees, J., & Pearson, A. (2021). "Masking is life": Experiences of masking in autistic and nonautistic adults. *Autism in Adulthood: Challenges and Management, 3*(4), 330–338. DOI: 10.1089/aut.2020.0083 PMID: 36601640

Nolan, C., Doyle, J. K., Lewis, K., & Treanor, D. (2023). Disabled students' perception of the sensory aspects of the learning and social environments within one higher education institution. *British Journal of Occupational Therapy*, *86*(5), 367–375. https://journals.sagepub.com/doi/pdf/10.1177/03080226221126895?download=true. DOI: 10.1177/03080226221126895 PMID: 40336521

Osifo, O., & Terashima, M. (2024). Addressing barriers in the university campus environment for neurodivergent students. *Studies in Health Technology and Informatics*, *29*(319), 293–306. DOI: 10.3233/SHTI240952 PMID: 39618368

Peña, E. V., Gassner, D., & Brown, K. R. (2020). Autistic-centered program development and assessment practices. *Journal of Postsecondary Education and Disability*, *33*(3), 233–240. https://eric.ed.gov/?id=EJ1280846

Story, M. F., Mueller, J. L., & Mace, R. L. (1998). *The universal design file: Designing for people of all ages and abilities* (Revised edition). Center for Universal Design. https://files.eric.ed.gov/fulltext/ED460554.pdf

Van Hees, V., Moyson, T., & Roeyers, H. (2015). Higher education experiences of students with Autism Spectrum Disorder: Challenges, benefits, and support needs. *Journal of Autism and Developmental Disorders*, *45*(6), 1673–1688. DOI: 10.1007/s10803-014-2324-2 PMID: 25448918

Waisman, T., Williams, Z. J., Cage, E., Santhanam, S. P., Magiati, I., Dwyer, P., Stockwell, K. M., Kofner, B., Brown, H., Davidson, D., Herrell, J., Shore, S. M., Caudel, D., Gurbuz, E., & Gillespie-Lynch, K. (2023). Learning from the experts: Evaluating a participatory autism and universal design training for university educators. *Autism*, *27*(2), 356–370. DOI: 10.1177/13623613221097207 PMID: 35652315

Waisman, T. C., Alba, L. A., & Green, S. A. (2022). Barriers to inclusive learning for autistic individuals. *Pediatrics*, *149*(4, Supplement 4), 1. DOI: 10.1542/peds.2020-049437Q PMID: 35363285

ADDITIONAL READING

Cook-Sather, A., Bovill, C., & Felten, P. (2014). *Engaging students as partners in learning and teaching: A guide for faculty* (1st ed.). Wiley.

Healey, M., Flint, A., & Harrington, K. (2014). *Engagement through partnership: Students as partners in learning and teaching in higher education*. Higher Education Academy. https://www.advance-he.ac.uk/knowledge-hub/engagement-through-partnership-students-partners-learning-and-teaching-higher

Mostafa, M. (2021). *The autism friendly university design guide*. Dublin City University. https://www.researchgate.net/publication/351936605_THE_AUTISM_FRIENDLY_UNIVERSITY_DESIGN_GUIDE#fullTextFileContent

Peña, E. V., Gassner, D., & Brown, K. R. (2020). Autistic-centered program development and assessment practices (Practice Brief). *Journal of Postsecondary Education and Disability*, *33*(3), 233–240. https://eric.ed.gov/?id=EJ1280846

Salisbury, Y., Foster, R., Hill, S., & Buck, G. (2024). Neurodiverse inclusive social work education considered through a student partnership. *Social Work Education*, •••, 1–16. DOI: 10.1080/02615479.2024.2378915

Sarrett, J. C. (2018). Autism and accommodations in higher education: Insights from the autism community. *Journal of Autism and Developmental Disorders*, *48*(3), 679–693. DOI: 10.1007/s10803-017-3353-4 PMID: 29243099

Takacs, S., Marom, L., Vanderveen, A., & Cruthers McNeney, A. (2024). *Storying Universal Design for Learning*. Kwantlen Polytechnic University. https://kpu.pressbooks.pub/storyingudl/

Toblin, J. T., & Behling, T. K. (2018). *Reach everyone, teach everyone: Universal Design for Learning in higher education*. West Virginia Press.

Epilogue

As we close this book, we reflect on the collective wisdom shared by our authors—researchers, educators, Neurodivergent individuals, and advocates from across the globe—who have illuminated the path toward inclusive, affirming post-secondary environments. We are reminded of the power of community in shaping meaningful change. Our scholar and practitioner authors have contributed to a richer understanding of what it means to support Neurodivergent learners holistically when we come together to uplift Neurodivergent students and reimagine our campuses as spaces of true belonging. This shared knowledge underscores a singular truth: Neurodivergent students bring unique strengths to higher education, and it is our shared responsibility to foster environments where they are not just accommodated but celebrated and empowered.

Creating truly inclusive campuses is an evolving process. It demands ongoing dialogue, reflection, and action. The questions raised during our initial conference presentation in 2019, which sparked this book, continue to resonate: How do we bridge the gaps between secondary and postsecondary education? How do we amplify Neurodivergent voices in shaping postsecondary institutional policies? How do we sustain momentum for change?

These questions, and the many others that have emerged, propel us toward the next phase of this work. Our forthcoming second text, *Collaborative Strategies for Designing Neuroinclusive College Campuses,* delves deeper into practical applications—offering actionable strategies for faculty training, specialized programming, extracurricular and orientation events, student-led advocacy, cross-campus partnerships, and inclusive course design, libraries, and residential life. We invite you, our readers, to join us in this ongoing exploration, to engage with the tools in *Collaborative Strategies for Designing Neuroinclusive College Campuses,* and to contribute to a global community committed to the educational and social success of Neurodivergent individuals.

Let this text serve not as an ending, but as a launching point for ongoing dialogue and action. Whether you are inspired to develop new campus programs, revise classroom practices, or advocate for systemic policy changes, know that your work matters deeply in embracing a cultural shift toward celebrating human diversity in all its forms. Welcoming all students to postsecondary education means embracing difference not as a barrier to overcome but as a valuable perspective that enriches our communities.

Editing this book has reaffirmed our belief that this work is never complete. The landscape of higher education and the understanding of neurodiversity will continue to evolve, and with it, our approaches must also evolve. Our hope is that the conversations and collaborations sparked by this book and *Collaborative Strategies for Designing Neuroinclusive College Campuses* will ripple outward, fostering new partnerships, research, and practices that center on the voices and needs of Neurodivergent students. Together, we can continue building spaces where every student feels seen, valued, and empowered to thrive. Our hope is that these books help others take steps toward a future where neurodiversity is not only accepted but celebrated as an essential part of our shared humanity.

As we move forward, we carry the inspiration of those we know and love in the neurodiversity community. Their resilience, creativity, and vision remind us that this work is not just about changing systems—it's about building a world where every learner is valued for who they are. Let this book be a stepping stone, and let us continue this journey together.

Glossary

Ableism: Ableism reflects a belief system that views people with disabilities as unequal to non-disabled individuals which may result in ableist actions that exclude people with disabilities from inclusion within systems and society. It is based on an assumption that there is a "correct" or "ideal" way for bodies and minds to function and those which do not are morally, physically, emotionally, psychologically, or otherwise inferior and in need of fixing; intentional and unintentional acts of discrimination stem from this assumption.

Access vs. Inclusion: Access refers to the ability to enter or approach a place, while inclusion focuses on ensuring that everyone, regardless of their characteristics or needs, can fully participate and benefit from that place or situation. In other words, access is about getting in, while inclusion is about belonging and thriving once one is invited inside.

Accessibility/Disability Support/Resource Office/Coordinator: These terms are often interchangeable and refer to the individuals or departments who are responsible for ensuring that people with disabilities have equal access to all aspects of an organization. In educational settings, this role involves identifying and removing barriers, providing accommodations, and advocating for inclusive practices.

Accommodation: Accommodations are changes made to the learning environment, curriculum, or instruction which allow an individual with disabilities to access the same content as their non-disabled peers. Accommodations are typically provided in any of the following areas: presentation (how content is presented, such as enlarged text), response (how an individual demonstrates their understanding or learning, such as allowing students to type or orally state responses instead of handwriting responses), setting (the environment in which learning or testing takes place, such as allowing a student to complete a quiz or exam in a separate, distraction free area or classroom), and/or timing (allowing for extended time for exams or quizzes to be completed, or providing flexible due dates).

Accreditation: Accreditation is the action or process of officially recognizing a particular status or qualification to perform a particular duty. In higher education, accrediting bodies provide guidelines to institutions to construct programs and then conduct thorough reviews to ensure all guidelines are met. If satisfactory evaluations are conducted, institutions are provided with accredited status, indicating that the institution has met all standards for that particular field.

Active Learning: Active learning is a student-centered pedagogy where students participate in the learning process rather than passively take in information imparted by instructors. Commonly used strategies include discussions, problem-solving projects, and practical applications of ideas presented.

Advocacy: By taking action, speaking out, and arguing in favor of a cause, an individual practices advocacy on behalf of themselves and/or others. Advocacy strives to amplify and provide space for voices that are often not heard. It works to protect individual and group rights.

Allyship: In a relationship described as allyship, an individual in possession of authority and privilege from a dominant group supports individuals in a marginalized group. An ally works for social justice against oppressive systems and promotes empowering others. Allies advocate for those with less power.

Andragogy: The term andragogy was coined by Malcolm Knowles in the late 1960s to differentiate between the teaching of children (pedagogy) and the teaching of adults (andragogy. Andragogy argues that adult learners bring several personal attributes to the adult education classroom, including their self-directed approach, their life experiences, a readiness to learn, an orientation to learning that offers immediate applications of new knowledge, strong internal motivation, and a clear perspective to what they need to know.

Americans with Disabilities Act (ADA): The Americans with Disabilities Act of 1990 is a U.S. civil rights law which prohibits discrimination based on disability. It ensures that people with disabilities have equal opportunities in the following areas: employment, transportation, and public accommodations, which includes institutions of higher education. This law was revised in 2009 to the ADA Amendments Act which broadened the definition of disability and strengthened the protections of individuals with disabilities.

Arts, Science, and Inclusive Applied Practice (ASIAP) Ireland: The Certificate in Arts, Science, and Inclusive Applied Practice (ASIAP) is a two-year, full-time program offered by Trinity College Dublin's Trinity Centre for People with Intellectual Disabilities (TCPID). It is designed for students with intellectual disabilities, providing them with a level 5 accredited certificate and opportunities to develop a broad range of skills for both employment and independent living.

Assistive Technology: Assistive technology is any device or service that aids individuals to increase, maintain, or improve their current capabilities. Assistive technology can come in many forms from "low tech" (paper with large spacing lines, cups with enlarged handles), "mid tech" (audio versions of textbooks, switch operated devices), and "high tech" (specific applications for tablets or computers, designed to aid communication). For example, speech to text options on cell phones provide users with the ability to transmit text messages to others without the need for visual processing or manual dexterity to type on small screens, and it also provides the user with the ability to have words spelled for them.

Autistic Burnout: Autistic individuals experiencing prolonged masking of autism characteristics or challenges navigating inaccessible environments can experience physical and mental exhaustion. The inability to function effectively with daily tasks and the increase in sensitivity to light and sound stimuli are representative of Autistic burnout.

Belonging: Belonging is a feeling of connectedness and acceptance by a group or community where individuals feel understood and accepted by others. When students identify with their university, feel socially accepted, and possess the cultural capital necessary to fit into their environment, they feel like they belong. Their sense of belonging can increase academic success, retention, and greater satisfaction with college attendance.

Biopsychosocial Model of Assessment: This holistic approach to assessment considers biological (physical attributes and conditions), psychological (thoughts, emotions, actions, and mental health indicators), and social factors (family interactions, SES, culture, and support networks). The interconnectedness of these elements affects well-being.

Collaboration: Collaboration is the act of working with other individuals to construct an action, item, or plan/program. Effective collaborators are known to have strong listening and communication skills, the ability to be empathetic, and communicate clearly and frequently with others.

Collaborative Learning: An educational approach where students work together in groups to solve problems, complete tasks, or learn new concepts is referred to as collaborative learning. Emphasizes interaction and shared responsibility, allowing students to leverage each other's resources and skills.

Collaborative Mentorship: In a traditional mentoring relationship, there is one person who has experiences, knowledge, and skills that they share with the less informed and less powerful mentee. Collaborative mentorship is a partnership whereby a mentor and mentee equally contribute to a relationship, sharing responsibilities to meet a mutually determined goal.

College Student Supports (CSS): CSS refers to assistance available to college students in multiple areas. These may include accommodations offered through the disability or accessibility office, writing and tutoring centers, as well as supports designed for specific student populations such as TRIO services for students from low socio-economic backgrounds, first-generation students, and those with disabilities. Inclusive Postsecondary Education (IPSE) programs provide more extensive support designed for students with intellectual disabilities.

Communication Modalities: Communication is the process of encoding and decoding information. This exchange of information can take on many forms from two major categories: verbal communication and non-verbal communication. Verbal communication consists of both spoken language (including computer aided auditory output via assistive technology) and written language while non-verbal communication includes gestures, sign language (or manual language), visual communication, and some forms of assistive technology such as the use of Picture Exchange Communication (PECS) systems.

Community-Informed Approaches: Community-Informed Approaches consider the context (where individuals reside, study, and work), the community members (the types of people one interacts with), and the permanent or temporary conditions present (social, cultural, economic, political, or environmental situations). A community-informed approach in education seeks feedback from and involvement of Neurodivergent individuals in every aspect of developing and implementing supports and systems that are meant to benefit Neurodivergent students. Community-informed approaches may be contrasted with more expert-focused or hierarchical approaches, which often fail to represent or reflect the priorities of the individuals whom the approaches will impact.

Compassionate Pedagogy: Compassionate pedagogy is an educational approach that emphasizes the emotional and physical well-being of students by cultivating a nurturing and supportive learning environment. Instructors actively listen to students' experiences, offer flexibility to accommodate individual challenges, and prioritize building genuine human connections. This approach seeks to remove barriers to learning, promote inclusivity, and address students' needs holistically—recognizing the importance of empathy and care alongside academic achievement.

Comprehensive Transition Program (CTP): Comprehensive Transition Program is a certified classification given to Inclusive Postsecondary Education (IPSE) programs that comply with a set of standards developed through research and administered by the Department of Education. Academic instruction, career training, and teaching independent living skills are all elements of CTP programming where students with Intellectual Disabilities (ID) attend college courses and participate in campus activities. One benefit of receiving CTP certification is that students in the program can access federal student financial aid to help pay for program attendance.

Coping: Coping refers to an individual's ability to effectively manage or deal with various situations or actions. Individuals often experience anxiety due to stressful life situations such as feeling the need to mask their neurodivergence. They may employ a variety of strategies to cope including exercise, mindfulness activities, yoga, aromatherapy, writing in a journal, or relaxing in a natural setting. Stable coping responses are self-regulation mechanisms that become consistent over time due to their production of effective outcomes.

Cultural Competency: People who acknowledge the differences between cultures and understand, accept, and respect those differences in values, beliefs, and actions are culturally competent. This acknowledgement enables individuals to successfully interact with people from diverse cultural backgrounds, including neurodiversity. It is important to recognize that not only is it essential to have knowledge about different cultures, but also to develop the skills to effectively communicate and engage with others.

Culturally Responsive: The act of being culturally responsive requires an individual to acknowledge and appreciate cultures other than one's own, including the neurodiverse community. This process reflects a respect and understanding for differing values, beliefs, behaviors, and communication styles. Being culturally responsive to a Neurodivergent student includes recognizing and valuing their cognitive differences.

Developmental Disability: Legally, developmental disability is an umbrella term for many different diagnoses made before the age of 22 which may be physical or cognitive, or a combination of both. Autism Spectrum Disorder, Cerebral Palsy, learning disabilities, and Down Syndrome are examples of developmental disabilities. Inclusive Post Secondary Education (IPSE) programs may serve students with developmental disabilities on college campuses.

Diagnosis: A diagnosis is the identification of an illness, injury, or disability through the examination and assessment of symptoms. The diagnosis of various conditions can only be made by highly trained professionals. A diagnosis for specific conditions (e.g. cancer) can only be made by a medical professional, whereas a diagnosis of specific learning disabilities (e.g. dyslexia) can be made by a school psychologist, clinical psychologist, or medical doctor.

Diagnostic Overshadowing: Diagnostic overshadowing occurs when the presence of one diagnosis leads clinicians to overlook other co-occurring conditions, often resulting in misdiagnosis. For example, a student may receive a diagnosis of anxiety disorder rather than autism which might be the correct diagnosis because both diagnoses can relate to social interaction.

Disability Access Route to Education (DARE) In education systems in Ireland, Disability Access Route to Education (DARE) is an alternative admissions process for students with disabilities whose schooling has been negatively impacted by their disability, requiring additional supports, accommodations, and/or adjustments to attendance and participation. DARE increases access to college for students with disabilities or specific learning difficulties.

Disability Models: The models of disability provide different definitions of disability and offer ways for people to analyze how disability works within society.

Three common perspectives include the medical, social and relational models. The medical model emphasizes abnormality and focuses on the part of the body that generated the disability rather than on the whole person. This model frames disability through a deficit lens and assumes non-disabled individuals as the standard to which others are compared. In a professional or educational setting, the disability is diagnosed by outside experts, rehabilitation is prescribed with the aim to cure people with disabilities or diminish the effects of the impairment to the greatest extent possible. The social model views disability and impairment as separate terms where disability is socially constructed. This model conceptualizes disability as resulting from inaccessible or ableist environments. The social model of disability defines people with disabilities as an oppressed group that is victimized by society through discrimination, isolation, dependence, exclusion, and institutionalization. The relational model refers to the link between disability and culture. This framework defines disability as not merely the product of an individual, nor just the imposition of a barrier by society but sees it as a result of the relationship between the two. The effects of impairment and society both play a role in this interpretation.

Disclosure: Disclosure is the act of sharing private information with others. In terms of disability, disclosure refers to individuals disclosing that they have a disability. The decision to disclose is a personal choice. One may disclose privately to close associates where they mention that they are disabled without giving the details about the specific impairment or they can disclose one of their disabilities but not another or they can disclose in some settings and not in others. To receive accommodations in higher education, students must formally disclose their disability through a disability disclosure process. Students may choose to avoid stigmatization by masking their disability and avoiding disclosure.

Double-Empathy Problem: This theory argues that communication breakdowns between individuals with and without autism is a two-way issue. The theory posits that both parties have difficulty understanding each other, and it is not the fault of one party or the other. This challenges the idea that Autistic individuals lack empathy or social skills and draws attention to the differences in neurological experiences and challenges in understanding others' perspectives.

Ecological Systems Theory: Introduced by Urie Bronfenbrenner, this theory argues that human development is shaped by interconnected environmental systems. The first and closest to a developing child is the immediate environment with social and personal interactions between family, friends, and community members (microsystem); then there are the connections between environments such as ways the family and the school environments may interact (mesosystem) and the indirect systems that do not directly touch the child but may affect those around them (exosystem). Broader cultural contexts including cultural and social values (macrosystem) follows, and finally there are changes over time (chronosystem).

Education for All Handicapped Children Act: The Education for All Handicapped Children Act was written into law in the U.S. in 1975 and provided the first legal protection of educational rights to students with disabilities. This act opened public school access to all students through the provision of free appropriate public education (FAPE) and was later revised and renamed to the Individuals with Disabilities Education Act (IDEA) of 1990.

Education for Persons with Special Educational Needs Act (2004) Ireland: In Ireland, the Education for Persons with Special Educational Needs (EPSEN) Act of 2004 mandates that children with disabilities that affect their education are educated in inclusive environments whenever possible. The education of children up to 18 years of age with special educational needs is covered by Act, and it ensures that students with special needs receive the skills necessary to participate fully in society and are prepared to live independently. The Act also established the National Council for Special Education (NCSE) to improve the delivery of education services.

Engagement: Engagement is the process in which an individual participates with other persons and/or within their environment. The level of engagement can be restricted by barriers to accessibility (physical access), communication, understanding (cognitive engagement) or other factors such as bias and stigma (emotional engagement).

Evidenced-Based: Evidence-based is a term which emphasizes the application of an approach which has been found to have positive outcomes through research. It provides a connection between theory and practice when educators use the results of reliable research studies to guide their teaching strategies and techniques.

Equality Act 2010 UK: The Equality Act 2010 of the United Kingdom is legislation requiring public institutions (including universities) to make reasonable adjustments to prevent discrimination against people with disabilities. It prohibits discrimination in employment, education, services, and public functions for those with disabilities. The Act also imposes a legal duty on public bodies to consider equality when making decisions.

Executive Functioning Skills: Executive functioning skills are a group of processes that help an individual to manage and/or complete tasks such as planning, organizing, and problem solving. Some examples of executive functioning skills include: attention, working memory, inhibition, cognitive flexibility, task initiation, time management, emotional control (self-control, self-monitoring), problem solving, and metacognition.

Exceptional/Twice Exceptional: An exceptional learner is one who requires specially designed instruction to meet their full human potential. To be designated as an exceptional learner, an individual must have a documented disability and assessments demonstrating the need for specially designed instruction. An individual who is categorized as twice exceptional is said to have exceptional strengths and challenges, for example an individual with a diagnosis of Gifted and a specific learning disability.

Experiential Learning: A teaching method where students learn through direct experience and reflection, rather than solely through traditional instruction. This method encourages forming new ideas based on reflection, and then testing those ideas in new contexts.

Family Educational Rights and Privacy Act (FERPA): The Family Educational Rights and Privacy Act of 1974 provides specific protections of privacy to student education records in the United States. For any student over the age of 18, express written permission must be provided to allow denoted others access to education records and other education information.

Hidden curriculum: The hidden curriculum is the unspoken, often implicit rules or practices that individuals are expected to intuit or learn from their context. These rules are not overtly identified nor easily accessed.

Higher Education Institutions (HEI): Higher Education Institutions include all postsecondary or tertiary education options offered by schools such as colleges, universities, vocational or trade schools, and community colleges. They provide degrees, certifications, or other qualifications to individuals who complete their programs over various lengths of time. These schools can also be referred to by using the acronym HE.

Higher Education Commission Of Pakistan (HEC): In Pakistan, The Higher Education Commission (HEC) oversees higher education. It was formed by the government of Pakistan and is in charge of funding and accrediting higher education institutions in the country. It develops policies and quality standards. It also supports research and development in higher education.

Higher Education Opportunity Act (HEOA): The Higher Education Opportunity Act of 2008 is a reauthorization of the Higher Education Act of 1965 in the United States. This law was designed to oversee the administration of federal higher education programs including financial assistance to students such as the Pell grants and transition services for students with disabilities; its provisions increase access to higher education.

Inclusive Postsecondary Education (IPSE): Programming identified as Inclusive Postsecondary Education refers to college campus based continuing education opportunities for students with intellectual disabilities. It frequently includes additional training in employment and independent living skills with the aid of support staff. IPSE provides students with intellectual disabilities the chance to attend college and participate in academic courses, social organizations and activities, athletics, and employment or internship opportunities with peers with and without disabilities.

Inclusive Practices: Activities, programs, and approaches that ensure all students are treated fairly and respectfully, regardless of their differences, reflect inclusive practices. For students with disabilities, inclusive practices allow them to succeed in the least restrictive environment at school. Inclusive practices promote belonging for all students. Collaborative learning in which students work together in groups to learn from each other and complete tasks can be an inclusive practice. Implementing Universal Design for Learning is an approach that demonstrates inclusive practices.

Individuals with Disabilities Education Act (IDEA): The Individuals with Disabilities Education Act (IDEA) of 1990 amended and effectively replaced the Education for All Handicapped Children Act of 1975. IDEA added additional protections for students with disabilities including: Individualized Education Programming (IEP), Non-Discriminatory Evaluation, Free Appropriate Public Education for all students regardless of disability type, Least Restrictive Environment, Parent and Student Participation, and Procedural Due Process.

Individualized Education Programs (IEP): Individualized Education Programs (IEP) are legally binding documents created for students with disabilities which outline a student's current educational and functional performance (Present Levels), measurable annual goals, specific services a student is to receive that supports their learning and participation within the school setting, any accommodations or modification the student is to receive, a description of how their progress will be monitored throughout the duration of the IEP, and a statement of the student's involvement in the general education setting (least restrictive environment).

Intellectual Disability (ID): Describing a student as having an Intellectual Disability (ID) refers to an individual with limitations in intellectual and cognitive functions and adaptive behaviors expressed in conceptual, social, and practical adaptive skills. A person with an intellectual disability needs additional time and support to achieve the same outcomes as a neuromajority individual.

Internalized Ableism: The tendency for people who are disabled to internalize damaging beliefs about what they "should" be able to do is referred to as internalized ableism. It can lead to negative self-concept, masking, anxiety, depression, meltdowns, shutdowns, and/or burnout.

Learning Centered Teaching (LCT): An educational approach that prioritizes the needs and active participation of students in the learning process. LCT shifts the focus from the instructor's delivery of information to the students' construction of knowledge and development of skills, emphasizes student engagement, collaboration, and reflection, fostering a more dynamic and personalized learning experience

Learned Helplessness Theory: Learned helplessness is a psychological condition where individuals stop attempting to overcome challenges due to repeated failures. It is rooted in the work of Martin Seligman. His theory explains that when an individual is repeatedly exposed to adverse events, they can develop a perceived lack of control over their own lives and a lack of motivation to attempt to make changes.

This can lead to an individual no longer trying to change their own circumstances, even if they have the capability to do so.

Life Skills: Life skills is a term used to describe daily living or functional skills individuals perform which include communication and social skills. Examples of specific skills include (but are not limited to) the ability to dress, toilet, and feed themselves, navigate their environment, socially engage in recreation of choice, adapt to environmental changes, and demonstrate resilience. Some Neurodivergent individuals need support and training to efficiently manage daily life skills.

Marginalization: The term marginalization refers to the treatment of an individual or group who is seen by the majority to be insignificant or deficient in some way as compared to the larger majority. People who are marginalized face stigmatization and discrimination; they are made to feel powerless and unimportant.

Masking: The conscious or unconscious compensation strategy used by some Neurodivergent individuals to hide their neurodivergence to fit in with the group or to avoid experiencing ableism from others is called masking. Descriptors such as high masking or low masking reflect the degree that an individual suppresses their neurodiverse traits. High masking individuals may appear neuromajority externally but experience significant internal stress. Low masking is less frequent and less intense. Many high-masking individuals struggle with internalized ableism, often being unable to advocate for their own needs and experiencing a lack of understanding and support from others.

Modification: Modifications are changes made to the curriculum in terms of complexity or amount of content. Modifications change what a person is required or expected to learn. Examples include (but are not limited to): allowing a student to use a calculator instead of mastering math facts/using mental math, reduced spelling words or reducing the number of questions on an assessment, and providing alternate materials for a student that does not contain the same amount of content as the general education curriculum.

Multidimensional Support: This term refers to the idea that support is not one-dimensional but rather consists of multiple areas of a person's life. For example, a Neurodivergent college student may have both academic and life skills support.

Multiply Neurodivergent: Multiply neurodivergent refers to an individual's neurocognitive functioning and how that differs from what is considered to be typical by the majority. This term can be used to describe an individual who has multiple diagnoses such as autism and anxiety or ADHD and depression.

National Access Plan 2022–2028 Ireland: The National Access Plan 2022–2028 is a strategic action plan for Ireland's higher education system that includes a focus on equity of access, participation, and success for all students.

Neuroaffirming: This term refers to an approach that recognizes and respects the unique differences in function and cognitive style characterized by neurodivergence. It views neurodiversity in more positive terms than using a deficit lens.

Neuroconforming: Neuroconforming refers to an individual whose cognitive and functional traits are considered to be "normal" or "average" for a given cultural or age group.

Neurodifference: This term refers to a variation in how a person's brain functions and/or processes information, acknowledging that there is no right or wrong way for a brain to work.

Neurodivergent/Neurodivergence: These terms describe a person or people who have a difference that affects the way in which the brain processes information, how a person learns, or how a person behaves that is considered to be atypical by the majority. It is a natural human variation and describes individuals who have a less typical cognitive variation such as Autism, ADHD, dyslexia, dyspraxia, or other cognitive differences. Neurodivergent is also more identity based rather than medically determined through a diagnosis that can reinforce the idea of neurodivergence as a disorder or deficit to be cured or remediated rather than accepted as human variation.

Neurodiversity/Neurodiverse: The noun neurodiversity and the adjective neurodiverse refer to the differences in brain function and cognitive characteristics. They are broader descriptors that refer to a population, a concept, a project, or research for example.

Neuroinclusive: This term refers to the creation of environments, policies and/or practices that support and embrace individuals with neurodifferences. Academic and social spaces that are created based on universal design principles are more neuroinclusive than settings geared toward neuromajority individuals only.

Neuromajority: Brains which learn and process information in what is often assumed the "standard" way are considered to be the neuromajority. A group of individuals who possess neurological functioning consistent with the majority of humans are sometimes referred to as neurotypical; however, whereas neurotypical may be a value laden term, neuromajority is a neutral term reflecting the proportion within the human population. This may be contrasted with the neurominority also referred to as Neurodivergent individuals who can be viewed as abnormal by the majority.

Neuronormativity: The assumption that there exists a "standard" or "superior" pattern of brain functioning and behavior by extension, is described as neuronormativity.

Neurotypes: Broader categories or labels of brains that, while not identical to one another, share common features in how they may communicate, process, think, remember, and/or experience the world are given labels to reflect their commonalities. These neurotypes can be described as neurotypical, autistic, ADHD, obsessive compulsive disorder, Tourette's syndrome, etc.

Orientation: Orientation is the organized introduction to college life, expectations, and resources offered by the higher education institution for incoming college students. This generally takes place during the period before classes begin and allows students to become familiar with options for academic, extracurricular, and social opportunities and support.

Participatory Methods: Work done in partnership or collaboration with the population being studied or served uses participatory methods that seek, value, and disseminate the experiences and viewpoints of those at the center of the research. Rather than conducting a study "on" a particular population, participatory methods include members of the population as full contributors who help design the study, drive the process, conduct the data collection, analyze the data, and disseminate the results.

Peer Mentoring: Peer mentoring is an education term that describes individuals with similar learning characteristics who support one another's growth and development through sharing information, skills, and support. They are members of the same group such as students or faculty members who share their own experiences to guide their peers. One peer is often more experienced such as an upper level student who mentors a beginning student.

Person-In-Environment (PIE): This is a social work theory that focuses on understanding individuals within their social, cultural, and physical environments. It recognizes that a person's environment significantly impacts their behavior and affects their well-being. The term is used to designate the importance of the interaction with the person-in-environment in determining engagement, assessment, and intervention in social work.

Pedagogy: Pedagogy is often described as the act of teaching. The pedagogy adopted by teachers shapes their actions, judgments, and teaching strategies by taking into consideration theories of learning, understandings of students and their needs, and the backgrounds and interests of individual students.

Phenomenology: A philosophical viewpoint and a method of research that examines an individual's experience, such as of an event or context, is called phenomenology. It focuses on understanding the lived experiences of individuals who encounter a particular phenomenon such as having a disability in postsecondary education or who come up against stigma in a social setting due to their disability.

Phenomenological Variant of Ecological Systems Theory (PVEST): PVEST is a framework that connects individual experience with the ecological systems theory of Urie Bronfenbrenner. This approach looks at human development in terms of how an individual is influenced by feedback from their surrounding environments, including the microsystem, mesosystem, exosystem, macrosystem, and chronosystem described by Bronfenbrenner.

Process, Person, Context, and Time (PPCT) Framework: PPCT is a model within Bronfenbrenner's ecological systems theory. The process includes interactions with others within the levels of ecological systems theory; the person refers to individual traits such as cognitive abilities that are impacted by the environment; the context includes the family, school, community, and cultural layers of the environment; and time examines how individuals develop over time and throughout history.

Problem-Centered Learning: Teachers who use problem-centered learning techniques provide students with real world problems to solve to learn about specific content. Critical thinking, collaboration, and self-direction are elements of problem-centered learning where the proposed problems are designed to engage students actively at a high level; the students do not passively receive information in problem-centered learning.

Professional Learning Community (PLC): In education, a PLC is a group of professional educators who come together to learn from each other. They meet to discuss problems they experience, solutions for those problems, and strategies to improve teaching and learning. The goal of the professional collaboration is to share expertise that will generate positive student outcomes. Action research can be at the center of the collaborative inquiry.

Reactive Coping Processes: Reactive coping processes are specific adaptive or maladaptive self-regulation mechanisms that individuals use in the moment to respond to challenges. After a stressful event has occurred, individuals react to the situation, whether positively or negatively. Reactive coping offers strategies for dealing with the problem, the emotions produced, and/or the complications of social relational interactions that result.

Reasonable Adjustments: In the United Kingdom, the term for learning accommodations offered to ensure students with disabilities are not substantially disadvantaged is called reasonable adjustments; the US equivalent is reasonable accommodations.

Rehabilitation Act of 1973 Section 504: In the United States, Section 504 of the Rehabilitation Act of 1973 provides protections to students who have disabilities whether they are in K12 schools or postsecondary education. It prohibits discrimination within all programs and activities that are federally funded including healthcare, public education, and transportation; it applies to service availability, accessibility, delivery, employment, and administrative activities and responsibilities. It is pertinent to students with disabilities who do not require special education services under IDEA but who still need accommodations.

Retention: In higher education, retention refers to the ability for institutions to keep students enrolled after they begin postsecondary study. The goal of retention initiatives is to maintain student progress through graduation, and it is a significant factor in the evaluation of an institution's effectiveness and success.

Russell Group: The Russell Group is a self-selected association of 24 public research universities in the United Kingdom, similar in prestige to the Ivy League in the United States. The group works to advocate for policies and practices supported by their research.

Salamanca Statement on Special Needs Education (UNESCO, 1994): The Salamanca Statement was written at the World Conference on Special Needs Education: Access and Quality in 1994. Its premise is that all children have a fundamental right to education and must be provided with the opportunity to achieve a reasonable level of education. It recognizes the uniqueness of each child in terms of individual traits, interests, and abilities, which may or may not require specific support. Details can be found at https://unesdoc.unesco.org/ark:/48223/pf0000098427

Scaffolding: In education, scaffolding is a teaching method or approach whereby instructors provide temporary support to learners to aid in the understanding of new skills. This temporary support is gradually taken away as a student becomes more proficient with the skill.

Self-Advocacy: Self-advocacy is the ability one has and the actions one takes to represent their own views or interests. Self-advocating requires an individual to speak for themselves and express their own unique interests, wants, and needs. Developing self-advocacy skills is important for Neurodivergent college students because of the structure of the disclosure process and system to obtain accommodations.

Self-Awareness: Self-awareness is the ability for individuals to recognize how they think, feel, act, and view themselves.

Self-Concept: Self-concept is the ability to understand oneself broadly, taking into account personal beliefs, personality traits, talents, weaknesses, and skills. It includes recognition of their roles within society.

Self-Determination: Self-determination is a term used to describe an individual's ability to make their own choices and decisions without interference from others. Self-determined individuals have the opportunity to set their own goals, make their own choices, and take responsibility for their life.

Self-Directed Learning: Self-directed learning is exhibited when students decide what they want to learn, come up with a way to learn, go through the process of learning, and evaluate their own success. It does not mean that they are learning in isolation; they can make a choice to learn within a group or classroom setting while they retain a degree of control over the process. Self-directed students typically learn through various networks and through consultation with others, often peers. The significant element in self-directed learning is that it is the individual student's choice how to go about learning; they take the initiative for their education. Self-directed learners are autonomous and directed by their personal goals.

Self-Management/Self-Regulation: For individuals to learn, they must be able to self-manage or self-regulate their behavior so that they can focus on the learning task. Students need self-management to be able to pay attention without becoming distracted, recognize what needs to be done, make a plan to accomplish the task, and move through the steps of the plan. They also need to be able to self-regulate their emotional responses in a learning environment and demonstrate resilience when faced with significant challenges that may cause disappointment if not easily achieved.

Sensory-Friendly: Sensory-Friendly is a term used to describe an environment or activity that has been altered to be accommodating to individuals with sensory sensitivities. For example, a sensory friendly dance may include the option of headphones instead of a traditional DJ or band, adjusted lighting (dimmed lighting and/or the avoidance of use of flashing lights), the provision of quiet spaces, and the limiting of scents within the environment by providing food and drink in a separate room.

Sensory Sensitivity: Sensory sensitivity is a common term for sensory processing sensitivity (SPS). This condition refers to a person's heightened awareness and response to sensory stimuli such as light, sound, smell, taste, or touch.

Social Constructivist Learning: Social constructivists view learning as occurring through social interaction with others where learners construct new knowledge together rather than merely absorbing information. Psychologist Lev Vygotsky (1896-1934) articulated its principles in his sociocultural theory. Cooperative learning and collaborative projects exemplify social constructivist learning.

Social Learning Theory: Albert Bandura's social learning theory emphasizes learning through observation and imitation. Students viewing others who model particular behaviors and skills can recognize the consequences of gaining skills and knowledge and learn to adopt them.

Sociocultural Theory: Sociocultural Theory/Zone of Proximal Development (ZPD) is Lev Vygotsky's framework that highlights how learning is shaped by social interaction and cultural context. The Zone of Proximal Development is the area in learning between what students can do on their own and what they can do with guidance from others such as teachers, peers, and/or learning specialists. The ZPD highlights the skills learners can achieve and the tasks they can accomplish with support.

Social-Emotional Construct: This construct argues that social and emotional development is a complex, ongoing, interconnected process. Its elements consist of all individuals acquiring varied skills and abilities within different timelines and levels of instruction and support.

Special Education: Special Education is a broad term used to describe the specially designed instruction and individualized supports and services provided to exceptional learners such as those who are neurodivergent. Special Education is a service, not a location or specific professionals, and it includes various evidence-based teaching methods, specialized materials and/or equipment, and adapted environments.

Standard Rules on the Equalization of Opportunities for Persons with Disabilities (UNESCO, 1993): The Standard Rules on the Equalization of Opportunities for Persons with Disabilities were adopted by the United Nations General Assembly in 1993. They represent a commitment to providing individuals with physical and cognitive disabilities equal opportunities and can guide policy-making. They reflect a human rights approach to inclusion and contain 4 specific sections on "preconditions for equal participation, target areas for equal participation, implementation measures, and the monitoring mechanism – and cover all aspects of life of persons with disabilities." Details can be found at https://www.un.org/development/desa/disabilities/standard%20rules-on-the-equalization-of-opportunities-for-persons-with-disabilities.html

Stigma: It is a negative view and perception of other people in society based on certain characteristics. Stigma results when human differences are viewed as abnormal and are present in a minority group of individuals who do not meet standards developed by the majority group. Neurodivergent learners are stigmatized and experience exclusions due to their cognitive differences. *Stigma: Notes on the Management of Spoiled Identity* by Erving Goffman is a seminal work on the topic.

Strengths, Weaknesses, Opportunities, and Threats Analysis (SWOT): Analyzing the strengths, weaknesses, opportunities and threats of an institution or organization can guide strategic planning and decision-making on policies and practices. First developed as a tool for business, it can also be applied in education by administrators, departments, faculty members, and students to identify problems and design solutions

Strength-Based Perspective: This framework concentrates on an individual's strengths, abilities, and resources rather than their weaknesses or deficits. It is person-centered and sees an individual as having the decision-making power to take charge of their own life and determine a path to accomplish their goals. It focuses on strengths, provides hope, builds resilience, and nurtures growth as a person moves within the community and interacts with others and uses available resources.

Student Engagement: On the postsecondary levels, student engagement includes not just attending classes but becoming actively involved and showing motivation to succeed. It creates an enhanced sense of belonging, and leads to increased learning, better grades, and higher graduation rates.

Students as Partners: This is a teaching approach that fosters collaboration between students and educators as equal partners in the learning process. For example, students actively contribute to curriculum development and course design. This creates a more inclusive and engaging learning environment.

Sustainability: Sustainable development are the goals established by the United Nations for appropriate future development for countries in the world. It focuses on how to meet present needs without damaging the prospects for meeting needs in the future. Sustainability can be studied and practiced in the areas of the environment, the economy, and the social construction of society.

Systems Change/Think Systems Theory: Systems thinking and systems change represents widespread shifts within an organization's functioning, processes, procedures, and environments. This may be contrasted with more targeted, less comprehensive change occurring in one office within a HEI, for example. Systems theory emphasizes understanding complex systems by focusing on how different parts interact and influence each other, rather than just analyzing individual components. It is a holistic approach that recognizes the interconnectedness of things and the dynamic nature of systems, where the whole is greater than the sum of its parts.

Think College: In the United States, Think College is the national coordinating center for Transition and Postsecondary Programs for Students with Intellectual Disability (TPSID) programs; it provides technical assistance and training for IPSE program development and carries on extensive IPSE research and evaluation.

Transition Planning: Transition planning is required under IDEA for students with disabilities as they move from K12 to post school in employment, postsecondary education and/or training, and independent living. The objective is for the student to become an independent, gainfully employed adult. Goals in each area are developed through the secondary school IEP team that describes what services are needed during the process, what activities will occur, what courses support an effective transition, and where, when, how often, and under whom the transition steps will occur.

Transition and Postsecondary Programs for Students with Intellectual Disabilities (TPSID): Transition and Postsecondary Programs for Students with Intellectual Disabilities (TPSID) is a federally funded grant in the United States that supports the development and operation of programs for individuals with Intellectual Disabilities to attend higher education and gain employment skills.

Universal Accessibility: Universal accessibility is the design and implementation of environments, products, and services to be usable by all people, regardless of their abilities, disabilities, or other differences, without the need for adaptation or specialized design.

Universal Design (UD): Universal Design is a framework that aims to proactively identify and prevent barriers within the design of systems, procedures, processes, materials, and environments to promote the greatest usability and inclusion by all individuals. Although developed within architecture, Universal Design has been applied to a variety of domains such as education.

Universal Design for Learning (UDL): This educational framework provides flexible teaching methods and materials to accommodate diverse learning needs, ensuring all students have equal opportunities to succeed in the learning process. The implementation of UDL focuses on designing instruction, assessment, and educational interactions within the context of teaching and learning. Multiple means of engagement, representation, and expression are key features of UDL. It is an educational framework that aims to improve and optimize teaching for all people based on scientific insights into how humans learn. It was introduced by David Rose and Anne Meyer in the 1990s, applying Ron Mace's architectural universal design principles to learning, and further articulated by researchers at their Center for Applied Special Technology (CAST).

United Nations Convention on the Rights of People with Disabilities (2006): The UNCRPD human rights model affirms the right of all people, including those with physical and intellectual disabilities, to be included in educational opportunities. It mandates that countries who have signed the agreement provide equal access to information for all individuals. Neurodiversity is covered in Article 9 that mandates access to the physical environment, transportation, information, communication, and other public facilities and services for individuals with disabilities; Article 21 requires public information to be presented in accessible formats and technologies; Article 24 explains the requirements for accessibility to learning materials and methods for individuals with intellectual and cognitive disabilities.

United Nations Educational, Scientific and Cultural Organization (UNESCO): A subgroup of the United Nations, UNESCO focuses on encouraging worldwide peace and equality through communication and educational, scientific, and cultural initiatives.

Video modeling: This is a type of instruction that involves recording a model demonstrating a skill or behavior and showing the video recording to a target student, who then works to perform the skill or behavior with increasing independence.

Workforce Innovation and Opportunity Act (WIOA): Signed into law in the United States in 2014, this act is "designed to help job seekers access employment, education, training, and support services to succeed in the labor market and to match employers with the skilled workers they need to compete in the global economy." (U.S. Department of Labor). Details can be found at https://www.dol.gov/agencies/eta/wioa

Workforce Readiness: Workforce readiness refers to the degree to which individuals possess the skills, knowledge, and behaviors needed to successfully enter and contribute to the workplace. The degree of readiness encompasses a combination of technical skills, "soft skills" (e.g. communication, time management, teamwork), and the ability to adapt to the demands of the modern work environment.

Compilation of References

Accardo, A. L., Bomgardner, E. M., Rubinstein, M. B., & Woodruff, J. (2024). Valuing neurodiversity on campus: Perspectives and priorities of neurodivergent students, faculty, and professional staff. *Journal of Diversity in Higher Education.* Advance online publication. https://doi-org.DOI: 10.1037/dhe0000571

Accardo, A. L., Bean, K., Cook, B., Gillies, A., Edgington, R., Kuder, S. J., & Bomgardner, E. M. (2019). College access, success and equity for students on the autism spectrum. *Journal of Autism and Developmental Disorders*, *49*(12), 4877–4890. DOI: 10.1007/s10803-019-04205-8 PMID: 31482372

ADA Amendments Act, Pub. L. No. 110-325, 42 U.S.C. 12101 et seq. (2008).

Adam, M. (2021). *A grounded theory of overcommitment in undergraduate college students* (Doctoral dissertation, Florida Atlantic University). https://www.proquest.com/docview/2621326323/abstract/3B0BDB12600C4E3EPQ/1

Adams, M., & Brown, S. (Eds.). (2006). *Towards inclusive learning in higher education: Developing curricula for disabled students.* Routledge. DOI: 10.4324/9780203088623

Aftab, R., Pirani, S., Mansoor, M., & Nadeem, T. (2023). Caregiver strain and its associated factors in Autism Spectrum Disorder in Karachi, Pakistan. *Journal of the College of Physicians and Surgeons—Pakistan*, *33*(7), 784–788. DOI: 0.29271/jcpsp.2023.07.784 PMID: 37401221

Aguilar, O., & Lipson, S. K. (2021). A public health approach to understanding the mental health needs of college students with disabilities: Results from a national survey. *Journal of Postsecondary Education and Disability*, *34*(3), 273–285. https://eric.ed.gov/?id=EJ1325421

Ahmad, S., & Yousaf, M. (2011). Special education in Pakistan: Perspectives of educational policies and plans. *Academic Research International*, *1*(2), 228. http://www.savap.org.pk/journals/ARInt./Vol.1(2)/2011(1.2-21a).pdf

Ahmad, Z., Sanauddin, N., & Nawab, H. (2023). From hostage to host: The spirit possession, mediumship, and gender relations in Chitral, Pakistan. *Journal of Humanities. Social and Management Sciences, 4*(1), 28–40. DOI: 10.47264/idea.jhsms/4.1.3

Ahmed, N., Pasha, A. R., & Malik, M. (2021). The role of teacher training programs in optimizing teacher motivation and professional development skills. *Bulletin of Education and Research,43*(2), 17-37. ISSN- 0555-7747. https://eric.ed.gov/?id=EJ1338294

Akhtar, S., Ahmed, A., Ahmad, A., Ali, Z., Riaz, M., & Ismail, T. (2013). Iron status of the Pakistani population: Current issues and strategies. *Asia Pacific Journal of Clinical Nutrition, 22*(3), 340–347. DOI: 10.6133/apjcn.2013.22.3.17 PMID: 23945403

Aladin, S., Smith, T., Dufresne, S., & Crehan, E. T. (2022, April 14). *Increasing accessibility at Tufts for neurodiverse individuals.* Poster presented at the 29th Annual Fred Rothbaum Student Presentation Day, Medford, MA.

Ali, S. K., & Baig, L. A. (2012). Problems and issues in implementing an innovative curriculum in developing countries: The Pakistani experience. *BMC Medical Education, 12*(1), 1–8. DOI: 10.1186/1472-6920-12-31 PMID: 22591729

Alonso, H. H. (1995). Nobel peace laureates, Jane Addams and Emily Greene Balch: Two women of the Women's International League for Peace and Freedom. *Journal of Women's History, 7*(2), 6–26. DOI: 10.1353/jowh.2010.0337

Alqazlan, S., Alallawi, B., & Totsika, V. (2019). Post-secondary education for young people with intellectual disabilities: A systematic review of stakeholders' experiences. *Educational Research Review, 28*, 100295. DOI: 10.1016/j.edurev.2019.100295

Amend, D. J., Lein, A. E., Taylor, A. J., & Dinkins, E. G. (2024). Collaborative inclusion: IEP team perspectives on supporting students with extensive needs and the implications for teacher preparation programs. *Kentucky Teacher Education Journal: The Journal of the Teacher Education Division of the Kentucky Council for Exceptional Children, 11*(2), 6. DOI: 10.61611/2995-5904.1062

American Psychological Association. (2024). *For parents: Adjusting to college - a brief guide and frequently asked questions for parents of students with disabilities.* https://www.apa.org/pi/disability/resources/parent-college-guide

Americans with Disabilities Act, 42 U.S.C. § 12101 et seq. (1990).

Americans with Disabilities Act. (n.d.). *Introduction to the Americans with Disabilities Act.* https://www.ada.gov/topics/intro-to-ada/

Ames, M. E., Coombs, C. E. M., Duerksen, K., Vincent, J., & McMorris, C. A. (2022). Canadian mapping of autism-specific supports for postsecondary students. *Research in Autism Spectrum Disorders*, *90*, 101899. DOI: 10.1016/j.rasd.2021.101899

Amin, N., Tariq, M., Arshad, M., & Cheema, M. A. (2024). Frequency of visual impairment in autistic children at an autism school in Lahore, Pakistan. *British Journal of Visual Impairment*, *42*(2), 478–485. DOI: 10.1177/02646196221145367

Anderson, A. H., Carter, M., & Stephenson, J. (2018). Perspectives of university students with Autism Spectrum Disorder. *Journal of Autism and Developmental Disorders*, *50*(3), 935–946. DOI: 10.1007/s10803-017-3257-3 PMID: 28756552

Anderson, A. H., Stephenson, J., & Carter, M. (2017). A systematic literature review of the experiences and supports of students with autism spectrum disorder in post-secondary education. *Research in Autism Spectrum Disorders*, *39*, 33–53. DOI: 10.1016/j.rasd.2017.04.002

Anderson, A. H., Stephenson, J., Carter, M., & Carlon, S. (2019). A systematic literature review of empirical research on postsecondary students with Autism Spectrum Disorder. *Journal of Autism and Developmental Disorders*, *49*(4), 1531–1558. DOI: 10.1007/s10803-018-3840-2 PMID: 30536219

Andresen, J. (2024). How inclusive is inclusive postsecondary education? Over-and under-representation of individuals with intellectual disabilities in postsecondary education. *Journal of Inclusive Postsecondary Education*, *5*(2). Advance online publication. DOI: 10.13021/jipe.2024.3547

Anicha, C. L., Aragon, C., Bilen-Green, C., Blaser, B., & Burgstahler, S. (2024). A continuum of actions you can take now to ADVANCE disability equity: A report from the field. *Advance Journal (Corvallis, Ore.)*, *4*(2), 1–32. DOI: 10.5399/osu/ADVJRNL.4.2.9

Appleton, R., Connell, C., Fairclough, E., Tuomainem, H., & Singh, S. P. (2019). Outcomes of young people who reach the transition boundary of child and adolescent mental health services: A systematic review. *European Child & Adolescent Psychiatry*, *2019*(28), 1431–1446. DOI: 10.1007/s00787-019-01307-7 PMID: 30850925

Aquino, K. C., Cook, K. D., & Bittinger, J. (2025). A national look at shifts in disability self-identification for students enrolled in higher education. *AERA Open*, *11*, 23328584251322511. DOI: 10.1177/23328584251322511

Ardeleanu, K., Steinberg, H., Garfield, T., Voltaire, S., Shea, L., Brown, M., Chvasta, K., & Tan, C. D. (2024). Self-identification of autism: Why some autistic adults lack a clinical diagnosis and why this matters for inclusion. *Autism. Autism, 13623613241297222*, 13623613241297222. Advance online publication. DOI: 10.1177/13623613241297222 PMID: 39552426

Armstrong, T. (2010). *Neurodiversity: Discovering the extraordinary gifts of autism, ADHD, dyslexia, and other brain differences*. ReadHowYouWant.com.

ASAN. (2013). *Navigating college: A handbook on self advocacy written for autistic students from autistic adults*. The Autistic Press.

Ashinoff, B. K., & Abu-Akel, A. (2021). Hyperfocus: The forgotten frontier of attention. *Psychological Research, 85*(1), 1–19. DOI: 10.1007/s00426-019-01245-8 PMID: 31541305

Asian Development Bank. (2024). *Pakistan and ADB*. Asian Development Bank. https://www.adb.org/countries/pakistan/main

Association of Occupational Therapists of Ireland (AOTI). (2025). *What is occupational therapy?* https://www.aoti.ie/what-is-ot

Association on Higher Education And Disability. (2021). *AHEAD annual report 2021*. AHEAD. https://www.ahead.ie/userfiles/files/AHEAD_Report_2021_digital.pdf

Aston, D. (2019). *Higher education opportunities for students with intellectual disabilities in the Republic of Ireland: A national response*. Trinity College Dublin. https://cc.careersportal.ie/mce/plugins/filemanager/files/Claire/A-National-Response%20INHEF%20Repoert.pdf

Attwood, T. (2006). *The complete guide to Asperger's syndrome*. Jessica Kingsley Publishers.

Attwood, T. (2007). *Autism and girls*. Future Horizons.

Austin, R. D., & Pisano, G. P. (2017). Neurodiversity as a competitive advantage. *Harvard Business Review, 95*(3), 96–103. https://celebratingneurodiversity365.com/wp-content/uploads/2019/08/Neurodiversity-Is-a-Competitive-Advantage-article-in-Harvard-Biz-Review.pdf

Azeem, M. W., Imran, N., & Nazeer, A. (2021). Pakistan and autism. In *Encyclopedia of Autism Spectrum Disorders* (pp. 3260–3262). Springer International Publishing. DOI: 10.1007/978-3-319-91280-6_102029

Baglieri, S. (2023). *Disability studies and the inclusive classroom. Critical practices for embracing diversity in education* (3rd ed.). Routledge.

Baio, J., Wiggins, L., Christensen, D. L., Maenner, M. J., Daniels, J., Warren, Z., Kurzius-Spencer, M., Zahorodny, W., Robinson, C., Rosenberg, , White, T., Durkin, M. S., Imm, P., Nikolaou, L., Yeargin-Allsopp, M., Lee, L.-C., Harrington, R., Lopez, M., Fitzgerald, R. T., & Dowling, N. F. (2018). Prevalence of Autism Spectrum Disorder among children aged 8 years—Autism and developmental disabilities monitoring network, 11 sites, United States, 2014. *MMWR. Surveillance Summaries*, *67*(6), 1–23. DOI: 10.15585/mmwr.ss6706a1 PMID: 29701730

Baker, D. L. (2011). *The politics of neurodiversity: Why people policy matters*. Lynne Rienner Publishers. DOI: 10.1515/9781685851224

Bakker, T., Krabbendam, L., Bhulai, S., & Begeer, S. (2019). Background and enrollment characteristics of students with autism in higher education. *Research in Autism Spectrum Disorders*, *67*, 101424. Advance online publication. DOI: 10.1016/j.rasd.2019.101424

Bal, V. H., Kim, S. H., Cheong, D., & Lord, C. (2015). Daily living skills in individuals with autism spectrum disorder from 2 to 21 years of age. *Autism*, *19*(7), 774–784. DOI: 10.1177/1362361315575840 PMID: 25922445

Bandura, A. (1977). *Social learning theory*. Prentice Hall.

Bandura, A. (1986). *Social foundations of thought and action: A social cognitive theory*. Prentice Hall.

Banks, J., Aston, D., & Shevlin, M. (2022). Falling between two stools? Post-secondary transition planning for students with intellectual disabilities in the Republic of Ireland. In *Transition programs for children and youth with diverse needs* (pp. 143–158). Emerald Publishing Limited. DOI: 10.1108/S1479-363620220000018011

Barden, O. (2021). Getting inside histories of learning disabilities. *Educational Action Research*, *29*(4), 619–635. DOI: 10.1080/09650792.2021.1899952

Barden, O., & Walden, S. J. (2021). The metanarrative of learning disability. In Bolt, D. (Ed.), *Metanarratives of disability: Culture, assumed authority, and the normative social order* (pp. 77–93). Routledge.

Bargiela, S., Steward, R., & Mandy, W. (2016). The experiences of late-diagnosed women with autism spectrum conditions: An investigation of the female autism phenotype. *Journal of Autism and Developmental Disorders*, *46*(10), 3281–3294. DOI: 10.1007/s10803-016-2872-8 PMID: 27457364

Bashe, P. R., & Kirby, B. L. (2005). *The OASIS guide to Asperger syndrome: Advice, support, insight, and inspiration*. Crown Publishing.

Bashir, N., & Khanum, H. (2024). Autism in Pakistan: Understanding the challenges and seeking solutions. *Educational Research and Innovation*, *4*(1), 96–104. DOI: 10.61866/eri.v4i1.65

Bathmaker, A.-M. (2015). Thinking with Bourdieu: Thinking after Bourdieu. Using 'field' to consider in/equalities in the changing field of English higher education. *Cambridge Journal of Education*, *45*(1), 61–80. DOI: 10.1080/0305764X.2014.988683

Batool, H., Khan, A. M., & Khanum, S. (2019). Evaluation of quality of life of parents having children with sensory disabilities. *Pakistan Journal of Humanities & Social Sciences Research*, *2*(2), 33–44. DOI: 10.37605/pjhssr.2.2.4

Baumeister, R. F., & Leary, M. R. (1995). The need to belong: Desire for interpersonal attachments as a fundamental human motivation. *Psychological Bulletin*, *117*(3), 497–529. DOI: 10.1037/0033-2909.117.3.497 PMID: 7777651

Beck, T. J. (2023). Neurodivergent culture and embodied knowledge beyond neoliberal identity politics. *Culture & Psychology*, Article 1354067X231191489. DOI: 10.1177/1354067X231191489

Begeer, S., Mandell, D., Wijnker-Holmes, B., Venderbosch, S., Rem, D., Stekelenburg, F., & Koot, H. M. (2013). Sex differences in the timing of identification among children and adults with Autism Spectrum Disorders. *Journal of Autism and Developmental Disorders*, *43*(5), 1151–1156. DOI: 10.1007/s10803-012-1656-z PMID: 23001766

Bennett, M., & Carlson-Manathara, E. (2024). Introducing the special theme issue: Examining allyship with Indigenous peoples. *Canadian Social Work Review*, •••, 5–18. DOI: 10.7202/1114538ar

Beresford, B. (2004). On the road to nowhere? Young disabled people and transition. *Child: Care, Health and Development*, *30*(6), 581–587. DOI: 10.1111/j.1365-2214.2004.00469.x PMID: 15527469

Berg, L. A., Jirikowic, T., Haerling, K., & MacDonald, G. (2017). Navigating the hidden curriculum of higher education for postsecondary students with intellectual disabilities. *The American Journal of Occupational Therapy*, *71*(3), 7103100020. Advance online publication. DOI: 10.5014/ajot.2017.024703 PMID: 28422626

Bishop-Fitzpatrick, L., Minshew, N. J., & Eack, S. M. (2013). A systematic review of psychosocial interventions for adults with Autism Spectrum Disorders. *Journal of Autism and Developmental Disorders*, *47*(3), 1953–1967. DOI: 10.1007/s10803-012-1615-8 PMID: 22825929

Bisman, C. D. (2001). Teaching social work's bio-psycho-social assessment. *Journal of Teaching in Social Work, 21*(3–4), 75–89. DOI: 10.1300/J067v21n03_07

Black, J., & Fraser, R. (2019). Integration through collaboration: Building strategic faculty partnerships to shift minds and practices. In Bracken, S., & Novak, K. (Eds.), *Transforming higher education through universal design for learning: An international perspective* (pp. 244–257). Routledge. DOI: 10.4324/9781351132077-15

Black, K. Z., Hardy, C. Y., De Marco, M., Ammerman, A. S., Corbie-Smith, G., Council, B., Ellis, D., Eng, E., Harris, B., Jackson, M., Jean-Baptiste, J., Kearney, W., Legerton, M., Parker, D., Wynn, M., & Lightfoot, A. (2013). Beyond incentives for involvement to compensation for consultants. *Progress in Community Health Partnerships, 7*(3), 263–270. DOI: 10.1353/cpr.2013.0040 PMID: 24056508

Bliss, D. L., & Ginn, H. (2021). Expanding presence of social work advocacy on the national stage. *Journal of Social Work Education, 57*(3), 432–444. DOI: 10.1080/10437797.2019.1671266

Bolton, P. (2023). *Tuition fee statistics* (CBP-917). House of Commons Library. https://commonslibrary.parliament.uk/research-briefings/sn00917/

Boobis, S. (2016). *Evaluation of a dialogical psychologically informed environment (PIE) pilot: Addressing homelessness, re-offending, substance abuse, and mental illness*. Fulfilling Lives-Newcastle & Gateshead.

Botha, M., & Frost, D. M. (2020). Extending the minority stress model to understand mental health problems experienced by the autistic population. *Society and Mental Health, 10*(1), 20–34. DOI: 10.1177/2156869318804297

Bourke, B. (2020). Leaving behind the rhetoric of allyship. *Whiteness and Education, 5*(2), 179–194. DOI: 10.1080/23793406.2020.1839786

Boven, F. (2018). Special interests and inclusive academic learning: An autistic perspective. *Advances in Autism, 4*(4), 155–164. https://doi-org.DOI: 10.1108/AIA-05-2018-0020

Bowman, K. S., Suarez, V. D., & Weiss, M. J. (2021). Standards for interprofessional collaboration in the treatment of individuals with autism. *Behavior Analysis in Practice, 14*(4), 1191–1208. DOI: 10.1007/s40617-021-00560-0 PMID: 34868822

Bracken, S., & Novak, K. (2019). *Transforming higher education through Universal Design for Learning. An international perspective.* Routledge. DOI: 10.4324/9781351132077

Brandsen, S., Blackshear, K., Coleman, R., Hallur, S., & Chandrasekhar, T. (2024). Developing an inclusive campus for autistic students. *Journal of Diversity in Higher Education.* Advance online publication. https://doi-org.DOI: 10.1037/dhe0000551

Brandsen, T., & Honingh, M. (2018). Definitions of co-production and co-creation. In Brandsen, T., Steen, T., & Verschuere, B. (Eds.), *Co-production and co-creation: Engaging citizens in public services*. Routledge. DOI: 10.4324/9781315204956-2

Braun, V., & Clarke, V. (2006). Using thematic analysis in psychology. *Qualitative Research in Psychology*, *3*(2), 77–101. DOI: 10.1191/1478088706qp063oa

Bray, A., Devitt, A., Banks, J., Sanchez Fuentes, S., Sandoval, M., Riviou, K., Byrne, D., Flood, M., Reale, J., & Terrenzio, S. (2024). What next for Universal Design for Learning? A systematic literature review of technology in UDL implementations at second level. *British Journal of Educational Technology*, *55*(1), 113–138. DOI: 10.1111/bjet.13328

Brickhill, R., Atherton, G., Piovesan, A., & Cross, L. (2023). Autism, thy name is man: Exploring implicit and explicit gender bias in autism perceptions. *PLoS One*, *18*(8), e0284013. DOI: 10.1371/journal.pone.0284013 PMID: 37611041

Brisenden, S. J. (1986). Independent living and the medical model of disability. *Disability, Handicap & Society*, *1*(2), 173–178. DOI: 10.1080/02674648666780171

Bronfenbrenner, U. (1974). Developmental research, public policy, and the ecology of childhood. *Child Development*, *45*(1), 1–5. DOI: 10.2307/1127743

Bronfenbrenner, U. (1977). Toward an experimental ecology of human development. *The American Psychologist*, *32*(7), 513–531. DOI: 10.1037/0003-066X.32.7.513

Bronfenbrenner, U. (1979). *The ecology of human development: Experiments by nature and design*. Harvard University Press. DOI: 10.4159/9780674028845

Bronfenbrenner, U. (1989). Ecological systems theory. *Annals of Child Development*, *6*, 187–249.

Bronfenbrenner, U. (1994). Ecological models of human development. In Husen, T., & Postlethwaite, T. (Eds.), *The International Encyclopedia of Education* (2nd ed., Vol. 3, pp. 1643–1647). Pergamon.

Bronfenbrenner, U. (2001). The bioecological theory of human development. In Smelser, N. J., & Baltes, P. B. (Eds.), *International encyclopedia of the social and behavioral sciences* (Vol. 10, pp. 6963–6970). Elsevier., DOI: 10.1016/B0-08-043076-7/00359-4

Bronstein, L. R. (2003). A model for interdisciplinary collaboration. *Social Work*, *48*(3), 297–306. DOI: 10.1093/sw/48.3.297 PMID: 12899277

Brown, S. A., Silvera-Tawil, D., Gemeinboeck, P., & McGhee, J. (2016). The case for conversation: A design research framework for participatory feedback from autistic children. *OzCHI '16: The 28th Australian Conference on Computer-Human Interaction*, 605–613. DOI: 10.1145/3010915.3010934

Brownlow, C., Martin, N., Thompson, D.-M., Dowe, A., Abawi, D., Harrison, J., & March, S. (2023). Navigating university: The design and evaluation of a holistic support programme for autistic students in higher education. *Education Sciences*, *13*(5), 521. Advance online publication. DOI: 10.3390/educsci13050521

Brown, N., & Leigh, J. (2020). *Ableism in academia: Theorising experiences of disabilities and chronic illnesses in higher education*. UCL Press. DOI: 10.2307/j.ctv13xprjr

Buck, A. (2022). *Exploring the impact of EnvisionIT curriculum implementation on IEP transition goals and student participation in the transition planning process: A qualitative case study* (Order No. 29730322) [Doctoral dissertation, The Ohio State University]. ProQuest Dissertations & Theses Global. https://www.proquest.com/docview/2720903749

Bumble, J. L., Worth, C. R. J., Athamanah, L. S., Rooney-Kron, M., Regester, A., & Lidgus, J. (2021). "Messy inclusion": A call for dignity of risk in inclusive postsecondary education. *In Practice*, *1*(2), 64–69. DOI: 10.1177/27324745211050023

Burgstahler, S. (2024). *What are alternatives to disability-related simulations to promote disability awareness?* University of Washington, DO-IT (Disabilities, Opportunities, Internetworking, and Technology) Center. https://www.washington.edu/doit/what-are-alternatives-disability-related-simulations-promote-disability-awareness#:~:text=Another%20way%20to%20do%20this,for%20her%20live%20with%20autism

Burgstahler, S. (2015). *Universal design in higher education: From principles to practice* (2nd ed.). Harvard Education Press.

Burke, M. M., Mercer, C., Ramos-Torres, S., Lindsay, R., & Burakov, I. (2024). Frequently asked questions and answers for supporting students with Section 504 plans. *Intervention in School and Clinic*, *60*(4), 214–219. DOI: 10.1177/10534512241297322

Burns, A., Dannecker, E., & Austin, M. J. (2019). Revisiting the biological perspective in the use of biopsychosocial assessments in social work. *Journal of Human Behavior in the Social Environment*, *29*(2), 177–194. DOI: 10.1080/10911359.2018.1500505

Bury, S. M., Jellett, R., Spoor, J. R., & Hedley, D. (2020). "It defines who I am" or "It's something I have": What language do Autistic Australian adults on the autism spectrum prefer? *Disability & Society, 35*(9), 1514–1537. DOI: 10.1007/s10803-020-04425-3 PMID: 32112234

Butcher, L., & Lane, S. (2024). Neurodivergent (Autism and ADHD) student experiences of access and inclusion in higher education: An ecological systems theory perspective. *Higher Education: The International Journal of Higher Education Research,* 1–21. https://doi-org.DOI: 10.1007/s10734-024-01319-6

Byrne, D. (2022). A worked example of Braun and Clarke's approach to reflexive thematic analysis. *Quality & Quantity, 56*(3), 1391–1412. DOI: 10.1007/s11135-021-01182-y

Cage, E., De Andres, M., & Mahoney, P. (2020). Understanding the factors that affect university completion for autistic people. *Research in Autism Spectrum Disorders, 72*, 101519. DOI: 10.1016/j.rasd.2020.101519

Cage, E., Monaco, J., & Newell, V. (2018). Experiences of autism acceptance and mental health in autistic adults. *Journal of Autism and Developmental Disorders, 48*(2), 473–484. DOI: 10.1007/s10803-017-3342-7 PMID: 29071566

Cage, E., & Troxell-Whitman, Z. (2019). Understanding the reasons, contexts, and costs of camouflaging for autistic adults. *Journal of Autism and Developmental Disorders, 49*(5), 1899–1911. DOI: 10.1007/s10803-018-03878-x PMID: 30627892

Caiels, J. C., Milne, A., & Beadle-Brown, J. (2021). Strengths-based approaches in social work and social care: Reviewing the evidence. *Journal of Long-Term Care, 401-402*, 401–422. Advance online publication. DOI: 10.31389/jltc.102

Cai, R. Y., & Richdale, A. L. (2016). Educational experiences and needs of higher education students with Autism Spectrum Disorder. *Journal of Autism and Developmental Disorders, 46*(1), 31–41. DOI: 10.1007/s10803-015-2535-1 PMID: 26216381

Caldora, J. B.II, & Coghill, E. M. H. (2020). Self advocacy. In Coghill, E. M. H., & Coghill, J. G. (Eds.), *Supporting neurodiverse college student success: A guide for librarians, student support services, and academic learning environments* (pp. 8–22). Rowman & Littlefield.

Canadian University Survey Consortium. (June, 2024). *2024 Graduating student survey master report.* https://cusc-ccreu.ca/wordpress/?lang=en&download=3708&tmstv=1742270935

Cassidy, S., Bradley, L., Shaw, R., & Baron-Cohen, S. (2018). Risk markers for suicidality in autistic adults. *Molecular Autism*, *9*(1), 42. DOI: 10.1186/s13229-018-0226-4 PMID: 30083306

CAST. (2024). *Universal Design for Learning Guidelines version 3.0* [graphic organizer]. https://udlguidelines.cast.org/static/udlg3-graphicorganizer-digital-numbers-a11y.pdf

CAST. (2024). *Universal design for learning guidelines version 3.0.* CAST. Retrieved from https://udlguidelines.cast.org

CAST. (2024a). About CAST. https://www.cast.org/about/about-cast

CAST. (2024a). *Research evidence*. Universal Design for Learning Guidelines version 3.0. https://udlguidelines.cast.org/more/research-evidence/

CAST. (2024b). *The UDL Guidelines*. Universal Design for Learning Guidelines version 3.0. https://udlguidelines.cast.org

CAST. (2024b). Universal Design for Learning Guidelines version 3.0. https://udlguidelines.cast.org/

CAST. (n.d.). The UDL guidelines. *UDL Guidelines*. https://udlguidelines.cast.org/

Center for Applied Special Technology (CAST). (2018). *Universal Design for Learning Guidelines* version 2.2. http://udlguidelines.cast.org

Chadwick, D., Ågren, K. A., Caton, S., Chiner, E., Danker, J., Gómez-Puerta, M., Heitplatz, V., Johansson, S., Normand, C. L., Murphy, E., Plichta, P., Strnadová, I., & Wallén, E. F. (2022). Digital inclusion and participation of people with intellectual disabilities during COVID-19: A rapid review and international bricolage. *Journal of Policy and Practice in Intellectual Disabilities*, *19*(3), 242–256. DOI: 10.1111/jppi.12410

Chapman, R. (2021). Neurodiversity and the Social Ecology of Mental Functions. *Perspectives on Psychological Science*, *16*(6), 1360–1372. https://doiorg.ezproxy.lib.ucalgary.ca/10.1177/1745691620959833. DOI: 10.1177/1745691620959833 PMID: 33577400

Cheang, R. T. S., Skjevling, M., Blakemore, A. I. F., Kumari, V., & Puzzo, I. (2024). Do you feel me? Autism, empathic accuracy and the double empathy problem. *AUTISM*. Advance online publication. https://doi-org.DOI: 10.1177/13623613241252320

Chen, P., Chavez, O., Ong, D. C., & Gunderson, B. (2017). Strategic resource use for learning: A self-administered intervention that guides self-reflection on effective resource use enhances academic performance. *Psychological Science*, *28*(6), 774–785. DOI: 10.1177/0956797617696456 PMID: 28447894

Cherewick, M. (2024). Future directions for neurodiversity affirming autism interventions: Adolescence is a second sensitive period to support positive developmental trajectories. *Current Psychology: A Journal for Diverse Perspectives on Diverse Psychological Issues, 43*(10), 9191–9198. https://doi-org.DOI: 10.1007/s12144-023-05053-7

Children and Families Act. 2014, c. 6. (UK). https://www.legislation.gov.uk/ukpga/2014/6/contents/enacted

Chiwandire, D., & Vincent, L. (2019). Funding and inclusion in higher education institutions for students with disabilities. *African Journal of Disability*, *8*(0), 336. Advance online publication. DOI: 10.4102/ajod.v8i0.336 PMID: 30899686

Choudhry, F. R., Khan, N., & Munawar, K. (2023). Barriers and facilitators to mental health care: A systematic review in Pakistan. *International Journal of Mental Health*, *52*(2), 124–162. DOI: 10.1080/00207411.2021.1941563

Çivitci, A. (2015). Perceived stress and life satisfaction in college students: Belonging and extracurricular participation as moderators. *Procedia: Social and Behavioral Sciences*, *205*, 271–281. DOI: 10.1016/j.sbspro.2015.09.077

Clayburn, C. (2023, November 14). How to navigate college admissions with a learning disability. *U. S. News & World Report.* https://www.usnews.com/education/articles/how-to-navigate-college-as-a-neurodivergent-student

Clince, M., Connolly, L., & Nolan, C. (2016). Comparing and exploring the sensory processing patterns of higher education students with attention deficit hyperactivity disorder and Autism Spectrum Disorder. *The American Journal of Occupational Therapy*, *70*(2), 1–9. DOI: 10.5014/ajot.2016.016816 PMID: 26943106

Clouder, L., Karakus, M., Cinotti, A., Ferreyra, M. V., Fierros, G. A., & Rojo, P. (2020). Neurodiversity in higher education: A narrative synthesis. *Higher Education*, *80*(4), 757–778. DOI: 10.1007/s10734-020-00513-6

Cole, A. (2016). The 'three conversations' model: turning away from long-term care. *The Guardian*. https://www.theguardian.com/social-care-network/2016/nov/01/the-three-conversations-model-turning-away-from-long-term-care

Cole, J. Y., Graham, J., Norvell, S., & Schaber, P. (2024). Universal design for learning principles impact on students with neurodiverse learning styles. *Journal of Occupational Therapy Education*, *8*(2), 1–21. DOI: 10.26681/jote.2024.080204

College Autism Network (CAN). (2025). *College Autism Network advocacy, research, training*. https://collegeautismnetwork.org

College Autism Network. (n.d.). *Autism-specific College Support Programs (ASPs)*. Retrieved March 5, 2024, from https://can.softr.app/

Collier-Spruel, L. A., & Ryan, A. M. (2024). Are all allyship attempts helpful? An investigation of effective and ineffective allyship. *Journal of Business and Psychology*, *39*(1), 83–108. DOI: 10.1007/s10869-022-09861-9

Connell, J. P., Halpem-Felsher, B. L., Clifford, E., Crichlow, W., & Usinger, P. (1995). Hanging in there: Behavioral, psychological, and contextual factors affecting whether African American adolescents stay in high school. *Journal of Adolescent Research*, *10*(1), 41–63. DOI: 10.1177/0743554895101004

Connolly, S. E., Constable, H. L., & Mullally, S. L. (2023). School distress and the school attendance crisis: A story dominated by neurodivergence and unmet need. *Frontiers in Psychiatry*, *14*, 1237052. Advance online publication. DOI: 10.3389/fpsyt.2023.1237052 PMID: 37810599

Connor, D. J. (2012). Helping students with disabilities transition to college: 21 tips for students with LD and/or ADD/ADHD. *Teaching Exceptional Children*, *44*(5), 16–25. DOI: 10.1177/004005991204400502

Conrad, J. A. (2020). On intellectual and developmental disabilities in the United States: A historical perspective. *Journal of Intellectual Disabilities*, *24*(1), 85–101. DOI: 10.1177/1744629518767001 PMID: 29621909

Cook, A. (2024). Conceptualisations of neurodiversity and barriers to inclusive pedagogy in schools: A perspective article. *Journal of Research in Special Educational Needs, 24*(3), 627–636. https://doi-org.DOI: 10.1111/1471-3802.12656

Cook-Sather, A. (2018). Listening to equity-seeking perspectives: How students' experiences of pedagogical partnership can inform wider discussions of student success. *Higher Education Research & Development*, *37*(5), 923–936. DOI: 10.1080/07294360.2018.1457629

Cook-Sather, A., Bovill, C., & Felten, P. (2014). *Engaging students as partners in learning and teaching: A guide for faculty* (1st ed.). Wiley.

Cooper, P. C., Bilton, K., & Kakos, M. (2012). The importance of a biopsychosocial approach to interventions for SEBD. In Daniels, H., Cole, T., & Visser, J. (Eds.), *The Routledge International Companion to Emotional and Behavioural Difficulties*. Routledge.

Cooper, S. A., McLean, G., Guthrie, B., McConnachie, A., Mercer, S., Sullivan, F., & Morrison, J. (2015). Multiple physical and mental health comorbidity in adults with intellectual disabilities: Population-based cross-sectional analysis. *BMC Family Practice*, *16*(1), 110. Advance online publication. DOI: 10.1186/s12875-015-0329-3 PMID: 26310664

Corby, D., Taggart, L., & Cousins, W. (2020). The lived experience of people with intellectual disabilities in post-secondary or higher education. *Journal of Intellectual Disabilities*, *24*(3), 339–357. DOI: 10.1177/1744629518805603 PMID: 30301416

Coryell, J. E. (2024). Interactive lecture: Engaging active learning/interactive teaching and learning with lecture. In Coryell, J. E., Baumgartner, L. M., & Bohonos, J. W. (Eds.), *Methods for facilitating adult learning: Strategies for enhancing instruction and instructor effectiveness* (pp. 27–37). Routledge. DOI: 10.4324/9781003446019-3

Council for Opportunity in Education. (n.d.). *COE and TRIO programs*. https://coenet.org/coe-and-trio-programs/

Council on Social Work Education. (2022). *Educational policy and accreditation standards for baccalaureate and master's social work programs*. https://www.cswe.org/accreditation/policies-process/2022epas/

Cox, B. E., Edelstein, J., Brogdon, B., & Roy, A. (2021). Navigating challenges to facilitate success for college students with autism. *The Journal of Higher Education*, *92*(2), 252–278. DOI: 10.1080/00221546.2020.1798203

Cox, B. E., Mintz, A., Locks, T., Thompson, K., Anderson, A., Morgan, L., Edelstein, J., & Wolz, A. (2017). Academic experiences for college students with autism: Identity, disclosure, and accommodations. *Journal of College Student Development*, *58*(1), 71–87. DOI: 10.1353/csd.2017.0004

Craig, S. L., Gardiner, T., Eaton, A. D., Pang, N., & Kourgiantakis, T. (2022). Practicing alliance: An experiential model of teaching diversity and inclusion for social work practice and education. *Social Work Education*, *41*(5), 801–819. DOI: 10.1080/02615479.2021.1892054

Crane, L., Hearst, C., Ashworth, M., & Davies, J. (2023). Evaluating the online delivery of an autistic-led programme to support newly diagnosed or identified autistic adults. *Autism & Developmental Language Impairments*, *8*, 1–9. DOI: 10.1177/23969415231189608 PMID: 37529634

Crane, L., Hearst, C., Ashworth, M., Davies, J., & Hill, E. L. (2021). Supporting newly identified or diagnosed autistic adults: An initial evaluation of an autistic-led programme. *Journal of Autism and Developmental Disorders*, *51*(3), 892–905. DOI: 10.1007/s10803-020-04486-4 PMID: 32266684

Creaven, A. (2024). Considering the sensory and social needs of disabled students in higher education: A call to return to the roots of universal design. *Policy Futures in Education*, *23*(1), 259–266. DOI: 10.1177/14782103241240808

Crehan, E. T., Phillips, A., Ngo, A., Donaghue, A., Bartlett, N., Rothstein, D., & Dufresne, S. (in preparation). What's autism and neurodiversity got to do with it? How liberal arts campuses in the US are (or are not) discussing invisible disabilities. *Eliot Pearson Department of Child Study & Human Development. Tufts University.*

Crompton, C. J., Hallett, S., Ropar, D., Flynn, E., & Fletcher-Watson, S. (2020). 'I never realised everybody felt as happy as I do when I am around Autistic people': A thematic analysis of Autistic adults' relationships with autistic and neurotypical friends and family. *Autism*, *24*(6), 1438–1448. DOI: 10.1177/1362361320908976 PMID: 32148068

Croninger, R., & Lee, V. (2001). Social capital and dropping out of high school: Benefits to at-risk students of teachers. *Teachers College Record*, *103*(4), 548–581. DOI: 10.1111/0161-4681.00127

Cumin, J.. (2021). Positive and differential diagnosis of autism in verbal women of typical intelligence: A Delphi study. *Autism. Online First*, (1). Advance online publication. DOI: 10.1177/13623613211042719 PMID: 34514874

Cumming, T. M., & Rose, M. C. (2022). Exploring Universal Design for Learning as an accessibility tool in higher education: A review of the current literature. *Australian Educational Researcher*, *49*(5), 1025–1043. https://link.springer.com/article/10.1007/s13384-021-00471-7. DOI: 10.1007/s13384-021-00471-7

Custodio, R. J. P., Hengstler, J. G., Cheong, J. H., Kim, H. J., Wascher, E., & Getzmann, S. (2024). Adult ADHD: It is old and new at the same time - what is it? *Reviews in the Neurosciences*, *35*(2), 225–241. DOI: 10.1515/revneuro-2023-0071 PMID: 37813870

Dahunsi, O., Robinson, N., Parks, C., & Nittrouer, C. (2024). How a DEI climate can enable allies and support people who are neurodivergent. In Patton, E., & Santuzzi, A. M. (Eds.), *Neurodiversity and Work: Employment, Identity, and Support Networks for Neurominorities* (pp. 207–230). Springer. DOI: 10.1007/978-3-031-55072-0_10

Daley, T. C. (2004). From symptom recognition to diagnosis: Children with autism in urban India. *Social Science & Medicine*, *58*(7), 1323–1335. DOI: 10.1016/S0277-9536(03)00330-7 PMID: 14759679

Dalrymple, J., & Boylan, J. (2016). Effective advocacy in social work. *Sage*.

Davies, J., Heasman, B., Livesey, A., Walker, A., Pellicano, E., & Remington, A. (2022). Autistic adults' views and experiences of requesting and receiving workplace adjustments in the UK. *PLoS One*, *17*(8), e0272420. DOI: 10.1371/journal.pone.0272420 PMID: 35930548

Davis, R. A., Wolfe, J., & Heiman, N. (2023). Increasing utilization of student mental health services on a college campus: Eight actionable tips. *Journal of American College Health*, *71*(3), 655–659. DOI: 10.1080/07448481.2021.1909035 PMID: 33891531

Day, M., Wood, C., Corker, E., & Freeth, M. (2024). Understanding the barriers to hiring autistic people as perceived by employers in the United Kingdom. *Autism*. Advance online publication. DOI: 10.1177/13623613241301493 PMID: 39629787

Dean, L. (2019). *Building employability: An exploratory study of the experiences and perceptions of autistic higher education students in preparing for graduate work* [Doctoral thesis, University of Sheffield]. White Rose eTheses Online. https://etheses.whiterose.ac.uk/id/eprint/27441/

den Houting, J. (2019). Neurodiversity: An insider's perspective. *Autism*, *23*(2), 271–273. DOI: 10.1177/1362361318820762 PMID: 30556743

den Houting, J., Higgins, J., Isaacs, K., Mahony, J., & Pellicano, E. (2021). 'I'm not just a guinea pig': Academic and community perceptions of participatory autism research. *Autism*, *25*(1), 148–163. DOI: 10.1177/1362361320951696 PMID: 32854511

DeRuy, E. (2016, March 23). How to graduate more black students. *The Atlantic*. https://www.theatlantic.com/education/archive/2016/03/how-to-graduate-more-black-students/475077/

Devitt, M., & Ringwood, B. (n.d.). *Business partnerships with Trinity Centre for People with Intellectual Disabilities*. Trinity College Dublin. https://www.tcd.ie/tcpid/business-partners/tcpid-business-partners-booklet-sept-2023.pdf

Dexter, S., Grace, K., Quinnell, S.-L., Surrey, A., & Crane, L. (2024). Towards 'a level playing field': A participatory study of autistic university students' experiences with academic support in England. *International Journal of Disability Development and Education, 72*(1), 26–41. DOI: 10.1080/1034912X.2024.2317475

Dijkhuis, R., de Sonneville, L., Ziermans, T., Staal, W., & Swaab, H. (2020). Autism symptoms, executive functioning and academic progress in higher education students. *Journal of Autism and Developmental Disorders, 50*(4), 1353–1363. DOI: 10.1007/s10803-019-04267-8 PMID: 31939082

Dillon, S., Armstrong, E., Goudy, L., Reynolds, H., & Scurry, S. (2021). Improving special education service delivery through interdisciplinary collaboration. *Teaching Exceptional Children, 54*(1), 36–43. DOI: 10.1177/00400599211029671

Disability Access Route to Education (DARE). (2025). *What is DARE?* Access College. https://accesscollege.ie/dare/

Dixon, A. (2023). *"I want to say that disabled people also want to live as human beings": Stigma experiences of women with disabilities in Pakistan* (Doctoral dissertation, University College London). UCL Discovery. https://discovery.ucl.ac.uk/id/eprint/10177028/

Dixon, S., Smith, C., & Touchet, A. (2018). *The disability perception gap.* Scope. https://www.scope.org.uk/campaigns/disability-perception-gap

Dolmage, J. (2017). *Academic ableism: Disability and higher education.* University of Michigan Press. https://muse.jhu.edu/book/57058

Doyle, N. (2020). Neurodiversity at work: A biopsychosocial model and the impact on working adults. *British Medical Bulletin, 135*(1), 108–125. DOI: 10.1093/bmb/ldaa021 PMID: 32996572

Drader-Mazza, N., Lopez-Kidwell, V., Kanwal, F., Reger, R. K., & Vogus, T. J. (2024). The double empathy problem and person-environment fit: Mutual understanding and bidirectional adjustment in autistic talent acquisition. *Human Resource Management.* Advance online publication. https://doi-org.DOI: 10.1002/hrm.22258

Dragoo, K. E., & Cole, J. P. (2019). *Laws affecting students with disabilities:Preschool through postsecondary education.* Congressional Research Service, Rep. No. R45595. https://files.eric.ed.gov/fulltext/ED597875.pdf

Dufresne, S. R. (2024). *Navigating Tufts for Neurodivergent Students: Developing, implementing, and evaluating a workshop series at a U.S. university* [Doctoral dissertation, Tufts University]. ProQuest Dissertations & Theses Global. https://www.proquest.com/docview/3059316104/abstract/EA60821E016B4156PQ/1

Duncan, E. A. (2021). *Foundations for practice in occupational therapy* (6th ed.). Elsevier Health Sciences.

DuPaul, G. J., Franklin, M. K., Pollack, B. L., Stack, K. S., Jaffe, A. R., & Gormley, M. J. Anastopoulos, A. D., & Weyandt, L. L. (2018). Predictors and trajectories of educational functioning in college students with and without attention-deficit/hyperactivity disorder. *Journal of Postsecondary Education and Disability, 31*(2), 161–178. https://pmc.ncbi.nlm.nih.gov/articles/PMC6586431/

DuPaul, G. J., Gormley, M. J., Anastopoulos, A. D., Weyandt, L. L., Labban, J., Sass, A. J., Busch, C. Z., Franklin, M. K., & Postler, K. B. (2021). Academic trajectories of college students with and without ADHD: Predictors of four-year outcomes. *Journal of Clinical Child and Adolescent Psychology*, *50*(6), 828–843. DOI: 10.1080/15374416.2020.1867990 PMID: 33529049

DuPaul, G. J., Weyandt, L. L., O'Dell, S. M., & Varejao, M. (2009). College students with ADHD: Current status and future directions. *Journal of Attention Disorders, 13*(3), 234–250. DOI: 10.1177/1087054709340650 PMID: 19620623

Dupree, D., Spencer, T. R., & Spencer, M. B. (2015). Stigma, stereotypes and resilience identities: The relationship between identity processes and resilience processes among Black American adolescents. In Theron, L. C., Liebenberg, L., & Ungar, M. (Eds.), *Youth Resilience and Culture: Commonalities and Complexities* (pp. 117–129). Springer Netherlands., DOI: 10.1007/978-94-017-9415-2_9

Durgungoz, F. C., & Durgungoz, A. (2025). "Interactive lessons are great, but too much is too much": Hearing out neurodivergent students, Universal Design for Learning and the case for integrating more anonymous technology in higher education. *Higher Education*. Advance online publication. DOI: 10.1007/s10734-024-01389-6

Dutcher, J. M., Lederman, J., Jain, M., Price, S., Kumar, A., Villalba, D. K., Tumminia, M. J., Doryab, A., Cresswell, K. G., Riskin, E., Sefdigar, Y., Seo, W., Mankoff, J., Cohen, S., Dey, A., & Creswell, J. D. (2022). Lack of belonging predicts depressive symptomatology in college students. *Psychological Science*, *33*(7), 1048–1067. DOI: 10.1177/09567976211073135 PMID: 35735353

Dwyer, P. (2022). The neurodiversity approach (es): What are they and what do they mean for researchers? *Human Development*, *66*(2), 73–92. DOI: 10.1159/000523723 PMID: 36158596

Dwyer, P. (2024). Autonomy and inclusion. In Halder, S., Goldstein, T., & Caudel, D. (Eds.), *Inclusion and Autism* (pp. 39–59). Routledge. DOI: 10.4324/9781003559276-3

Dwyer, P., Mineo, E., Mifsud, K., Lindholm, C., Gurba, A., & Waisman, T. C. (2023). Building neurodiversity-inclusive postsecondary campuses: Recommendations for leaders in higher education. *Autism in Adulthood: Challenges and Management*, *5*(1), 1–14. https://www.liebertpub.com/doi/pdf/10.1089/aut.2021.0042 PMID: 36941859

Edgewick, P.. (2021). Gender differences in mental health prevalence in autism. *Advances in Autism*, *7*(3), 17. DOI: 10.1108/AIA-01-2020-0007

Education For All Handicapped Children Act, Public Law 142, U.S. Statutes at Large 89 (1975): 773-796.

Education for Persons with Special Educational Needs Act. 2004. (2004). Irish Statute Book. https://www.irishstatutebook.ie/eli/2004/act/30/enacted/en/html

Educational Advocates. (2024). *Learning Disabilities and the College Process: Navigating Admissions and Support Services*. https://educationaladvocates.com/college-student-with-learning-disabilities/

Eide, B. L., & Eide, F. F. (2023). *The dyslexic advantage (revised and updated): Unlocking the hidden potential of the dyslexic brain*. Penguin.

Eisenmenger, A. (2019, December 12). *Ableism 101*. Access Living. https://www.accessliving.org/newsroom/blog/ableism-101/

Ejaz, N., & Mallawaarachchi, T. (2023). Disparities in economic achievement across the rural–urban divide in Pakistan: Implications for development planning. *Economic Analysis and Policy*, *77*, 487–512. DOI: 10.1016/j.eap.2022.11.023

Eki, A., & Isaksoon, G. (2013). How adults with ADHD get engaged in and perform everyday activities. *Scandinavian Journal of Occupational Therapy*, *20*(4), 282–291. DOI: 10.3109/11038128.2013.799226 PMID: 23713791

Elias, R., & White, S. W. (2018). Autism goes to college: Understanding the needs of a student population on the rise. *Journal of Autism and Developmental Disorders*, *48*(3), 732–746. DOI: 10.1007/s10803-017-3075-7 PMID: 28255760

Elmore, K., Saia, T., & Thomson, E. A. (2018). *Special feature: An introduction to disability cultural centers in U.S. higher education, part I*. AHEAD - Association on Higher Education And Disability. https://www.ahead.org/professional-resources/publications/hub/hub-nov-2018/hub-nov-2018-special-feature-disability-cultural-centers

Eng, S., & Onysko, M. (2025, March 25). Tufts accepts 10.5% of applicants to the Class of 2029. *The Tufts Daily*. https://www.tuftsdaily.com/article/2025/03/tufts-accepts-105-of-applicants-to-the-class-of-2029

Engel, G. L. (1977). The need for a new medical model: A challenge for biomedicine. *Science, 196*(4286), 129–136. DOI: 10.1126/science.847460 PMID: 847460

Equality Act. 2010, c. 15. (UK). https://www.legislation.gov.uk/ukpga/2010/15/contents

Ernst & Young. (2022). *Engage. enable. empower: Creating meaningful employment for persons with intellectual disabilities.* https://www.ey.com/content/dam/ey-unified-site/ey-com/en-ie/campaigns/documents/ey-ireland-engage-enable-empower.pdf

Evans, D., Granson, M., Langford, D., & Hirsch, S. (2023). Autism spectrum disorder: Reconceptualising support for neurodiverse students in higher education. *Journal of Higher Education Policy and Management, 45*(2), 243–257. https://doi-org.DOI: 10.1080/1360080X.2023.2180168

Evans, N. J., Broido, E. M., Brown, K. R., & Wilke, A. K. (2017). *Disability in higher education: A social justice approach.* John Wiley & Sons.

Fabricant, M., & Fisher, R. (2008). *Settlements and neighborhood centers. Encyclopedia of Social Work.* Oxford University Press. https://www.oxfordreference.com/view/10.1093/oi/authority.20110803100457433

Fabri, M., Andrews, P. C. S., & Pukki, H. K. (2016). Using design thinking to engage autistic students in participatory design of an online toolkit to help with transition into higher education. *Journal of Assistive Technologies, 10*(2), 102–114. DOI: 10.1108/JAT-02-2016-0008

Farrant, F., Owen, E., Hunkins-Beckford, F. L., & Jacksa, M. (2022). Celebrating neurodiversity in higher education. *The Psychologist, 35*, 2–3. https://www.bps.org.uk/psychologist/celebrating-neurodiversity-higher-education

Feuer, D., & Geber, B. (1988). Uh-oh... Second thoughts about adult learning theory. *Training (New York, N.Y.), 25*(12), 31–39.

Fisher, A. G. (1998). Uniting practice and theory in an occupational framework. *The American Journal of Occupational Therapy, 52*(7), 509–521. DOI: 10.5014/ajot.52.7.509 PMID: 9693695

Flegenheimer, C., & Scherf, K. S. (2022). College as a developmental context for emerging adulthood in autism: A systematic review of what we know and where we go from here. *Journal of Autism and Developmental Disorders, 52*(5), 2075–2097. DOI: 10.1007/s10803-021-05088-4 PMID: 34060001

Fletcher-Watson, S., Adams, J., Brook, K., Charman, T., Crane, L., Cusack, J., Leekam, S., Milton, D., Parr, J. R., & Pellicano, E. (2019). Making the future together: Shaping autism research through meaningful participation. *Autism, 23*(4), 943–953. DOI: 10.1177/1362361318786721 PMID: 30095277

Florian, L. (2007). *The SAGE handbook of special education.* SAGE., DOI: 10.4135/9781848607989

Foote, L. S. (2015). Re-storying life as a means of critical reflection: The power of narrative learning. *Christian Higher Education, 14*(3), 116–126. DOI: 10.1080/15363759.2015.1028580

Fovet, F. (2020). *Exploring the potential of universal design for learning with regards to mental health issues in higher education*. [conference proceedings]. Pacific Rim International Conference on Disability and Diversity. University of Hawai'i at Mānoa, Honolulu, Hawai'i. http://hdl.handle.net/10125/69333

Fovet, F. (2024) Accommodations 2.0: Reflecting on the future of post-secondary accommodations in a UDL landscape. *AHEAD Journal*, 17.

Francisco, M. P. B., Hartman, M., & Wang, Y. (2020). Inclusion and special education. *Education Sciences, 10*(9), 238. https://www.mdpi.com/2227-7102/10/9/238. DOI: 10.3390/educsci10090238

Franz, D. J., Lenhard, W., Marx, P., & Richter, T. (2023). Here I sit, making men in my own image: How learning disorder labels affect teacher student's expectancies. *Current Psychology: A Journal for Diverse Perspectives on Diverse Psychological Issues, 42*(12), 9795–9809. https://doi-org./DOI: 10.1007/s12144-021-02250-0

Fraser Butlin, S. (2011). The UN Convention on the Rights of Persons with Disabilities: Does the Equality Act 2010 measure up to UK international commitments? *Industrial Law Journal, 40*(4), 428–438. DOI: 10.1093/indlaw/dwr015

Freddolino, P. P., Moxley, D., & Hyduk, C. (2004). A differential model of advocacy in social work practice. *Families in Society, 85*(1), 119–128. DOI: 10.1606/1044-3894.241

Friedman, Z. L., & Nash-Luckenbach, D. (2024). Has the time come for heutagogy? Supporting neurodivergent learners in higher education. *Higher Education, 87*(6), 1905–1920. https://doi-org.DOI: 10.1007/s10734-023-01097-7

Frost, K. M., Bailey, K. M., & Ingersoll, B. R. (2019). "I just want them to see me as…me": Identity, community, and disclosure practices among college students on the autism spectrum. *Autism in Adulthood: Challenges and Management, 1*(14), 268–275. DOI: 10.1089/aut.2018.0057 PMID: 36601323

Fundación Indígena [FSI], & Kothari, B. (2008). Rights to the benefits of research: Compensating indigenous peoples for their intellectual contribution. *Human Organization, 56*(2), 127–137. DOI: 10.17730/humo.56.2.j63678502x782100

Furrukh, J., & Anjum, G. (2020). Coping with Autism Spectrum Disorder (ASD) in Pakistan: A phenomenology of mothers who have children with ASD. *Cogent Psychology*, *7*(1), 1728108. DOI: 10.1080/23311908.2020.1728108

Galbraith, M. W., & Jones, M. S. (2008). First things first in becoming a teacher of adults. *Journal of Adult Education*, *37*(1), 1–12. https://eric.ed.gov/?id=EJ891070

Gale, L. (2022). Biopsychosocial-spiritual assessment: An overview. *Social Work Practice & Skill.* Cinahl Information Systems. https://www.ebsco.com/sites/g/files/nabnos191/files/acquiadam-assets/Social-Work-Reference-Center-Skill-Biopsychosocial-Spiritual-Assessment.pdf

Garratt, D., Johnson, K., Millear, A., Picken, S., Slattery, J., & Walmsley, J. (2022). Celebrating thirty years of inclusive research. *Social Sciences (Basel, Switzerland)*, *11*(9), 385. DOI: 10.3390/socsci11090385

Gasker, J. (2023). *Generalist social work practice* (2nd ed.). Sage.

Gauthier-Boudreault, C., Couture, M., & Gallagher, F. (2021). Obstacles to the transition to adulthood of people with severe to profound intellectual disability and potential solutions: Perspectives of professionals in one region of Quebec. *Journal of Intellectual & Developmental Disability*, *46*(3), 239–249. DOI: 10.3109/13668250.2021.1873753 PMID: 39818552

Gavín-Chocano, Ó., García-Martínez, I., & de la Rosa, A. L. (2024). Self-regulated learning as an inherent factor of academic self-concept in university students. *Current Psychology (New Brunswick, N.J.)*, *43*(34), 27469–27480. DOI: 10.1007/s12144-024-06352-3

Gelbar, N. W., Shefyck, A., & Reichow, B. (2015). A comprehensive survey of current and former college students with Autism Spectrum Disorders. *The Yale Journal of Biology and Medicine*, *88*(1), 45–68. https://pmc.ncbi.nlm.nih.gov/articles/PMC4345538/ PMID: 25745374

Gelbar, N. W., Smith, I., & Reichow, B. (2014). Systematic review of articles describing experience and supports of individuals with autism enrolled in college and university programs. *Journal of Autism and Developmental Disorders*, *44*(10), 2593–2601. DOI: 10.1007/s10803-014-2135-5 PMID: 24816943

Gensic, J., & Brunton, J. (2022). *The actually autistic guide to advocacy: Step-by-step advice on how to ally and speak up with autistic people and the autism community*. Jessica Kingsley Publishers. https://www.google.com/books/edition/The_ActuallyAutistic_Guide_to_Advocacy/7RJJEAAAQBAJ?hl=en&gbpv=1&dq=neurodiversity+allyship&pg=PP1&printsec=frontcover

Germain, C. B. (1973). An ecological perspective in casework practice. *Social Casework, 54*(6), 323–330. DOI: 10.1177/104438947305400601

Getzel, E. E., & Thoma, C. A. (2008). Experiences of college students with disabilities and the importance of self-determination in higher education settings. *Career Development for Exceptional Individuals, 31*(2), 77–84. DOI: 10.1177/0885728808317658

Giarelli, E., Wiggins, L. D., Rice, C. E., Levy, S. E., Kirby, R. S., Pinto-Martin, J., & Mandell, D. (2010). Sex differences in the evaluation and diagnosis of Autism Spectrum Disorders among children. *Journal of the American Academy of Child and Adolescent Psychiatry, 49*(8), 789–800. DOI: 10.1016/j.dhjo.2009.07.001 PMID: 21122776

Gibson, S. (2012). Narrative accounts of university education: Sociocultural perspectives on the learning experiences of students with disabilities. *Disability & Society, 27*(3), 353–369. DOI: 10.1080/09687599.2012.654987

Gillen-O'Neel, C., & Fuligni, A. (2013). A longitudinal study of school belonging and academic motivation across high school. *Child Development, 84*(2), 678–692. DOI: 10.1111/j.1467-8624.2012.01862.x PMID: 23002809

Gillespie-Lynch, K., Brooks, P. J., Someki, F., Obeid, R., Shane-Simpson, C., Kapp, S. K., Daou, N., & Smith, D. S. (2015). Changing college students' conceptions of autism: An online training to increase knowledge and decrease stigma. *Journal of Autism and Developmental Disorders, 45*(8), 2553–2566. DOI: 10.1007/s10803-015-2422-9 PMID: 25796194

Gillespie-Lynch, K., Bublitz, D., Donachie, A., Wong, V., Brooks, P. J., & D'Onofrio, J. (2017). "For a long time our voices have been hushed": Using student perspectives to develop supports for neurodiverse college students. *Frontiers in Psychology, 8*. Advance online publication. DOI: 10.3389/fpsyg.2017.00544 PMID: 28458645

Gillespie-Lynch, K., Daou, N., Obeid, R., Reardon, S., Khan, S., & Goldknopf, E. J. (2021). What contributes to stigma towards autistic university students and students with other diagnoses? *Journal of Autism and Developmental Disorders, 51*(2), 459–475. DOI: 10.1007/s10803-020-04556-7 PMID: 32504342

Gillespie-Lynch, K., Dwyer, P., Constantino, C., Kapp, S. K., Hotez, E., Riccio, A., DeNigris, D., Kofner, B., & Endlich, E. (2020). Can we broaden the neurodiversity movement without weakening it? Participatory approaches as a framework for cross-disability alliance building. In Carey, A. C., Ostrove, J. M., & Fannon, T. (Eds.), *Disability alliances and allies: Opportunities and challenges* (pp. 189–223). Emerald Publishing Limited. DOI: 10.1108/S1479-354720200000012013

Giri, A., Aylott, J., Giri, P., Ferguson-Wormley, S., & Evans, J. (2022). Lived experience and the social model of disability: Conflicted and inter-dependent ambitions for employment of people with a learning disability and their family carers. *British Journal of Learning Disabilities*, *50*(1), 98–106. DOI: 10.1111/bld.12378

Gitterman, A., Knight, C., & Germain, C. B. (2021). *The life model of social work practice: Advances in theory and practice* (4th ed.). Columbia University Press.

Gobbo, K., & Shmulsky, S. (2012). Classroom needs of community college students with Asperger's disorder and Autism Spectrum Disorders. *Community College Journal of Research and Practice*, *37*(1), 40–51. DOI: 10.1080/10668920903381813

Goffman, E. (1963). *Stigma: Notes on the Management of Spoiled Identity*. Simon and Schuster.

Goodenow, C. (1993). Classroom belonging among early adolescent students: Relationships to motivation and achievement. *The Journal of Early Adolescence*, *13*(1), 21–43. DOI: 10.1177/0272431693013001002

Goode, R. W., Cowell, M., McMillan, D., Van Deinse, T., & Cooper-Lewter, C. (2021). Preparing social workers to confront social injustice and oppression: Evaluating the role of social work education. *Social Work*, *66*(1), 39–48. DOI: 10.1093/sw/swaa018 PMID: 32793955

Goodley, D. (2014). *Dis/ability Studies: Theorising disablism and ableism*. Routledge. DOI: 10.4324/9780203366974

Goodley, D. (2024). *Disability studies: An interdisciplinary introduction*. Sage Publications Ltd.

Gould, R., Harris, S. P., & Mullin, C. (2019). Higher education and the ADA: An ADA knowledge translation center research brief. *ADA National Network*. https://adata.org/research_brief/higher-education-and-ada

Gould, J., & Ashton-Smith, J. (2011). Missed diagnosis or misdiagnosis? Girls and women on the autism spectrum. [GAP]. *Good Autism Practice*, *12*(1), 34–41.

Government of Pakistan, Ministry of Federal Education and Professional Training. (2018). *National education policy for persons with disabilities*. Government of Pakistan.

Government of Pakistan, Ministry of Federal Education and Professional Training. (2020). *Achievements in adult literacy*. Government of Pakistan.

Grace, A. P. (1996). Taking a critical pose: Andragogy—missing links, missing values. *International Journal of Lifelong Education, 15*(5), 382–392. DOI: 10.1080/0260137960150506

Gragoudas, S. (2014). Preparing students with disabilities to transition from school to work through self-determination training. *Work (Reading, Mass.), 48*(3), 407–411. DOI: 10.3233/WOR-131782 PMID: 24284673

Green, J. C., Buck, A., & Izzo, M. (2024). Evaluating Ohio's postsecondary programs for students with intellectual disability: A survey of program directors. *DADD Online Journal, 11*(1), 114–130. https://daddcec.com/sites/default/files/2025-01/doj_2024_final.pdf

Grigal, M., Hart, D., & Weir, C. (2011). *Think college standards quality indicators, and benchmarks for inclusive higher education.* University of Massachusetts Boston, Institute for Community Inclusion. https://www.mass.edu/strategic/maicei/documents/think-college-standards.pdf

Grigal, M., & Hart, D. (2010). *Think College. Postsecondary education options for students with intellectual disabilities*. Brookes Publishing.

Grigal, M., Hart, D., & Weir, C. (2012). A survey of postsecondary education programs for students with intellectual disabilities in the United States. *Journal of Policy and Practice in Intellectual Disabilities, 9*(4), 223–233. DOI: 10.1111/jppi.12012

Grigal, M., Soldovieri, S. J., Myers, B., Papay, C., & Bukaty, C. A. (2024). Benefits of postsecondary education experiences for adults with intellectual and developmental disability. *International Review of Research in Developmental Disabilities, 66*, 1–31. Advance online publication. DOI: 10.1016/bs.irrdd.2024.09.003

Grow, G. (1991). Teaching learners to be self-directed. *Adult Education Quarterly, 41*(3), 125–149. DOI: 10.1177/0001848191041003001

Grummt, M. (2024). Sociocultural perspectives on neurodiversity-An analysis, interpretation and synthesis of the basic terms, discourses and theoretical positions. *Sociology Compass, 18*(8), 1–17. DOI: 10.1111/soc4.13249

Gupta, A., Chaplot, I., Detamore, B., Thakkar, S., Nguyen, K., Camilli, S., & Nguyen, D. (2023). Individualized Education Program (IEP) under examination: A literature review of systemic flaws in education for students with disabilities. *Social Science Research Network*. DOI: 10.2139/ssrn.4508281

Gu, Q., & Schweisfurth, M. (2015). Transnational connections, competences, and identities: Experiences of Chinese international students after their return "home.". *British Educational Research Journal*, *41*(6), 947–970. DOI: 10.1002/berj.3175

Gurbuz, E., Hanley, M., & Riby, D. M. (2019). University students with autism: The social and academic experiences of university in the UK. *Journal of Autism and Developmental Disorders*, *49*(2), 617–631. DOI: 10.1007/s10803-018-3741-4 PMID: 30173311

Gustavsson, A., Wendelborg, C., & Tøssebro, J. (2021). Educated for welfare services—The hidden curriculum of upper secondary school for students with intellectual disabilities. *British Journal of Learning Disabilities*, *49*(4), 424–432. DOI: 10.1111/bld.12418

Haber, M. G., Mazzotti, V. L., Mustian, A. L., Rowe, D. A., Bartholomew, A. L., Test, D. W., & Fowler, C. H. (2016). What works, when, for whom, and with whom: A meta-analytic review of predictors of postsecondary success for students with disabilities. *Review of Educational Research*, *86*(1), 123–162. DOI: 10.3102/0034654315583135

Haegele, J. A., & Hodge, S. (2016). Disability discourse: Overview and critiques of the medical and social models. *Quest*, *68*(2), 193–206. DOI: 10.1080/00336297.2016.1143849

Halder, S., & Squires, G. (2023). *Inclusion and diversity: Communities and practices across the world*. Routledge. DOI: 10.4324/9781003379034

Hallahan, D. P., Kauffman, J. M., & Pullen, P. (2022). *Exceptional Learners: An introduction to special education* (15thed.). Pearson Publishing.

Hamblet, E. C. (2023). *Seven steps to college success: A pathway for students with disabilities* (3rd ed.). Rowman & Littlefield Publishers., https://www.ldadvisory.com/high-school-to-college/ DOI: 10.5771/9781475864458

Hamilton, L. G., & Petty, S. (2023). Compassionate pedagogy for neurodiversity in higher education: A conceptual analysis. *Frontiers in Psychology*, *14*, 1093290. Advance online publication. DOI: 10.3389/fpsyg.2023.1093290 PMID: 36874864

Hamilton, L. G., & Petty, S. (2024). Corrigendum: Compassionate pedagogy for neurodiversity in higher education: A conceptual analysis. *Frontiers in Psychology*, *14*, 1–2. DOI: 10.3389/fpsyg.2023.1345256 PMID: 38444880

Han, E., Scior, K., Grace, K., Heath, E., Dufresne, S., & Crane, L. (2024). 'Who, When, How to Share': Pilot study of a new disclosure decision-making programme for autistic adults. *Autism*, *28*(8), 2090–2104. Advance online publication. DOI: 10.1177/13623613231221685 PMID: 38339979

Hansan, J. E. (2011). Settlement houses: An introduction. *Social Welfare History Project.* https://socialwelfare.library.vcu.edu/settlement-houses/settlement-houses/

Harris, J. C. (2006). *Intellectual disability: Understanding its development, causes, classification, evaluation, and treatment.* Oxford University Press.

Harrison, M., Rowlings, J., & Aivaliotis-Martinez, D. (2024). Supporting neurodivergent players. In *Press B to Belong* (pp. 65–77). Emerald Publishing Limited. DOI: 10.1108/978-1-80455-926-020241005

Hart, D., Grigal, M., Sax, C., Martinez, D., & Will, M. (2006). Research to practice: Postsecondary education options for students with intellectual disabilities. *Research to Practice Series, Institute for Community Inclusion, 6*(45). https://scholarworks.umb.edu/ici_researchtopractice/6

Hasselkus, B. R., & Dickie, V. (2021). *The meaning of everyday occupation* (3rd ed.). Routledge., DOI: 10.4324/9781003525035

Hayes, N., O'Toole, L., & Halpenny, A. (2017). *Introducing Bronfenbrenner: A guide for practitioners and students in early years education.* Routledge. DOI: 10.4324/9781315646206

Healey, M., Flint, A., & Harrington, K. (2014). *Engagement through partnership: Students as partners in learning and teaching in higher education.* Higher Education Academy. https://www.advance-he.ac.uk/knowledge-hub/engagement-through-partnership-students-partners-learning-and-teaching-higher

Heiman, T., & Shemesh, D. O. (2012). Students with LD in higher education: Use and contribution of assistive technology and website courses and their correlation to students' hope and well-being. *Journal of Learning Disabilities*, *45*(4), 308–318. DOI: 10.1177/0022219410392047 PMID: 21252373

Hennessy, T., McMahon, J., & Doody, O. (2024). How people with an intellectual disability experience inclusive third-level education: A scoping review. *British Journal of Learning Disabilities*, 1–34. DOI: 10.1111/bld.12626

Henning, C., Summerfeldt, L. J., & Parker, J. D. (2022). ADHD and academic success in university students: The important role of impaired attention. *Journal of Attention Disorders, 26*(6), 893–901. DOI: 10.1177/10870547211036758 PMID: 34384265

Hesjedal, E., Hetland, H., & Iversen, A. C. (2015). Interprofessional collaboration: Self-reported successful collaboration by teachers and social workers in multidisciplinary teams. *Child & Family Social Work, 20*(4), 437–445. DOI: 10.1111/cfs.12093

Heyer, K. (2015). *Rights enabled: The Disability Revolution, from the US, to Germany and. Japan, to the United Nations.* University of Michigan Press.

Higher Education Authority (HEA). (2024). *PATH 4 Phase 2 - Course provision for students with intellectual disabilities*. Department of Further and Higher Education, Research, Innovation, and Science. https://hea.ie

Higher Education Commission. (2021). *HEC policy for students with disabilities at higher education institutions in Pakistan*. Higher Education Commission of Pakistan.

Higher Education Commission. (2021). *Policy for students with disabilities at higher education institutions in Pakistan*. Higher Education Commission of Pakistan. https://www.hec.gov.pk/english/services/universities/pages/policy.aspx

Higher Education Opportunity Act. 20 U.S.C. §1140 (2008). https://www.govinfo.gov/content/pkg/PLAW-110publ315/pdf/PLAW-110publ315.pdf

Higher Education Statistics Agency (HESA). (2022). *Where do HE students come from?* https://www.hesa.ac.uk/data-and-analysis/students/where-from

Hillier, A., Goldstein, J., Tornatore, L., Byrne, E., & Johnson, H. M. (2019). Outcomes of a peer mentoring program for university students with disabilities. *Mentoring & Tutoring, 27*(5), 487–508. DOI: 10.1080/13611267.2019.1675850

Hills, M., Overend, A., & Hildebrandt, S. (2022). Faculty perspectives on UDL: Exploring bridges and barriers for broader adoption in higher education. *The Canadian Journal for the Scholarship of Teaching and Learning, 13*(1), 1–18. DOI: 10.5206/cjsotlrcacea.2022.1.13588

Hilton, S. (2023, September 25). The net of overcommitment: How we keep each other overburdened. *The Wesleyan Argus.* https://wesleyanargus.com/2023/09/25/the-net-of-overcommitment-how-we-keep-each-other-overburdened/

Hirota, T., Cheon, K.-A., & Lai, M.-C. (2024). Neurodiversity paradigms and their development across cultures: Some reflections in East Asian contexts. *Autism, 28*(11), 2685–2689. DOI: 10.1177/13623613241285678 PMID: 39370696

Hollomotz, A. (2018). Successful interviews with people with intellectual disability. *Qualitative Research, 18*(2), 153–170. DOI: 10.1177/1468794117713810

Holzberg, D. (2017). Differences between secondary and postsecondary education. *National Technical Assistance Center on Transition.* https://transitionta.org/wp-content/uploads/docs/Highschool_vs_College_list.pdf

Hope, E. C., & Spencer, M. B. (2017). Civic engagement as an adaptive coping response to conditions of inequality: An application of Phenomenological Variant of Ecological Systems Theory (PVEST). In Cabrera, N. J., & Leyendecker, B. (Eds.), *Handbook on Positive Development of Minority Children and Youth* (pp. 421–435). Springer International Publishing., DOI: 10.1007/978-3-319-43645-6_25

Horlin, C., Hronska, B., & Nordmann, E. (2024). I can be a "normal" student: The role of lecture capture in supporting disabled and neurodivergent students' participation in higher education. *Higher Education: The International Journal of Higher Education Research,* 1–18. https://doi-org.DOI: 10.1007/s10734-024-01201-5

Hosking, D. L. (2008). *Critical disability theory*. [Paper presentation]. 4th Biennial Disability Studies Conference, Lancaster University. https://www.lancaster.ac.uk/fass/events/disabilityconference_archive/2008/papers/hosking2008.pdf

Hotez, E., Rava, J., & Kuo, A. A. (2023). Brief research report: Investigating neurodiversity acceptance in the college classroom: An exploratory study. *Frontiers in Education, 8*, 1223175. Advance online publication. DOI: 10.3389/feduc.2023.1223175

Hotez, E., Rosenau, K. A., Fernandes, P., Eagan, K., Shea, L., & Kuo, A. A. (2022). A national cross-sectional study of the characteristics, strengths, and challenges of college students with Attention Deficit Hyperactivity Disorder. *Cureus, 14*(1), e21520. DOI: 10.7759/cureus.21520 PMID: 35223296

Hotez, E., Shane-Simpson, C., Obeid, R., DeNigris, D., Siller, M., Costikas, C., Pickens, J., Massa, A., Giannola, M., D'Onofrio, J., & Gillespie-Lynch, K. (2018). Designing a summer transition program for incoming and current college students on the autism spectrum: A participatory approach. *Frontiers in Psychology, 9*, 46. DOI: 10.3389/fpsyg.2018.00046 PMID: 29487547

Hull, L., Levy, L., Lai, M.-C., Petrides, K. V., Baron-Cohen, S., Allison, C., Smith, P., & Mandy, W. (2020). Is social camouflaging associated with anxiety and depression in autistic adults? *Molecular Autism, 12*(1), 13. Advance online publication. DOI: 10.1186/s13229-021-00421-1 PMID: 33593423

Hull, L., Petrides, K. V., Allison, C., Smith, P., Baron-Cohen, S., Lai, M.-C., & Mandy, W. (2017). 'Putting on my best normal': Social camouflaging in adults with autism spectrum conditions. *Journal of Autism and Developmental Disorders*, *47*(8), 2519–2534. DOI: 10.1007/s10803-017-3166-5 PMID: 28527095

Hull, L., Petrides, K. V., & Mandy, W. (2020). The female autism phenotype and camouflaging: A narrative review. *Review Journal of Autism and Developmental Disorders*, *7*(4), 306–317. DOI: 10.1007/s40489-020-00197-9

Hurtado, S., & Carter, D. F. (1997). Effects of college transition and perceptions of the campus racial climate on Latino college students' sense of belonging. *Sociology of Education*, *70*(4), 324–345. DOI: 10.2307/2673270

Hussain, S., Alam, A., & Ullah, S. (2023). Persons with disabilities and the profession of social work in Pakistan: A review of literature. *Pakistan Journal of Society, Education and Language (PJSEL)*, *10*(1), 282–290. https://pjsel.jehanf.com/index.php/journal/article/view/1304

Hussain, S., Munir, A., & Ibrar, M. (2020). Children with disability: Problems and challenges in Pakistan. *Journal of the Humanities and Social Sciences*, *28*(1), 87–99. http://ojs.uop.edu.pk/jhss/article/view/387

Hussain, S., Shahzadi, U., & Khan, I. (2020). Challenges to learners with disabilities in higher education institutions in Pakistan: A review. [RJSSER]. *Research Journal of Social Sciences and Economics Review*, *1*(3), 12–19. DOI: 10.36902/rjsser-vol1-iss3-2020(12-19)

Imran, M., Oad, L., Jat, Z. G., Hafeez, A., & Sultana, Z. (2024). Enhancing support for slow learners evaluating inclusive education models in contemporary classrooms. *Research Journal for Societal Issues*, *6*(3), 156–177. DOI: 10.56976/rjsi.v6i3.268

Imran, N., Chaudry, M. R., Azeem, M. W., Bhatti, M. R., Choudhary, Z. I., & Cheema, M. A. (2011). A survey of autism knowledge and attitudes among healthcare professionals in Lahore, Pakistan. *BMC Pediatrics*, *11*(1), 1–6. DOI: 10.1186/1471-2431-11-107 PMID: 22107951

Inclusion. (2021). UNESCO. https://education-profiles.org/central-and-southern-asia/pakistan/~inclusion

Individuals with Disabilities Education Act, 20 U.S.C. § 1400 et seq. (2004). https://sites.ed.gov/idea/statute-chapter-33/subchapter-i/1400

Ingold, T. (2018). *Anthropology and/as education*. Routledge.

Irvine, B., & MacLeod, A. (2022). What are the challenges and successes reported by Autistic students at university? A literature review. *Good Autism Practice, 23*(1), 49–59. https://discovery.ucl.ac.uk/id/eprint/10157822/1/GAP_Spring_2022_ARTICLE_6_%28IRVINE_MACLEOD%29.pdf

Irvine, B., & MacLeod, A. (2022). What are the challenges and successes reported by autistic students at university?: A literature review. *Good Autism Practice.*, *23*(1), 49–59.

Jackson, P. (1968). *Life in classrooms*. Teachers College Press.

Jackson, S. L. J., Hart, L., Brown, J. T., & Volkmar, F. R. (2018). Brief report: Self-reported academic, social, and mental health experiences of post-secondary students with Autism Spectrum Disorder. *Journal of Autism and Developmental Disorders*, *48*(2), 643–650. DOI: 10.1007/s10803-017-3315-x PMID: 29022149

Jacob, S. V., Pillay, J., Adeoye, O. E., & Kelinde Oni, T. (2023). Barriers to employment of people with intellectual disability. *Work (Reading, Mass.)*, *74*(1), 207–218. DOI: 10.3233/WOR-211097 PMID: 36214017

Jacobs, P., MacMahon, K., & Quayle, E. (2020). Who decides? Transitions from school to adult services for and with young people with severe intellectual disabilities. *Disability & Society*, *35*(7), 1058–1084. DOI: 10.1080/09687599.2019.1669435

Jaird, M. A. (2022). Mapping out student support: An exploration of student disability programs and practices at selective higher education institutions. University of Vermont. *Graduate College Dissertations and Theses*. 1506. https://scholarworks.uvm.edu/graddis/1506

Jamil, B. R. (2009, August). Curriculum reforms in Pakistan: A glass half full or half empty. In *Seminar on School Curriculum Policies and Practices in South Asian Countries* (pp. 10–12). NCERT., https://itacec.org/document/nep09/NCERT%20Pakistan%20paper%20BRJ.pdf

Jarrow, J. (2022). *An open letter to parents of students with disabilities about to enter college*. https://daisclasses.com/wp-content/uploads/2022/01/OpenLetterParents.pdf

Jenkins, T. (2009). A seat at the table that I set: Beyond social justice allies. *About Campus: Enriching the Student Learning Experience*, *14*(5), 27–29. DOI: 10.1002/aca.305

Jobe, L. E., & Williams White, S. (2007). Loneliness, social relationships, and a broader autism phenotype in college students. *Personality and Individual Differences*, *42*(8), 1479–1489. DOI: 10.1016/j.paid.2006.10.021

Jones, D. R., Botha, M., Ackerman, R. A., King, K., & Sasson, N. J. (2024). Non-autistic observers both detect and demonstrate the double empathy problem when evaluating interactions between autistic and non-autistic adults. *Autism: The International Journal of Research and Practice, 28*(8), 2053–2065. https://doi-org.DOI: 10.1177/13623613231219743

Jurgens, A. (2020). Neurodiversity in a neurotypical world: An enactive framework for investigating autism and social institutions. In Vecchi, D. J. (Ed.), *Neurodiversity studies: A new critical paradigm* (pp. 73–88). Routledge. DOI: 10.4324/9780429322297-8

Kalina, P. (2020). Performative allyship. *Technium Social Science Journal, 11*, 478. https://heinonline.org/HOL/Page?collection=journals&handle=hein.journals/techssj11&i

Karpicz, J. R. (2020). Just my being here is self-advocacy. *Journal Committed to Social Change on Race and Ethnicity*, *6*(1), 138–163. https://www.jstor.org/stable/48644514

Keating, C. T. (2021). Participatory autism research: How consultation benefits everyone. *Frontiers in Psychology*, *12*, 713982. DOI: 10.3389/fpsyg.2021.713982 PMID: 34504463

Kelly, E. (2021). *Higher education funding in England* (CBP-7973). House of Commons Library. https://commonslibrary.parliament.uk/research-briefings/cbp-7973/

Kentrou, V., Livingston, L. A., Grove, R., Hoekstra, R. A., & Begeer, S. (2024). Perceived misdiagnosis of psychiatric conditions in autistic adults. *EClinicalMedicine*, *71*, 102586. DOI: 10.1016/j.eclinm.2024.102586 PMID: 38596613

Kerschbaum, S., Eisenman, L., & Jones, J. (Eds.). (2017). *Negotiating disability: Disclosure and higher education*. University of Michigan Press. DOI: 10.3998/mpub.9426902

Khalid, M., & Anjum, G. (2019). Use of remedial teaching approaches for dyslexic students: Experiences of remedial teachers working in urban Pakistan. *Cogent Psychology*, *6*(1), 1580181. Advance online publication. DOI: 10.1080/23311908.2019.1580181

Khan, N. H., Ju, Y., & Hassan, S. T. (2019). Investigating the determinants of human development index in Pakistan: An empirical analysis. *Environmental Science and Pollution Research International*, *26*(19), 19294–19304. DOI: 10.1007/s11356-019-05271-2 PMID: 31073836

Kickett, G., Hendrick, A., & Young, S. (2024). Ally work at the intersections: Theorising for practice and practicing for theory. In Baines, D., Rasool, S., Harms-Smith, L., Muñoz-Arce, G., & Noble, C. (Eds.), *The Routledge International Handbook of Feminisms in Social Work* (pp. 485–497). Routledge. DOI: 10.4324/9781003317371-48

Kimball, E. W., Wells, R. S., Ostiguy, B. J., Manly, C. A., & Lauterbach, A. A. (2016). Students with disabilities in higher education: A review of the literature and an agenda for future research. In Paulsen, M. (Ed.), *Higher education: Handbook of theory and research* (pp. 91–156). Springer., DOI: 10.1007/978-3-319-26829-3_3

Knowles, M. (1980). *Andragogy*, not pedagogy. *Adult Leadership*, *17*(1), 350–352.

Knowles, M. S. (1970). *The modern practice of adult education: Andragogy versus pedagogy*. The Association Press.

Knowles, M. S. (1990). *The adult learner: A neglected species* (4th ed.). Gulf.

Knox, K. (2024). Meeting the need of students and families: Adapting service delivery of Special Education Social Workers during a pandemic. *Children & Schools*, *46*(2), 107–116. DOI: 10.1093/cs/cdae002

Koenig, T., Spano, R., & Thompson, J. (2020). Human behavior theory for social work practice. *Sage (Atlanta, Ga.)*.

Kondrat, M. E. (2013). *Person-in-environment. Encyclopedia of Social Work*. National Association of Social Workers Press and Oxford University Press. DOI: 10.1093/acrefore/9780199975839.013.285

Kopp, S., & Gillberg, C. (1997). Selective mutism: A population-based study: A research note. *Journal of Child Psychology and Psychiatry, and Allied Disciplines*, *38*(2), 257–262. DOI: 10.1111/j.1469-7610.1997.tb01859.x PMID: 9232472

Kopp, S., Kelly, K. B., & Gillberg, C. (2009). Girls with social and/or attention deficits: A descriptive study of 100 clinic attenders. *Journal of Attention Disorders*, *14*(2), 167–181. DOI: 10.1177/1087054709332458 PMID: 19541882

Kranke, D., Jackson, S. E., Taylor, D. A., Anderson-Fye, E., & Floersch, J. (2013). College student disclosure of non-apparent disabilities to receive classroom accommodations. *Journal of Postsecondary Education and Disability*, *26*(1), 35–51. https://eric.ed.gov/?Id=EJ1026808

Krause, K. L., & Armitage, L. (2014). Australian student engagement, belonging, retention and success: A synthesis of the literature. *The Higher Education Academy, 2014*, 1-45. https://www.newcastle.edu.au/__data/assets/pdf_file/0007/558871/Australian_student_engagement_lit_syn_2.pdf

Kubiak, J. (2017). Using 'voice' to understand what college students with intellectual disabilities say about the teaching and learning process. *Journal of Research in Special Educational Needs*, *17*(1), 41–48. DOI: 10.1111/1471-3802.12098

Kuder, S. J., Accardo, A., & Woodruff, J. (2023). *College success for students on the autism spectrum: A neurodiversity perspective*. Taylor & Francis. DOI: 10.4324/9781003443452-2

Kutlaca, M., & Radke, H. R. (2023). Towards an understanding of performative allyship: Definition, antecedents and consequences. *Social and Personality Psychology Compass, 17*(2), e12724. DOI: 10.1111/spc3.12724

Lai, , Anagnostou, E., Wiznitzer, M., Allison, C., & Baron-Cohen, S. (2020). Lai, M. C., Anagnostou, E., Wiznitzer, M., Allison, C., & Baron-Cohen, S. (2020). Evidence-based support for autistic people across the lifespan: Maximising potential, minimising barriers, and optimising the person–environment fit. *Lancet Neurology*, *19*(5), 434–451. DOI: 10.1016/S1474-4422(20)30034-X PMID: 32142628

Lai, M.-C., Lombardo, M. V., Ruigrok, A. N., Chakrabarti, B., Auyeung, B., Szatmari, P., Happé, F., & Baron-Cohen, S.MRC AIMS Consortium. (2015). Quantifying and exploring camouflaging in men and women with autism. *Autism*, *21*(6), 690–702. DOI: 10.1177/1362361316671012 PMID: 27899710

Lanford, M. (2021). In pursuit of respect: The adult learner attending community college in the "new economy.". *The Educational Forum*, *85*(1), 34–48. DOI: 10.1080/00131725.2020.1775329

Lawson, J. (2010). An investigation into behaviours which challenge at university: The impact of neurotypical expectations on Autistic students. *Good Autism Practice, 11*(1), 45–51. https://citeseerx.ist.psu.edu/document?repid=rep1&type=pdf&doi=ccb1d460781375d98835c76525c4e6fac3c87d37#page=46

Laxton, S., Moriarty, C., Sapiets, S., Hastings, R., & Totsika, V. (2024). Neighbourhood deprivation and access to early intervention and support for families of children with intellectual and developmental disabilities. *Journal of Policy and Practice in Intellectual Disabilities*, *21*(1), 1–10. DOI: 10.1111/jppi.12486

Leake, D. W., & Stodden, R. A. (2014). Higher education and disability: Past and future of underrepresented populations. *Journal of Postsecondary Education and Disability*, *27*(4), 399–408. https://files.eric.ed.gov/fulltext/EJ1059990.pdf

Learning Disabilities Association of America (LDAA). (2024, December 12). *Modifications vs. accommodations: High school vs. college*. LDAAmerica.org. https://ldaamerica.org/lda_today/modifications-vs-accommodations-high-school-vs-college/

Learning Disabilities Association of America. (n.d.). The adult learning disability assessment process. https://ldaamerica.org/info/adult-learning-disability-assessment-process/

Lee, A. M. I. (2024). *Accommodations: What they are and how they work*. Understood.org. https://www.understood.org/en/articles/accommodations-what-they-are-and-how-they-work

Lee, C. E., & Taylor, J. L. (2022). A review of the benefits and barriers to postsecondary education for students with intellectual and developmental disabilities. *The Journal of Special Education*, *55*(4), 234–245. DOI: 10.1177/00224669211013354

Leedham, A., Thompson, A. R., Smith, R., & Freeth, M. (2019). 'I was exhausted trying to figure it out': The experiences of females receiving an autism diagnosis in middle to late adulthood. *Autism*, *24*(1), 135–146. DOI: 10.1177/1362361319853442 PMID: 31144507

Legault, M., Bourdon, J. N., & Poirier, P. (2021). From neurodiversity to neurodivergence: The role of epistemic and cognitive marginalization. *Synthese*, *199*(5-6), 12843–12868. DOI: 10.1007/s11229-021-03356-5

Lei, J., Calley, S., Brosnan, M., Ashwin, C., & Russell, A. (2020). Evaluation of a transition to university programme for students with Autism Spectrum Disorder. *Journal of Autism and Developmental Disorders*, *50*(7), 2397–2411. DOI: 10.1007/s10803-018-3776-6 PMID: 30315485

LeMaire, K. L., Miller, M., Skerven, K., & Nagy, G. A. (2020). Allyship in the academy. *Susan Bulkeley Butler Center for Leadership Excellence and ADVANCE Working Paper Series, 3* (1), 6-26. https://www.purdue.edu/butler/documents/5-WPS_Spring-2020_Allyship-in-the-Academy.pdf

Leng, L. L., Zhu, Y. W., & Zhou, L. G. (2023). Explaining differences in autism detection timing: Age of diagnosis and associated individual and socio-familial factors in Chinese children. *Autism*, *28*(4), 896–907. DOI: 10.1177/13623613231187184 PMID: 37491952

Lewis, L. F. (2016a). Exploring the experience of self-diagnosis of Autism Spectrum Disorder in adults. *Archives of Psychiatric Nursing*, *30*(5), 575–580. DOI: 10.1016/j.apnu.2016.03.009 PMID: 27654240

Lewis, L. F. (2016b). Realizing a diagnosis of Autism Spectrum Disorder as an adult. *International Journal of Mental Health Nursing*, *25*(4), 346–354. DOI: 10.1111/inm.12200 PMID: 26940281

Lin, X. (2024). Chinese teachers' perspective on integrating autistic children in mainstream primary school classes. *SHS Web of Conferences*, 187, 03006. DOI: 10.1051/shsconf/202418703006

Lindeman, E. C. (1926). *The meaning of adult education*. New Republic, Inc.

Lindsay, B. L., Bernier, E., Bowman, J. & Boyce, M. (2022). Understanding the connection between student wellbeing and teaching and learning at a Canadian research university: A qualitative student perspective. *Pedagogy in Health Promotion: The Scholarship of Teaching and Learning,* 1-12. DOI: 10.1177/23733799221089578

Lipscomb, S., Haimson, J., Liu, A. Y., Burghardt, J., Johnson, D. R., & Thurlow, M. L. (2017). *Preparing for life after high school: The characteristics and experiences of youth in special education. Findings from the National Longitudinal Transition Study 2012*; *Comparisons across disability groups: Full report (NCEE 2017–4018).* Department of Education, Institute of Education Sciences, National Center for Education Evaluation and Regional Assistance: Volume 2. https://ies.ed.gov/ncee/projects/evaluation/disabilities_nlts2012.asp

Locke, J., Osuna, A., Myrvold, R. J., & Closson, J. S. (2023). Supporting Autistic college students: Examining the Mentoring, Organization and Social Support for Autism Inclusion on Campus (MOSSAIC) program. *Journal of Autism and Developmental Disorders*. Advance online publication. DOI: 10.1007/s10803-023-05969-w PMID: 37017864

Loeng, S. (2018). Various ways of understanding the concept of andragogy. *Cogent Education*, *5*(1), 1496643. Advance online publication. DOI: 10.1080/2331186X.2018.1496643

Lollini, A. (2021). Brain Equality: Legal Implication of Neurodiversity in a Comparative Perspective. *New York University Journal of International Law & Politics. New York University. International Law Society*, *51*, 70–133. http://hdl.handle.net/11585/817387

Loomes, R., Hull, L., & Mandy, W. P. L. (2017). What is the male-to-female ratio in Autism Spectrum Disorder? A systematic review and meta-analysis. *Journal of the American Academy of Child and Adolescent Psychiatry*, *56*(6), 466–474. DOI: 10.1016/j.jaac.2017.03.013 PMID: 28545751

Lorenz, T., & Heinitz, K. (2014). Aspergers – different, not less: Occupational strengths and job interests of individuals with Asperger's syndrome. *PLoS One*, *9*(6), e100358. DOI: 10.1371/journal.pone.0100358 PMID: 24950060

Lubicz-Nawrocka, T., & Bovill, C. (2023). Do students experience transformation through co-creating curriculum in higher education? *Teaching in Higher Education*, *28*(7), 17441760. DOI: 10.1080/13562517.2021.1928060

Lucas, R., & James, A. I. (2018). An evaluation of specialist mentoring for university students with Autism Spectrum Disorders and mental health conditions. *Journal of Autism and Developmental Disorders*, *48*(3), 694–707. DOI: 10.1007/s10803-017-3303-1 PMID: 28918532

Madaus, J., & Shaw, S. (2010). College as a realistic option for students with learning disabilities. *InfoSheets*. Council for Learning Disabilities. http://www.council-for-learning-disabilities.org/wp-content/uploads/2013/11/College-Realistic-Option-for-Students-with-Learning-Disabilities.pdf

Madaus, J. W., Kowitt, J. S., & Lalor, A. R. (2012). The higher education opportunity act: Impact on students with disabilities. *Rehabilitation Research, Policy, and Education*, *26*(1), 33–41. DOI: 10.1891/216866512805000893

Maestas, R., Vaquera, G. S., & Zehr, L. M. (2007). Factors impacting sense of belonging at a Hispanic-serving institution. *Journal of Hispanic Higher Education*, *6*(3), 237–256. DOI: 10.1177/1538192707302801

Mandy, W. (2019). Social camouflaging in autism: Is it time to lose the mask? *Autism*, *23*(8), 1879–1881. DOI: 10.1177/1362361319878559 PMID: 31552745

Mandy, W. (2023). The old and the new way of understanding autistic lives: Reflections on the life of Donald Triplett, the first person diagnosed as autistic. *Autism*, *27*(7), 1853–1855. DOI: 10.1177/13623613231194476 PMID: 37665266

Manett, J. (2022). The Social Association for Students with Autism: Principles and practices of a social group for university students with ASD. *Social Work with Groups*, *45*(2), 157–171. DOI: 10.1080/01609513.2021.1994511

Marginson, S. (2019). Higher education in the global knowledge economy. *Procedia: Social and Behavioral Sciences*, *2*(5), 6962–6980. DOI: 10.1016/j.sbspro.2010.05.049

Martin, F., Budhrani, K., Kumar, S., & Ritzhaupt, A. (2019). Award-winning faculty online teaching practices: Roles and competencies. *Online Learning : the Official Journal of the Online Learning Consortium, 23*(1), 184–205. https://eric.ed.gov/?id=EJ1211042. DOI: 10.24059/olj.v23i1.1329

Marwat, A. (2023). Studying dyslexia and cognitive deficits in a global context to investigate learning difficulties in primary school students. *Journal of International Relations and Social Dynamics, 2*(1), 1–10.

Masataka, N. (2017). Implications of the idea of neurodiversity for understanding the origins of developmental disorders. *Physics of Life Reviews, 20*, 85–108. DOI: 10.1016/j.plrev.2016.11.002 PMID: 27876343

Mattila, M. L., Kielinen, M., Jussila, K., Linna, S. L., Bloigu, R., Ebeling, H., & Moilanen, I. (2007). An epidemiological and diagnostic study of Asperger syndrome according to four sets of diagnostic criteria. *Journal of the American Academy of Child and Adolescent Psychiatry, 46*(5), 636–646. DOI: 10.1097/chi.0b013e318033ff42 PMID: 17450055

Ma, Y., Siu, A., & Tse, W. S. (2018). The role of high parental expectations in adolescents' academic performance and depression in Hong Kong. *Journal of Family Issues, 39*(9), 2505–2522. DOI: 10.1177/0192513X18755194

Mazzotti, V. L., Rowe, D. A., Kwiatek, S., Voggt, A., Chang, W.-H., Fowler, C. H., Poppen, M., Sinclair, J., & Test, D. W. (2021). Secondary transition predictors of postschool success: An update to the research base. *Career Development and Transition for Exceptional Individuals, 44*(1), 47–64. DOI: 10.1177/2165143420959793

Mazzotti, V. L., Rowe, D. A., Sinclair, J., Poppen, M., Woods, W. E., & Shearer, M. L. (2016). Predictors of post-school success: A systematic review of NLTS2 secondary analyses. *Career Development and Transition for Exceptional Individuals, 39*(4), 196–215. https://psycnet.apa.org/doi/10.1177/2165143415588047. DOI: 10.1177/2165143415588047

Mc Guckin, C., & Minton, S. J. (2014). From theory to practice: Two ecosystemic approaches and their applications to understanding school bullying. *Australian Journal of Guidance & Counselling, 24*(1), 36–48. DOI: 10.1017/jgc.2013.10

McDowall, A., Doyle, N., & Kisleva, M. (2023). *Neurodiversity at work: A supply and demand gap analysis.* Neurodiversity in Business. https://neurodiversityinbusiness.org/research/neurodiversity-in-business-research-report-2023/

McDowall, A., & Kiseleva, M. (2024). A rapid review of supports for neurodivergent students in higher education. Implications for research and practice. *Neurodiversity*, *2*, 27546330241291769. Advance online publication. DOI: 10.1177/27546330241291769

McGrath, J. (2023). *Curriculum, accreditation and transition pathways: Pupils with intellectual disability in special schools (Ireland)*. Trinity College Dublin https://www.tcd.ie/tcpid/assets/docs/2024/Curriculum-Accreditation-and-Transition-Pathways-Pupils-with-Intellectual-Disability-in-Special-Schools-Ireland.pdf

McGrath, V. (2009). Reviewing the evidence on how adult students learn: An examination of Knowles' model of andragogy. *Adult Learner: The Irish Journal of Adult and Community Education,* 99–110.

McKee, T. E. (2017). Peer relationships in undergraduates with ADHD symptomatology: Selection and quality of friendships. *Journal of Attention Disorders*, *21*(12), 1020–1029. DOI: 10.1177/1087054714554934 PMID: 25359763

McLeod, J. D., Meanwell, E., & Hawbaker, A. (2019). The experiences of college students on the autism spectrum: A comparison to their neurotypical peers. *Journal of Autism and Developmental Disorders*, *49*(6), 2320–2336. DOI: 10.1007/s10803-019-03910-8 PMID: 30734173

McNaught, J., Biegun, D., & Swartzentruber, K. (2024). Student-led Individualized Education Programs: A gateway to self-determination. *Language, Speech, and Hearing Services in Schools*, *55*(2), 276–302. DOI: 10.1044/2023_LSHSS-23-00079 PMID: 38266231

Mercer-Mapstone, L., Dvorakova, S. L., Matthews, K. E., Abbot, S., Cheng, B., Felten, P., Knorr, K., Marquis, E., Shammas, R., & Swaim, K. (2017). A systematic literature review of students as partners in higher education. *International Journal for Students as Partners*, *1*(1), 15–37. DOI: 10.15173/ijsap.v1i1.3119

Mercier, H., & Sperber, D. (2018). *The Enigma of Reason. A New Theory of Human Understanding*. Penguin Books.

Merriam, S. B., & Bierema, L. L. (2014). *Adult learning: Linking theory and practice* (1st ed.). Jossey-Bass.

Meyer, A., Rose, D. H., & Gordon, D. (2014). *Universal Design for Learning: Theory and practice.* CAST Professional Publishing. https://www.cast.org/books-media/universal-design-for-learning-meyer-rose-gordon

Miclea, B. (2024). Neurodiversity and mental disorders. *BRAIN: Broad Research in Artificial Intelligence & Neuroscience, 15*(2), 225–233. https://doi-org.DOI: 10.18662/brain/15.2/574

Migliore, A., Butterworth, J., & Hart, D. (2009). Postsecondary education and employment outcomes for youth with intellectual disabilities. *Institute for Community Inclusion, Data Note Series, 21*. https://www.communityinclusion.org/pdf/DN21.pdf

Miller, D., Rees, J., & Pearson, A. (2021). "Masking is life": Experiences of masking in autistic and nonautistic adults. *Autism in Adulthood: Challenges and Management, 3*(4), 330–338. DOI: 10.1089/aut.2020.0083 PMID: 36601640

Milligan, F. (1995). In defence of andragogy. *Nurse Education Today, 15*(1), 22–27. DOI: 10.1016/S0260-6917(95)80074-3 PMID: 7708024

Milner, V., McIntosh, H., Colvert, E., & Happé, F. (2019). A qualitative exploration of the female experience of Autism Spectrum Disorder (ASD). *Journal of Autism and Developmental Disorders, 49*(6), 2389–2402. DOI: 10.1007/s10803-019-03906-4 PMID: 30790191

Milton, D. (2014). Autistic expertise: A critical reflection on the production of knowledge in autism studies. *Autism, 18*(7), 794–802. DOI: 10.1177/1362361314525281 PMID: 24637428

Milton, D. E. M. (2012). On the ontological status of autism: The 'double empathy problem.'. *Disability & Society, 27*(6), 883–887. DOI: 10.1080/09687599.2012.710008

Mitchell, D. T., & Snyder, S. L. (2015). *The biopolitics of disability: Neoliberalism, ablenationalism, and peripheral embodiment*. The University of Michigan Press. DOI: 10.3998/mpub.7331366

Moll, I. (2024). A psychological critique of Knowles' andragogy as a theory of learning. *Andragoška spoznanja/Studies in Adult Education and Learning, 30*(1), 151–170. DOI: 10.4312/as/16396

Moore, T. (2022). Relationships and reciprocity: Where next for strengths-based social work in adult social care? *Journal of Social Work Practice, 36*(4), 451–463. DOI: 10.1080/02650533.2022.2119946

Morin, A., & Kirchner-Morris, E. (2023) Is your school welcoming to neurodiverse students? *The Learning Professional, 44*(5), 46-48. https://learningforward.org/journal/reaching-all-learners/is-your-school-welcoming-to-neurodiverse-students/

Moriña, A. (2017). Inclusive education in higher education: Challenges and opportunities. *European Journal of Special Needs Education*, *32*(1), 3–17. DOI: 10.1080/08856257.2016.1254964

Moriña, A., Sandoval, M., & Carnerero, F. (2020). Higher education inclusivity: When the disability enriches the university. *Higher Education Research & Development*, *39*(6), 1202–1216. DOI: 10.1080/07294360.2020.1712676

Morningstar. M., & Clavenna-Deane, B. (2018). *Your complete guide to transition planning and services*. Brookes Publishing.

Morsanyi, K., Hamilton, J., Stamenković, D., & Holyoak, K. J. (2022). Linking metaphor comprehension with analogical reasoning: Evidence from typical development and autism spectrum disorder. *British Journal of Psychology (London, England: 1953)*, *113*(2), 479–495. https://doi-org.libproxy.txstate.edu/10.1111/bjop.12542

Morton, T. R., & Parsons, E. C. (2018). #BlackGirlMagic: The identity conceptualization of Black women in undergraduate STEM education. *Science Education*, *102*(6), 1363–1393. DOI: 10.1002/sce.21477

Muneeb, S. (2024). *Establishing the design space for educational technologies to support autistic children in the context of Pakistan* (Doctoral dissertation, Queensland University of Technology). Queensland University of Technology.

Naasko, R. T. (2022). *The social work role in higher education: A systematic review.* [Doctoral dissertation University of Alabama]. UA Repository. https://ir-api.ua.edu/api/core/bitstreams/0e0782f3-0f2f-40b6-8e32-9d8f3e9b9f91/content

Nachman, B. R. (2020). Enhancing transition programming for college students with autism: A systematic literature review. *Journal of Postsecondary Education and Disability*, *33*(1), 81–95. https://eric.ed.gov/?id=EJ1273654

Nachman, B. R., McDermott, C. T., & Cox, B. E. (2022). Brief report: Autism-specific college support programs: Differences across geography and institutional type. *Journal of Autism and Developmental Disorders*, *52*(2), 863–870. DOI: 10.1007/s10803-021-04958-1 PMID: 33770324

Nadeau, K. (2006). *Survival guide for college students with ADHD or LD*. Magination Press.

Nafukho, F., Amutabi, M., & Otunga, R. (2005). *Foundations of adult education in Africa*. Pearson; UNESCO Institute for Education.

Najmi, S. (2021). *A communicative assessment of mental health literacy in Pakistan* (Master's thesis, Texas Southern University). Texas Southern University.

Nash-Luckenbach, D. M., & Friedman, Z. L. (2024). The neurodivergent college learner: Faculty Perceptions of supporting individuals with ADHD in higher education. *Quality Assurance in Education: An International Perspective, 32*(4), 597–610. https://doi-org.DOI: 10.1108/QAE-01-2024-0014

National Association of Social Workers. (2021). *Code of ethics.* https://www.socialworkers.org/About/Ethics/Code-of-Ethics/Code-of-Ethics-English

National Autistic Society (NAS). (2021). *Left waiting: The crisis in autism diagnosis and employment outcomes.* https://www.autism.org.uk

National Autistic Society. (2022). Now I Know Campaign. https://www.autism.org.uk/what-we-do/acceptance-and-awareness/now-i-know-campaign

National Autistic Society. (2023). Autism facts and history. https://www.autism.org.uk/advice-and-guidance/what-is-autism/autism-facts-and-history

National Center for College Students with Disabilities. (n.d.). *Future College Students.* University of Minnesota. https://nccsd.ici.umn.edu/clearinghouse/audience-specific-resources/future-college-students

National Center for Education Statistics [NCES]. (2017). *Bachelor's degree attainment at first institution through June 2017 by disability* (Beginning Postsecondary Students: 2012/2017). https://nces.ed.gov/datalab/powerstats/71-beginning-postsecondary-students-2012-2017/percentage-distribution

National Coordinating Center Accreditation Workgroup and Inclusive Higher Education Accreditation Council. (2024). The 2024 guide to accreditation for higher education programs for students with intellectual disability. University of Massachusetts Boston, Institute for Community Inclusion. https://thinkcollege.net/sites/default/files/files/resources/PDF%202024%20accreditation%20guide%20.pdf

National Institute for Health and Care Excellence (NICE). (2016). *Autism Spectrum Disorder in adults: Diagnosis and management.* https://www.nice.org.uk/guidance/cg142

National Technical Assistance Center on Transition, & the The Collaborative. (NTACT:C). (2024). *Differences between high school and postsecondary education.* https://transitionta.org/differences-between-hs-postsecondary-education/

Naylor, C. (2023). *'Much better set up to do my best work': What does 'neurodiversity-affirming practice' mean to the autistic community?* [Thesis, University of Nottingham]. https://eprints.nottingham.ac.uk/76179/

Nazim, A., & Khalid, R. (2019). Assessment of temperament in children with autism spectrum disorder. *JPMA. The Journal of the Pakistan Medical Association, 69*(10), 1437–1441. DOI: 10.5455/JPMA.290521 PMID: 31622293

Naz, S., Majeed, Z., & Sulman, N. (2024). The challenges of accessibility and equity for students with disabilities in higher education institutions with special reference to the University of Karachi, Pakistan. *Siazga Research Journal, 3*(3), 313–322. DOI: 10.58341/srj.v3i3.97

NCLD. (2023, March 30). *Remove barriers for college students with disabilities by supporting the RISE Act.* National Center for Learning Disabilities. https://www.ncld.org/news/policy-and-advocacy/bi-partisan-rise-act-opens-new-doors-for-students-with-disabilities/

Neuman, W. L. (2011). *Social research methods: Qualitative and quantitative approaches* (7th ed.). Pearson.

Neurodiversity Hub. (n.d.). *Changing the narrative about autism and neurodiversity through awareness, education, and engagement.* https://www.neurodiversityhub.org/

Newman, L., Wagner, M., Cameto, R., Knokey, A.-M., & Shaver, D. (2010). Comparisons across time of the outcomes of youth with disabilities up to 4 years after high school: A report of findings from the National Longitudinal Transition Study (NLTS) and the National Longitudinal Transition Study-2 (NLTS2). In *National Center for Special Education Research.* National Center for Special Education Research. https://eric.ed.gov/?id=ED512149

Newman, L., Wagner, M., Knokey, A. M., Marder, C., Nagle, K., Shaver, D., & Schwarting, M. (2011). *The post-high school outcomes of young adults with disabilities up to 8 years after high school: A report from the National Longitudinal Transition Study-2 (NLTS-2).* SRI International. https://eric.ed.gov/?id=ED524044

Newman, L., Madaus, J. W., Lalor, A. R., & Javitz, H. S. (2019). Support receipt: Effect on postsecondary success of students with learning disabilities. *Career Development and Transition for Exceptional Individuals, 42*(1), 6–16. DOI: 10.1177/2165143418811288

Newman, L., Wagner, M., Knokey, A.-M., Marder, C., Nagle, K., Shaver, D., Wei, X., Cameto, R., Contreras, E., Ferguson, K., Greene, S., & Schwarting, M. (2011). *The post-high school outcomes of young adults with disabilities up to 8 years after high school: A report from the National Longitudinal Transition Study-2 (NLTS2) (NCSER 2011-3005).* SRI International.

Ng, C. S. M., & Ng, S. S. L. (2022). A qualitative study on the experience of stigma for Chinese parents of children with Autism Spectrum Disorder. *Scientific Reports*, *12*(1), 19885. Advance online publication. DOI: 10.1038/s41598-022-23978-0 PMID: 36379973

Nisar, A., Bashir, I., & Naseem, A. (2023). Special needs students' lived experiences of support practices in higher educational institutes in Pakistan. *Journal of Asian Development Studies*, *12*(3), 1487–1497.

Nixon, S. A. (2019). The coin model of privilege and critical allyship: Implications for health. *BMC Public Health*, *19*(1), 1637. DOI: 10.1186/s12889-019-7884-9 PMID: 31805907

Nizamani, M. K., & Nizamani, A. (2022). Dyslexia: Emotional and psychological effects in relation to the social behavior of caretakers in Sindh, Pakistan. [LASSIJ]. *Liberal Arts and Social Sciences International Journal*, *6*(2), 43–62. DOI: 10.47264/idea.lassij/6.2.3

Nolan, C., Doyle, J. K., Lewis, K., & Treanor, D. (2023). Disabled students' perception of the sensory aspects of the learning and social environments within one higher education institution. *British Journal of Occupational Therapy*, *86*(5), 367–375. https://journals.sagepub.com/doi/pdf/10.1177/03080226221126895?download=true. DOI: 10.1177/03080226221126895 PMID: 40336521

Noor, H., Khan, I. N., & Humara, B. (2023). Effectiveness of self-regulation training plan for the treatment of adolescents with Attention Deficit Hyperactivity Disorder *Pakistan Journal of Social Sciences, 43*(2),177-189. https://pjss.bzu.edu.pk/index.php/pjss/article/view/1254

Note, N., De Backer, F., & Donder, L. D. (2021). A novel viewpoint on andragogy: Enabling moments of community. *Adult Education Quarterly, 71*(1), 3-19. https://doi-org.DOI: 10.1177/0741713620921361

O'Bryant, J. M., & Schaffzin, K. T. (2017). First-generation students in law school: A proven success model. *Arkansas Law Review*, *70*(4), 913–958. https://heinonline.org/HOL/LandingPage?handle=hein.journals/arklr70&div=36&id=&page=

Office for Students. (2022). *Funding for higher education providers*. https://www.officeforstudents.org.uk/advice-and-guidance/funding-for-providers/

Onwumelu, R. (2024) How you can support Neurodiverse students at Xavier. *Xavier University* https://www.xavier.edu/now/2024/how-to-support-neurodiverse-students

Osifo, O., & Terashima, M. (2024). Addressing barriers in the university campus environment for neurodivergent students. *Studies in Health Technology and Informatics, 29*(319), 293–306. DOI: 10.3233/SHTI240952 PMID: 39618368

Overton, G. L., Marsà-Sambola, F., Martin, R., & Cavenagh, P. (2024). Understanding the self-identification of autism in adults: A scoping review. *Review Journal of Autism and Developmental Disorders, 11*(4), 682–702. DOI: 10.1007/s40489-023-00361-x

Ozaki, C. C., Olson, A. B., Johnston-Guerrero, M. P., & Pizzolato, J. E. (2020). Understanding persistence using a Phenomenological Variant of Ecological Systems Theory. *Community College Review, 48*(3), 252–276. DOI: 10.1177/0091552120906884

Pakistan Bureau of Statistics. (2023). *Announcement of results of 7th Population and Housing Census–2023.* Pakistan Bureau of Statistics. https://www.pbs.gov.pk

Pakistan Curriculum. (2025). Department of Education and Knowledge, https://www.adek.gov.ae/en/Education-System/Private-Schools/Curriculum/Pakistani-Curriculum

Palmer, S. B., Wehmeyer, M. L., & Shogren, K. A. (2017). The development of self-determination during childhood. In Wehmeyer, M., Shogren, K., Little, T., & Lopez, S. (Eds.), *Development of Self-Determination Through the Life-Course* (pp. 71–88). Springer., DOI: 10.1007/978-94-024-1042-6_6

Park, T. W., Sheward, K. L., & Rogers-Shaw, C. (2023). Tips for supporting students with social skill, mental health, and communication disabilities in digital settings. *eLearn, 2023*(2023). DOI: 10.1145/3596691.3596515

Park, T., Sheward, K., & Rogers-Shaw, C. *(2023).* Tips for supporting students with social skill, mental health & communication disabilities in digital settings. *eLearn. 5*(2023). https://dl.acm.org/doi/fullHtml/10.1145/3596691.3596515

Patel, D. R., & Brown, K. A. (2017). An overview of the conceptual framework and definitions of disability. *International Journal of Child Health and Human Development, 10*(3), 247–252. https://www.proquest.com/scholarly-journals/overview-conceptual-framework-definitions/docview/1999052730/se-2

Patel, D. R., Cabral, M. D., Ho, A., & Merrick, J. (2020). A clinical primer on intellectual disability. *Translational Pediatrics, 9*(S1, Suppl. 1), S23–S35. https://tp.amegroups.org/article/view/36118/28320. DOI: 10.21037/tp.2020.02.02 PMID: 32206581

Patton, L. D. (Ed.). (2023). *Culture centers in higher education: Perspectives on identity, theory, and practice.* Routledge. DOI: 10.4324/9781003443971

Paul, M., Street, C., Wheeler, N., & Singh, S. P. (2015). Transition to adult services for young people with mental health needs: A systematic review. *Clinical Child Psychology and Psychiatry*, *20*(3), 436–457. DOI: 10.1177/1359104514526603 PMID: 24711585

Pellicano, E., Dinsmore, A., & Charman, T. (2021). What should autism research focus upon? Community views and priorities. *Autism*, *25*(3), 756–770. DOI: 10.1177/1362361314529627 PMID: 24789871

Peña, E. V., Gassner, D., & Brown, K. R. (2020). Autistic-centered program development and assessment practices. *Journal of Postsecondary Education and Disability*, *33*(3), 233–240. https://eric.ed.gov/?id=EJ1280846

Petcu, S. D., Van Horn, M. L., & Shogren, K. A. (2017). Self-determination and the enrollment in and completion of postsecondary education for students with disabilities. *Career Development and Transition for Exceptional Individuals*, *40*(4), 225–234. DOI: 10.1177/2165143416670135

Peterson, C., Maier, S. F., & Seligman, M. E. P. (1993). *Learned helplessness: A theory for the age of personal control.* Oxford University Press. DOI: 10.1093/oso/9780195044669.001.0001

Petri, G., Beadle-Brown, J., & Bradshaw, J. (2021). 'Even a self-advocate needs to buy milk': Economic barriers to self-advocacy in the autism and intellectual disability movement. *Scandinavian Journal of Disability Research*, *23*(1), 180–191. DOI: 10.16993/sjdr.738

Picault, J. (2021). Structure, flexibility, and consistency: A dynamic learning approach for an online asynchronous course. *Applied Economics Teaching Resources (AETR), 3*(4), 30-43. https://ageconsearch.umn.edu/record/316503/?v=pdf

Pietri, E. S., Moser, C. E., Derricks, V., & Johnson, I. R. (2024). A framework for understanding effective allyship. *Nature Reviews Psychology*, *3*(10), 1–15. DOI: 10.1038/s44159-024-00359-0

Pratt, D. D. (2002). Good teaching: One size fits all? *New Directions for Adult and Continuing Education, 2002*(93), 5-16. https://doi-org.DOI: 10.1002/ace.45

Pratt, D. D. (1993). Andragogy after twenty-five years. *New Directions for Adult and Continuing Education*, *57*(57), 15–23. DOI: 10.1002/ace.36719935704

Price, D. (2022). *Unmasking autism: Discovering the new faces of neurodiversity.* Harmony Books.

Public Services Committee. (2024). *Think work first: The transition from education to work for young disabled people.* House of Lords. https://publications.parliament.uk/pa/ld5901/ldselect/pubserv/12/12.pdf

Purchase College. (n.d.). *Assistive technology.* Office of Disability Resources. https://www.purchase.edu/offices/disability-resources/assistive-technology/

Quirke, M., McGuckin, C., & McCarthy, P. (2024). *Adopting a UDL attitude within academia: Understanding and practicing inclusion across higher education*. Routledge. DOI: 10.4324/9781003137672

Rachal, J. R. (2014). Book review: Malcolm Shepherd Knowles: A history of his thought. *Adult Education Quarterly, 64*(1), 80-84. https://doi-org.DOI: 10.1177/0741713613496616

Radke, H. R., Kutlaca, M., Siem, B., Wright, S. C., & Becker, J. C. (2020). Beyond allyship: Motivations for advantaged group members to engage in action for disadvantaged groups. *Personality and Social Psychology Review*, *24*(4), 291–315. DOI: 10.1177/1088868320918698 PMID: 32390573

Rahbar, M. H., Ibrahim, K., & Assassi, P. (2011). Knowledge and attitude of general practitioners regarding autism in Karachi, Pakistan. *Journal of Autism and Developmental Disorders*, *41*(4), 465–474. DOI: 10.1007/s10803-010-1068-x PMID: 20632204

Raines, A. R., Francis, G. L., Fujita, M., & Macedonia, A. (2023). Belonging from the perspectives of individuals with disabilities: A scoping review. *Psychology in the Schools*, *60*(6), 2112–2127. DOI: 10.1002/pits.22864

Rando, H., Huber, M. J., & Oswald, G. R. (2016). An academic coaching model intervention for college students on the autism spectrum. *Journal of Postsecondary Education and Disability*, *29*(3), 257–262. https://files.eric.ed.gov/fulltext/EJ1123790.pdf

Rapp, C. A., & Chamberlain, R. (1985). Case management services for the chronically mentally ill. *Social Work*, *30*(5), 417–422. https://www.jstor.org/stable/23714362. DOI: 10.1093/sw/30.5.417 PMID: 10273981

Rapp, C. A., Saleebey, D., & Sullivan, W. P. (2005). The future of strength based social work. *Advances in Social Work*, *6*(1), 79–90. DOI: 10.18060/81

Rasch, E. V. (2022). The lights are too loud: Neurodivergence in the student affairs profession. *Vermont Connection*, *43*(1), 189–203.

Rasheed, H., Hashmi, N. U., Bhutta, M. H., & Chaudhry, A. G. (2023). Social inclusion of persons with disabilities: A right-based approach. *Pakistan Islamacus: An International Journal of Islamic & Social Sciences, 3*(2), 426–441. https://www.pakistanislamicus.com/index.php/home/article/view/74

Rathore, F. A., New, P. W., & Iftikhar, A. (2011). A report on disability and rehabilitation medicine in Pakistan: Past, present, and future directions. *Archives of Physical Medicine and Rehabilitation*, *92*(1), 161–166. DOI: 10.1016/j.apmr.2010.10.004 PMID: 21187218

Raymaker, D., & Nicolaidis, C. (2013). Participatory research with autistic communities. In J. Davidson & M. Orsini (Eds.), *Worlds of Autism* (pp. 169–188). University of Minnesota Press.

Raymaker, D. M., Teo, A. R., Steckler, N. A., Lentz, B., Scharer, M., Delos Santos, A., Kapp, S. K., Hunter, M., Joyce, A., & Nicolaidis, C. (2020). "Having all of your internal resources exhausted beyond measure and being left with no clean-up crew": Defining autistic burnout. *Autism in Adulthood: Challenges and Management*, *2*(2), 132–143. DOI: 10.1089/aut.2019.0079 PMID: 32851204

Razzak, J. A., Hyder, A. A., Akhtar, T., Khan, M., & Khan, U. R. (2008). Assessing emergency medical care in low-income countries: A pilot study from Pakistan. *BMC Emergency Medicine*, *8*(1), 8. Advance online publication. DOI: 10.1186/1471-227X-8-8 PMID: 18598353

Reeble, C. J., Lefler, E. K., Abu-Ramadan, T., Bodalski, E. A., & Canu, W. H. (2023). Social support in college students with ADHD symptoms: Quantity beats quality in moderating impairment. *Journal of College Student Psychotherapy*, *0*(0), 1–22. DOI: 10.1080/87568225.2023.2202351

Reiss, S., & Szyszko, J. (1983). Diagnostic overshadowing and professional experience with mentally retarded persons. *American Journal of Mental Deficiency*, *87*(4), 396–402. https://europepmc.org/article/med/6829617 PMID: 6829617

Richards, S. B., & Hulewicz, R. (2024). Historical concepts and perspectives. In Richards, S. B., Brady, M. P., & Taylor, R. L. (Eds.), *Understanding Intellectual Disabilities: Historical perspectives, current practices, and future directions* (3rd ed., pp. 3–37). Routledge. DOI: 10.4324/9781003345602-2

Richmond, M. E. (1917). *Social diagnosis*. Russell Sage Foundation. DOI: 10.2307/3406141

Rillotta, F., Arthur, J., Hutchinson, C., & Raghavendra, P. (2020). Inclusive university experience in Australia: Perspectives of students with intellectual disability and their mentors. *Journal of Intellectual Disabilities*, *24*(1), 102–117. DOI: 10.1177/1744629518769421 PMID: 29685066

Ringwood, B., & Devitt, M. (2022, October 22). *The TCPID graduate internship programme: The need for a pathway with a feedback loop to support graduates and businesses with an ever-evolving working world* [Conference proceedings]. European State-Of-The-Art Congress on Inclusive Post-Secondary Programmes for Students with Intellectual Disabilities, Salzburg, Austria. https://joinin.education/wp-content/uploads/2022/12/ESOTA-2022-conferenceproceedings.pdf

Ringwood, B., Banks, J., & Shevlin, M. (2024). Breaking new ground? An analysis of the use of embedded occupational therapy in a postsecondary education program for students with intellectual disabilities. *British Journal of Learning Disabilities*, *52*(2), 422–431. DOI: 10.1111/bld.12583

Rocco, T. S. (2005). From disability studies to critical race theory: Working towards critical disability theory. *Proceedings of the 46th Annual Adult Education Research Conference*. https://newprairiepress.org/aerc/2005/papers/17

Rodriguez, D. D., Menchaca, V. D., & Padilla, G. (2021). Social justice: School administrative staff perceptions of strengths, challenges, and training needs in Section 504-only services. *Journal of Leadership, Accountability and Ethics*, *18*(1), 89–101. http://www.na-businesspress.com/JLAE/JLAE18-1/7_MenchacaFinal.pdf

Rogers, A. T. (2022). *Human behavior and the social environment: Perspectives on development and the life course* (6th ed.). Routledge. DOI: 10.4324/9781003195542

Rogers-Shaw, C., Park, T. W., & Mohney, K. D. (2023). Strategies for supporting learners with disabilities in postsecondary education. *New Horizons in Adult Education and Human Resource Development*, *35*(4), 199–207. DOI: 10.1177/19394225231189136

Röhm, A., Grengel, M., Möhring, M., Zensen-Möhring, J., Nellen, C., & Hastall, M. R. (2022). Applying the mixed-blessings model and labeling theory to stigma in inclusive education: An experimental study of student and trainee teachers' perceptions of pupils with ADHD, DLD, and intellectual disability. *Frontiers in Psychology, 13*, 1-14. https://doi-org.DOI: 10.3389/fpsyg.2022.910702

Rosa, E. M., & Tudge, J. (2013). Urie Bronfenbrenner's theory of human development: Its evolution from ecology to bioecology. *Journal of Family Theory & Review*, *5*(4), 243–258. DOI: 10.1111/jftr.12022

Rosenau, K. A., Hotez, E., Fernandes, P., Gomez, C., Eagan, K., Shea, L., & Kuo, A. (2023). Anxiety and depression in autistic college students: The freshman survey results. *Cureus, 15*(3), e35820. Advance online publication. DOI: 10.7759/cureus.35820 PMID: 37033553

Ross-Gordon, J. M., & Procknow, G. (2021). Adult education and disability. In Rocco, T. S., Smith, M. C., Mizzi, R. C., Merriweather, L. R., & Hawley, J. D. (Eds.), *Handbook of adult and continuing education* (pp. 392–400). Stylus.

Ross-Gordon, J., Rose, A. D., & Kasworm, C. E. (2017). *Foundations of adult and continuing education.* Jossey-Bass.

Rourke, B., Bellur, S., & Nowak, K. (2024). All distractions are not equal: The moderating role of autistic traits and technology multitasking on academic performance among college students. *Atlantic Journal of Communication, 32*(3), 325–347. DOI: 10.1080/15456870.2023.2177292

Rowan, A. (2024). Beyond 'reasonable': Experiences of disabled international students in UK higher education. *Journal of Inclusive Practice in Further and Higher Education, 16*(1). https://nadp-uk.org/wp-content/uploads/2024/06/5.-A-Rowan-Beyond-Reasonable-Experiences-of-disabled-international-students-in-UK-Higher-Education.docx.pdf

Rowe, D. A., Alverson, C. Y., Unruh, D. K., Fowler, C. H., Kellems, R., & Test, D. W. (2015). A Delphi study to operationalize evidence-based predictors in secondary transition. *Career Development and Transition for Exceptional Individuals, 38*(2), 113–126. DOI: 10.1177/2165143414526429

Rowe, T., Charles, T., & DuBose, H. (2020). Supporting students with ASD on campus: What students may need to be successful (Practice Brief). *Journal of Postsecondary Education and Disability, 33*(1), 97–101. https://files.eric.ed.gov/fulltext/EJ1273702.pdf

Rowland, M. L., & ERIC Clearinghouse on Adult, Career, and Vocational Education, Columbus, OH (2000). African Americans and self-help education: The missing link in adult education. *ERIC Digest No. 222.*

Roy, R., & Jain, S. (2021). Global neurodiverse support systems: Primary research findings on key challenges and optimized solutions in Mumbai, India. *The Physician, 6*(3), 1–22. DOI: 10.38192/1.6.3.9

Ruedas-Gracia, N., Jiang, G., & Maghsoodi, A. H. (2023). Is belonging stable over time?: A four-year longitudinal examination of university belonging differences among students. *Emerging Adulthood, 11*(4), 1022–1038. DOI: 10.1177/21676968231181720

Rumberger, R. W., & Rotermund, S. (2012). The relationship between engagement and high school dropout. In S. L. Christenson, A. L. Reschly, & C. Wylie (Eds.), *Handbook of Research on Student Engagement* (pp. 491–513). Springer Science + Business Media. DOI: 10.1007/978-1-4614-2018-7_24

Russell, G., Stapley, S., Newlove-Delgado, T., Salmon, A., White, R., Warren, F., & Ford, T. (2020). Time trends in autism diagnosis in the UK: Evidence from primary care records. *Journal of Autism and Developmental Disorders*, *50*(12), 4358–4372. DOI: 10.1111/jcpp.13505 PMID: 34414570

Saleebey, D. (1996). The strengths of perspective in social work practice: Extensions and cautions. *Social Work*, *41*(3), 296–305. DOI: 10.1093/sw/41.3.296 PMID: 8936085

Salusky, I., Monjaras-Gaytan, L., Ulerio, G., Forbes, N., Perron, G., & Raposa, E. (2022). The formation and role of social belonging in on-campus integration of diverse first-generation college students. *Journal of College Student Retention: Research, Theory & Practice. Article, 15210251221092709.* Advance online publication. DOI: 10.1177/15210251221092709

Sánchez, B., Colón, Y., & Esparza, P. (2005). The role of sense of school belonging and gender in the academic adjustment of Latino adolescents. *Journal of Youth and Adolescence*, *34*(6), 619–628. DOI: 10.1007/s10964-005-8950-4

Sanderson, K. A., Goldman, S. E., & Rojas, A. (2021). A review and analysis of single-case research examining adolescent participation in IEP Meetings. *The Journal of Special Education*, *56*(2), 97–109. DOI: 10.1177/00224669211047232

Sandland, B., MacLeod, A., & Hall, N. (2023). Neurodiverse students within higher education: Initial thoughts from a collaborative project. *Good Autism Practice, 24(*2), 13–22. https://www.ingentaconnect.com/content/bild/gap/2023/00000024/00000002/art00004# Sandlin, J. A. (2005). Andragogy and its discontents: An analysis of andragogy from three critical perspectives. *PAACE Journal of Lifelong Learning, 14,* 25–42.

Santhanam, S. P., & Wilson, K. (2024). A comparison of autistic and non-autistic college students' perceived challenges and engagement in self-advocacy. *American Journal of Speech-Language Pathology*, *33*(3), 1471–1484. DOI: 10.1044/2024_AJSLP-22-00381 PMID: 38470839

Sapir, A., & Banai, A. (2024). Balancing attendance and disclosure: Identity work of students with invisible disabilities. *Disability & Society*, *39*(8), 2032–2052. DOI: 10.1080/09687599.2023.2181765

Sarrett, J. C. (2018). Autism and accommodations in higher education: Insights from the autism community. *Journal of Autism and Developmental Disorders, 48*(3), 679–693. https://doi-org.DOI: 10.1007/s10803-017-3353-4

Schaefer, J., & Sanchez, A. (2024). *Shining a light on neurodiversity in higher ed.* University of Wisconsin-Madison School of Education. https://education.wisc.edu/news/shining-a-light-on-neurodiversity-in-higher-ed/

Scheef, A., Caniglia, C., & Barrio, B. L. (2020). Disability as diversity: Perspectives of institutions of higher education in the U.S. *Journal of Postsecondary Education and Disability, 33*(1), 49–61. https://files.eric.ed.gov/fulltext/EJ1273652.pdf

Schelbe, L., Pryce, J., & Gaab, N. (2022). Dyslexia in the context of social work: Screening and early intervention. *Families in Society, 103*(3), 269–280. DOI: 10.1177/10443894211042323

Schmidt, E. K., Faieta, J., & Tanner, K. (2020). Scoping review of self-advocacy education interventions to improve care. *The Occupational Therapy Journal of Research, 40*(1), 50–56. DOI: 10.1177/1539449219860583 PMID: 31342850

Schneider, R., Lester, L., & Ochieng, J. (2008). *Advocacy. Encyclopedia of Social Work.* Oxford University Press., https://www-oxfordreference-com.proxy-commonwealthu.klnpa.org/view/10.1093/acref/9780195306613.001.0001/acref-9780195306613-e-10

Scott, M., Jacob, A., Hendrie, D., Parsons, R., Girdler, S., Falkmer, T., & Falkmer, M. (2017). Employers' perception of the costs and the benefits of hiring individuals with Autism Spectrum Disorder in open employment in Australia. *PLoS One, 12*(5), e0177607. DOI: 10.1371/journal.pone.0177607 PMID: 28542465

Seale, J. (2014). *E-learning and disability in higher education: Accessibility research and practice*. Routledge.

Section 504 of the Rehabilitation Act of 1973 (29 U.S.C. § 794).

Seelmeyer, L. (2024). Disability and neurodiversity in the academic library: Fostering new and continuing engagement. *Public Services Quarterly, 20*(3), 217–224. https://doi-org.DOI: 10.1080/15228959.2024.2367530

Seligman, M. (1975). *Helplessness: On depression, development, and death*. W. H. Freeman.

Shaewitz, D., & Crandall, J. R. (2020, October 19). Higher education's challenge: Disability inclusion on campus. *Higher Education Today*. https://www.higheredtoday.org/2020/10/19/higher-educations-challenge-disability-inclusion-campus/

Shallish, L. (2015). “Just how much diversity will the law permit?”: The Americans with Disabilities Act, diversity and disability in higher education. *Disability Studies Quarterly*, *35*(3). Advance online publication. DOI: 10.18061/dsq.v35i3.4942

Shattuck, P. T., Durkin, M., Maenner, M., Newschaffer, C., Mandell, D. S., Wiggins, L., & Yeargin-Allsopp, M. (2009). Timing of identification among children with an Autism Spectrum Disorder: Findings from a population-based surveillance study. *Journal of the American Academy of Child and Adolescent Psychiatry*, *48*(5), 474–483. DOI: 10.1097/CHI.0b013e31819b3848 PMID: 19318992

Shattuck, P. T., Narendorf, S. C., Cooper, B., Sterzing, P. R., Wagner, M., & Taylor, J. L. (2012). Postsecondary education and employment among youth with an autism spectrum disorder. *Pediatrics*, *129*(6), 1042–1049. DOI: 10.1542/peds.2011-2864 PMID: 22585766

Shefcyk, A. (2015). Count us in: Addressing gender disparities in autism research. *Autism*, *19*(2), 131–132. DOI: 10.1177/1362361314566585 PMID: 25789398

Shepherd, J., Sutton, B., Smith, S., & Szlenkier, M. (2024). ‘Sea-glass survivors’: Autistic testimonies about education experiences. *British Journal of Special Education*, *51*(2), 142–155. https://doi-org.DOI: 10.1111/1467-8578.12506

Shevlin, M., Kubiak, J., O’Donovan, M., Devitt, M., Ringwood, B., Aston, D., & Mc Guckin, C. (2020). *Effective practices for helping students transition to work*. Oxford University Press., DOI: 10.1093/acrefore/9780190264093.013.1234

Sheward, K., Rogers-Shaw, C., & Park, T. W. (2022). *Creating connection by design: Supporting adult learners by building inclusive online academic communities*. Proceedings of the Adult Education Research Conference, Virtual. https://newprairiepress.org/aerc/2022/papers/27

Shogren, K. A., Garnier Villarreal, M., Lang, K., & Seo, H. (2017). Mediating role of self-determination constructs in explaining the relationship between school factors and postschool outcomes. *Exceptional Children*, *83*(2), 165–180. DOI: 10.1177/0014402916660089

Shogren, K. A., Luckasson, R., & Schalock, R. L. (2021). Leveraging the power of context in disability policy development, implementation, and evaluation: Multiple applications to enhance personal outcomes. *Journal of Disability Policy Studies*, *31*(4), 230–243. DOI: 10.1177/1044207320923656

Shogren, K. A., Wehmeyer, M. L., Palmer, S. B., Soukup, J. H., Little, T. D., Garner, N., & Lawrence, M. (2007). Examining individual and ecological predictors of the self-determination of students with disabilities. *Exceptional Children*, *73*(4), 488–510. DOI: 10.1177/001440290707300406

Shukat, S. (2023). Challenges for education of children with disabilities *in Pakistan. Intervention in School and Clinic*, *59*(1), 75–80. DOI: 10.1177/10534512221130082

Sidjaja, F. F. (2024). The growing definition of autism. *International Journal of Disability Development and Education*, •••, 1–7. https://doi-org.libproxy.txstate.edu/10.1080/1034912X.2024.2393382. DOI: 10.1080/1034912X.2024.2393382

Skivington, K., Matthews, L., Simpson, S. A., Craig, P., Baird, J., Blazeby, J. M., Boyd, K. A., Craig, N., French, D. P., McIntosh, E., Petticrew, M., Rycroft-Malone, J., White, M., & Moore, L. (2021). A new framework for developing and evaluating complex interventions: Update of Medical Research Council guidance. *BMJ (Clinical Research Ed.)*, *374*, 2061. Advance online publication. DOI: 10.1136/bmj.n2061 PMID: 34593508

Smith, I., & Mueller, C. O. (2022). The importance of disability identity, self-advocacy, and disability activism. *In Practice*, *1*(2), 47–54. DOI: 10.1177/27324745211057155

Smith, P. S., & Myers, B. (2024). Instructor experiences providing accommodations and modifications for students with intellectual disability in inclusive higher education. *International Journal of Inclusive Education*, •••, 1–14. DOI: 10.1080/13603116.2024.2305653

Sohn, M. A., Zhao, L. M., & Tadros, E. (2024). Integrating structural and experiential family therapy in neurodivergent families: A case study. *Issues in Mental Health Nursing*, *45*(5), 477–487. DOI: 10.1080/01612840.2024.2328260 PMID: 38593465

Solomon, M., Miller, M., Taylor, S. L., Hinshaw, S. P., & Carter, C. S. (2012). Autism symptoms and internalizing psychopathology in girls and boys with Autism Spectrum Disorders. *Journal of Autism and Developmental Disorders*, *42*(1), 48–59. DOI: 10.1007/s10803-011-1215-z PMID: 21442362

Southon, C. (2022). The relationship between executive function, neurodevelopmental disorder traits, and academic achievement in university students. *Frontiers in Psychology*, *13*, 958013. Advance online publication. DOI: 10.3389/fpsyg.2022.958013 PMID: 36118426

Spaeth, E., & Pearson, A. (2023). A reflective analysis on how to promote a positive learning experience for neurodivergent students. *Journal of Perspectives in Applied Academic Practice*, *11*(2), 109–120. https://doi-org.DOI: 10.56433/jpaap.v11i2.517

Spain, D., Zıvralı Yarar, E., & Happé, F. (2020). Social anxiety in adults with autism: A qualitative study. *International Journal of Qualitative Studies on Health and Well-being, 15*(1), 1–15. DOI: 10.1080/17482631.2020.1803669 PMID: 32815779

Spencer, M. B. (2006). Phenomenology and ecological systems theory: Development of diverse groups. In Damon, W., & Lerner, R. (Eds.), *Theoretical models of human development* (6th ed., pp. 829–893). Handbook of child psychology. John Wiley & Sons Inc.

Spindler, C. M. (2008, March). You, me, and mom makes three: How academic advisors can capitalize on parental involvement. *Academic Advising Today, 31*(1). https://nacada.ksu.edu/Resources/Academic-Advising-Today/View-Articles/You-Me-and-Mom-Makes-Three-How-Academic-Advisors-Can-Capitalize-on-Parental-Involvement.aspx

Stanford University. (n.d.). *Assistive technology for online learning.* Office of Accessible Education. https://oae.stanford.edu/students/remote-learning-coping-during-covid-19/assistive-technology-online-learning

Staniland, L. (2011). *Public perceptions of disabled people. Evidence from the British Social Attitudes Survey, 2009.* Office for Disability Issues.

Ştefani, S. C. (2023). The role of advocacy in social work practice. *Social Work Review / Revista de Asistenta Sociala*, 4, 77–86. http://www.swreview.ro/index.pl/the_role_of_advocacy_in_social_work_practice

Steinberg, L. D. (2022). *Adolescence* (13th ed.). McGraw Hill.

Stice, L. V., & Lavner, J. A. (2019). Social connectedness and loneliness mediate the association between autistic traits and internalizing symptoms among young adults. *Journal of Autism and Developmental Disorders, 49*(3), 1096–1110. DOI: 10.1007/s10803-018-3812-6 PMID: 30406911

Stinnett, C. V., Lazo, R., & Pound, S. (2023). “Think higher. Think college.” A resource guide for inclusive postsecondary education for students with intellectual disability. *Think College.* University of Massachusetts Boston. https://thinkhighered.net/uploads/TCcampaign-resource-booklet_R-fixed.pdf

Stockwell, K. M., Bottini, S., Jaswal, V. K., & Gillis, J. M. (2021). Brief report: Social behavior and special interests in the stigmatization of autistic college students. *Journal of Autism & Developmental Disorders, 51*(9), 3356–3364. https://doi-org.DOI: 10.1007/s10803-020-04769-w

Stone, S., Austin, M. J., Berzin, A., & Taylor, S. (2007). Exploring the knowledge base of human behavior and the social environment using the concept of reciprocity. *Journal of Human Behavior in the Social Environment, 16*(3), 89–106. DOI: 10.1300/10911350802107769

Story, M. F., Mueller, J. L., & Mace, R. L. (1998). *The universal design file: Designing for people of all ages and abilities* (Revised edition). Center for Universal Design. https://files.eric.ed.gov/fulltext/ED460554.pdf

Stowers, S. (2022, June 4). *Types of neurodiversity and how to design learning experiences for them*. eLearning Industry. https://elearningindustry.com/types-of-neurodiversity-and-how-to-design-learning-experiences-for-them

Strayhorn, T. L. (2012). *College students' sense of belonging: A key to educational success for all students*. Routledge. DOI: 10.4324/9780203118924

Strunk, K., Hinkle, A. R., & Thurlow, M. L. (2022). Supporting IEP team decisions. *Journal of Special Education Leadership, 35*(2), 73–85. https://files.eric.ed.gov/fulltext/EJ1370360.pdf

Sturm, A., Huang, S., Bal, V., & Schwartzman, B. (2024). Psychometric exploration of the RAADS-R with autistic adults: Implications for research and clinical practice. *Autism, 28*(9), 2334–2345. DOI: 10.1177/13623613241228329 PMID: 38305196

Sullivan, J. (2024). Organisational neurotypicalness: Fighting unintentional ableism in working spaces. *Disability & Society, 1–4*. Advance online publication. DOI: 10.1080/09687599.2024.2373769

Sultan, M. A., Closser, S., Majidulla, A., Ahmed, S., Naz, F., Nayyab, S., & Sohail, A. (2023). How to eradicate polio in Pakistan: Insights from community health workers. *PLOS Global Public Health, 3*(8), e0002289. DOI: 10.1371/journal.pgph.0002289 PMID: 37643151

Sumerau, J. E., Forbes, T. D., Denise, E. J., & Mathers, L. A. (2021). Constructing allyship and the persistence of inequality. *Social Problems, 68*(2), 358–373. DOI: 10.1093/socpro/spaa003

Suppes, M. A., & Wells, C. C. (2018). *The social work experience: A case-based introduction to social work and social welfare* (7th ed.). Pearson.

Swift, K. D., Hall, C. L., Marimuttu, V., Redstone, L., & Hollis, C. (2013). Transition to adult mental health services for young people with Attention Deficit/Hyperactivity Disorder (ADHD): A qualitative analysis of their experiences. *BMC Psychiatry, 13*(74), 1–11. DOI: 10.1186/1471-244X-13-74 PMID: 23497082

Szulc, J. M., Davies, J., Tomczak, M. T., & McGregor, F. L. (2021). AMO perspectives on the well-being of neurodivergent human capital. *Employee Relations*, *43*(4), 858–872. DOI: 10.1108/ER-09-2020-0446

Taj, R. (2015). Mental health in Pakistan. In Bhurga, D., Tse, S., Ng, R., & Takei, N. (Eds.), *Routledge handbook of psychiatry in Asia* (pp. 101–114). Routledge.

Tarconish, E., Lombardi, A., & Taconet, A. (2023). Disability awareness & inclusive teaching online training videos for college instructors featuring students with disabilities. *Journal of Postsecondary Education and Disability*, *35*(4), 339–353.

Tarhirkeli, H. (2022). Special education in Pakistan: Hope for children with special needs. *socialprotection.org*. https://socialprotection.org/discover/blog/special-education-pakistan-hope-children-special-needs-0

Tariq, N. (2021). Health care challenges in Pakistan. *Journal of Islamabad Medical & Dental College.*, *10*(4), 190–191. DOI: 10.35787/jimdc.v10i4.826

Taylor, B., & Kroth, M. (2009). Andragogy's transition into the future: Meta-analysis of andragogy and its search for a measurable instrument. *Journal of Adult Education*, *38*(1), 1–11. https://eric.ed.gov/?id=EJ891073

Terry, K. (n. d.) *Neurodiversity: The new cultural competency in social work education*. University of Saint Thomas. https://www.nacsw.org/Convention/Resources2018/TerryKNeurodiversity.pdf

Test, D. W., Fowler, C. H., Wood, W. M., Brewer, D. M., & Eddy, S. (2005). A conceptual framework of self-advocacy for students with disabilities. *Remedial and Special Education*, *20*(1), 45–54. DOI: 10.1177/07419325050260010601

Test, D. W., Mazzotti, V. L., Mustian, A. L., Fowler, C. H., Kortering, L., & Kohler, P. (2009). Evidence-based secondary transition predictors for improving postschool outcomes for students with disabilities. *Career Development for Exceptional Individuals*, *32*(3), 160–181. https://psycnet.apa.org/doi/10.1177/0885728809346960. DOI: 10.1177/0885728809346960

Tharwani, Z. H., Bilal, W., Khan, H. A., Kumar, P., Butt, M. S., Hamdana, A. H., Essar, M. Y., Nashwan, A. J., Habib, Z., & Marzo, R. R. (2023). Infant & child mortality in Pakistan and its determinants: A review. *Inquiry : a Journal of Medical Care Organization, Provision and Financing*, *60*, 00469580231167024. Advance online publication. DOI: 10.1177/00469580231167024 PMID: 37085986

The Buckland Review of Autism Employment. (2023). *Report and recommendations*. GOV.UK. https://www.gov.uk/government/publications/the-buckland-review-of-autism-employment-report-and-recommendations/the-buckland-review-of-autism-employment-report-and-recommendations

The Care Act (2014). The National Archives of the United Kingdom. https://www.legislation.gov.uk/ukpga/2014/23/contents

Thelin, R., & Grigal, M. (2019). *Meeting the new requirements of WIOA through partnerships with institutions of higher education enrolling students with intellectual and developmental disabilities*. VR and Youth Rehabilitation Research and Training Center Practice Brief, Issue No. 02. TransCen, Inc.

Think College National Coordinating Center Accreditation Workgroup. (2021). Report on model accreditation standards for higher education programs for students with intellectual disability: Progress on the path to education, employment, and community living. University of Massachusetts Boston, Institute for Community Inclusion. https://thinkcollege.net/sites/default/files/files/resources/TCreport_Accred_full_F3.pdf

Think College. (2020). *Think college standards for inclusive higher education*. (Rev. ed.). University of Massachusetts Boston, Institute for Community Inclusion. https://thinkcollege.net/sites/default/files/files/tc_standards%2Bchecklists_draftFeb2020_0.pdf

Think College. (2025). *College search*. Institute for Community Inclusion. University of Massachusetts Boston. https://thinkcollege.net/college-search

Thomas, C. (2004). Rescuing a social relational understanding of disability. *Scandinavian Journal of Disability Research*, *6*(1), 22–36. DOI: 10.1080/15017410409512637

Thomas, G., & Loxley, A. (2022). *Deconstructing special education and constructing inclusion*. McGraw-Hill Education.

Thompson, A. C., & Lefler, E. K. (2016). ADHD stigma among college students. *Attention Deficit and Hyperactivity Disorders*, *8*(1), 45–52. DOI: 10.1007/s12402-015-0179-9 PMID: 26135022

Ting, J. Y., & Hwang, W. C. (2009). Cultural influences on help-seeking attitudes in Asian American students. *The American Journal of Orthopsychiatry*, *79*(1), 125–132. DOI: 10.1037/a0015394 PMID: 19290732

Tipton, W., & Wideman, S. (2021). Toward an invitational andragogy: Articulating a teaching philosophy for the andragogic classroom. *Journal of Communication Pedagogy*, *5*, 156–163. DOI: 10.31446/JCP.2021.2.16

Tovar, E. (2015). The role of faculty, counselors, and support programs on Latino/a community college students' success and intent to persist. *Community College Review, 43*(1), 46–71. DOI: 10.1177/0091552114553788

Trillingsgaard, A. (1999). The script model in relation to autism. *European Child & Adolescent Psychiatry, 8*(1), 45–49. DOI: 10.1007/s007870050082 PMID: 10367740

Tufts, O. I. R. (2023a). *First Year Experience Survey 2023* (Tufts University Office of Institutional Research). Tufts University.

Tufts, O. I. R. (2023b). *Sophomore Experience Survey 2023* (Tufts University Office of Institutional Research). Tufts University.

U. S. Department of Labor. (2024). *Disability Employment Statistics*. https://www.dol.gov/agencies/odep/research-evaluation/statistics

U.S. Department of Education. (2011a, September). *Students with disabilities preparing for postsecondary education: Know your rights and responsibilities*. https://www.ed.gov/higher-education/students-with-disabilities-preparing-for-postsecondary-education

U.S. Department of Education. (2011b, March). *Transition of students with disabilities to postsecondary education: A guide for high school educators*. https://www.ed.gov/teaching-and-administration/supporting-students/transition-of-students-with-disabilities-to-postsecondary-education-a-guide-for-high-school-educators

U.S. Department of Education. (2020). *A transition guide to postsecondary education and employment for students and youth with disabilities*. Washington, D.C., Office of Special Education and Rehabilitative Services. https://www.ed.gov/sites/ed/files/about/offices/list/osers/transition/products/postsecondary-transition-guide-08-2020.pdf

U.S. Department of Education. (2020, April). *The Family Educational Rights and Privacy Act: Guidance for parents*. https://studentprivacy.ed.gov/sites/default/files/resource_document/file/FERPAGuidanceForParents.pdf

UC Academic Senate. (2021). *Recommendations for making UC a more welcoming place for neurodivergent students*. University of California. https://senate.universityofcalifornia.edu/_files/reports/mg-mb-recs-neurodivergent-students.pdf

Uditsky, B., & Hughson, E. (2012). Inclusive postsecondary education: An evidence-based moral imperative. *Journal of Policy and Practice in Intellectual Disabilities, 9*(4), 298–302. DOI: 10.1111/jppi.12005

Unger, D. D., Li, J., Shreffler, A., Puleo, M., & Wyant, S. (2022). *The Ohio longitudinal transition study: Indicator 14 data collection and reporting*. Kent State University. https://www-s3-live.kent.edu/s3fs-root/s3fs-public/file/2022%20OLTS%20Annual%20State%20Report_0.pdf?VersionId=HfN1s3tL04m8UftIsGFUuXG_uN6AVNp7

United Kingdom Council for International Student Affairs. (2023). *Annual Policy Review 2022–23*. UKCISA. https://www.ukcisa.org.uk/Research--Policy/Resource-bank/resources/250/Annual-policy-review-2022-23

United Nations Educational, Scientific and Cultural Organization (UNESCO). (2005). *Guidelines for inclusion: Ensuring access to education for all.* United Nations Educational, Scientific and Cultural Organization. https://unesdoc.unesco.org/ark:/48223/pf0000140224

United Nations Educational, Scientific and Cultural Organization (UNESCO). (2010). *Implementing the right to education: A compendium of practical examples.* UNESCO Education Sector. https://unesdoc.unesco.org/ark:/48223/pf0000245196

United Nations. (1948). *Universal declaration of human rights.* United Nations Department of Public Information. https://www.un.org/en/about-us/universal-declaration-of-human-rights

United Nations. (2006). *Convention on the rights of persons with disabilities.* https://www.un.org/development/desa/disabilities/convention-on-the-rights-of-persons-with-disabilities.html

United States Department of Justice and Civil Rights Division. The American with Disabilities Act (2024). https://www.ada.gov/

University of Michigan. (n.d.). *Assistive technology resources.* Services for Students with Disabilities. https://ssd.umich.edu/article/assistive-technology-resources

University of Washington. (2025). *What is the difference between accommodation and modification for a student with a disability?* Disabilities, Opportunities, Internetworking, and Technology (DO-IT). https://doit.uw.edu/knowledge-base/what-is-the-difference-between-accommodation-and-modification-for-a-student-with-a-disability/

University of Washington. (n.d.). *About/overview.* Disabilities, Opportunities, Internetworking, and Technology (DO-IT) Center. https://www.washington.edu/doit/about/overview

US News & World Report. (2025). The best national universities in America. *US News & World Report*. https://www.usnews.com/best-colleges/rankings/national-universities?_sort=rank&_sortDirection=asc

Van Gaasbeek, E. (2024). *Examining the predictors of life satisfaction in college students with intellectual disability* [Unpublished doctoral dissertation]. The Ohio State University.

Van Gaasbeek, E. K., & Tassé, M. J. (2024). Constructing a preliminary model of school belonging for students with intellectual disability. *Journal of Intellectual Disabilities*, *28*(3), 591–614. DOI: 10.1177/17446295231164438 PMID: 37060351

Van Hees, V., Moyson, T., & Roeyers, H. (2015). Higher education experiences of students with Autism Spectrum Disorder: Challenges, benefits and support needs. *Journal of Autism and Developmental Disorders*, *45*(6), 1673–1688. DOI: 10.1007/s10803-014-2324-2 PMID: 25448918

Van Reusen, A. K., Bos, C. S., Schumaker, J. B., & Deshler, D. D. (2002). *The self-advocacy strategy for enhancing student motivation and self-determination: An education and transition planning process*. Edge Enterprises.

Van Wijngaarden-Cremers, P. J. M., van Eeten, E., Groen, W. B., Van Deurzen, P. A., Oosterling, I. J., & Van der Gaag, R. J. (2014). Gender and age differences in the core triad of impairments in Autism Spectrum Disorders: A systematic review and meta-analysis. *Journal of Autism and Developmental Disorders*, *44*(3), 627–635. DOI: 10.1007/s10803-013-1913-9 PMID: 23989936

Vaucher, C., Cudré-Mauroux, A., & Piérart, G. (2020). Environmental, personal, and relational barriers and facilitators to self-determination among adults with intellectual disabilities. *Scandinavian Journal of Disability Research*, *22*(1), 97–107. DOI: 10.16993/sjdr.624

Veesar, G. Y., Akhlaq, A., & Siddiqi, A. Q. (2023). The faces of deceptive healers: A scoping review of titles and traits associated with quacks across regions. *National Journal of Health Sciences*, *8*(4), 203–211. DOI: 10.21089/njhs.84.0203

Vella, J. (2002). *Learning to listen. Learning to teach. The power of dialogue in educating adults* (Revised ed.). Jossey-Bass.

Vincent, J., & Fabri, M. (2020). The ecosystem of competitive employment for university graduates with autism. *International Journal of Disability Development and Education*, *69*(6), 705–722. DOI: 10.1080/1034912X.2019.1626488

Vincent, J., & Ralston, K. (2024). Uncovering employment outcomes for autistic university graduates in the United Kingdom: An analysis of population data. *Autism*, *28*(3), 732–743. DOI: 10.1177/13623613231182756 PMID: 37353923

Voelker, D. M. (2013). Evidence of academic access in higher education: College programs that include students with intellectual disabilities [Doctoral dissertation, University of Florida]. https://www.proquest.com/openview/a7c7ad9b0b7a9f314824ab755167f47a/1?pq-origsite=gscholar&cbl=18750 [proquest.com]

Vygotsky, L. S. (1978). *Mind in society: The development of higher psychological processes*. Harvard University Press.

Waisman, T. C., Alba, L. A., & Green, S. A. (2022). Barriers to inclusive learning for autistic individuals. *Pediatrics*, *149*(4, Supplement 4), 1. DOI: 10.1542/peds.2020-049437Q PMID: 35363285

Waisman, T., Williams, Z. J., Cage, E., Santhanam, S. P., Magiati, I., Dwyer, P., Stockwell, K. M., Kofner, B., Brown, H., Davidson, D., Herrell, J., Shore, S. M., Caudel, D., Gurbuz, E., & Gillespie-Lynch, K. (2023). Learning from the experts: Evaluating a participatory autism and universal design training for university educators. *Autism*, *27*(2), 356–370. DOI: 10.1177/13623613221097207 PMID: 35652315

Wallerstein, N., Duran, B., Oetzel, J. G., & Minkler, M. (2018). *Community-based participatory research for health: Advancing social and health equity* (3rd ed.). Wiley.

Warraich, A., Rauf, N. K., Ingersoll, D. S. S. B., & Khan, M. (2024). Exploring maternal perspectives on autism spectrum disorder in Pakistan: Communication, stigma, and intervention. *Remittances Review, 9*(4), 924-950. https://remittancesreview.com/menu-script/index.php/remittances/article/view/2197

Wassell, C., & Burke, E. (2022). *Autism, girls, & keeping it all inside*. Autistic Girls Network. https://autisticgirlsnetwork.org/wp-content/uploads/2022/03/AGN-Report-Autism-Girls-Keeping-It-All-Inside.pdf

Watson, D., Lawless, M., & Maître, B. (2017). Employment transitions among people with disabilities in Ireland: An analysis of the quarterly national household survey, 2010–2015. *The Economic and Social Research Institute*. https://www.voced.edu.au/content/ngv:75674

Wehman, P., Sima, A. P., Ketchum, J., West, M. D., Chan, F., & Luecking, R. (2015). Predictors of successful transition from school to employment for youth with disabilities. *Journal of Occupational Rehabilitation*, *25*(2), 323–334. DOI: 10.1007/s10926-014-9541-6 PMID: 25240394

Wehmeyer, M. L. (2001). Self-determination and mental retardation. *International Review of Research in Mental Retardation, 24*, 1–48. DOI: 10.1016/S0074-7750(01)80004-5

Wehmeyer, M. L. (2005). Self-determination and individuals with severe disabilities: Re-examining meanings and misinterpretations. *Research and Practice for Persons with Severe Disabilities : the Journal of TASH, 30*(3), 113–120. DOI: 10.2511/rpsd.30.3.113

Wehmeyer, M. L. (2020). The importance of self-determination to the quality of life of people with intellectual disability: A perspective. *International Journal of Environmental Research and Public Health, 17*(19), 7121. DOI: 10.3390/ijerph17197121 PMID: 33003321

Wehmeyer, M. L., & Palmer, S. B. (2003). Adult outcomes for students with cognitive disabilities three-years after high school: The impact of self-determination. *Education and Training in Developmental Disabilities, 38*(2), 131–144. https://www.jstor.org/stable/23879591

Weick, A., Rapp, C., Sullivan, W. P., & Kisthardt, W. (1989). A strengths perspective for social work practice. *Social Work, 34*(4), 350–354. https://www.jstor.org/stable/23715838. DOI: 10.1093/sw/34.4.350

Wells, M. B. (2024). Supporting higher education students with attention deficit hyperactivity disorder through universal design for learning. *College Teaching, 72*(3), 227–230. https://doi-org.DOI: 10.1080/87567555.2022.2160959

Wenzler, S., & Keeley, J. (2024). The initiation or continuation of mental health services in the transition to college. *Journal of American College Health, 72*(6), 1768–1777. DOI: 10.1080/07448481.2022.2089851 PMID: 35728259

West Chester University. (n.d.). *Dub-C Autism program (D-CAP).* https://www.wcupa.edu/deputy-provost/dcap/

Westby, C. (2023). Promoting self-determination. *Word of Mouth, 34*(5), 13-15. https://journals.sagepub.com/doi/abs/10.1177/10483950231161474d

Whelpley, C. E., Holladay-Sandidge, H. D., Woznyj, H. M., & Banks, G. C. (2023). The biopsychosocial model and neurodiversity: A person-centered approach. *Industrial and Organizational Psychology: Perspectives on Science and Practice, 16*(1), 25–30. DOI: 10.1017/iop.2022.95

White, S. W., Richey, J. A., Gracanin, D., Coffman, M., Elias, R., LaConte, S., & Ollendick, T. H. (2016). Psychosocial and computer-assisted intervention for college students with autism spectrum disorder: Preliminary support for feasibility. *Education and Training in Autism and Developmental Disabilities*, *51*(3), 307–317. https://pmc.ncbi.nlm.nih.gov/articles/PMC5241080/pdf/nihms836993.pdf PMID: 28111607

Whittington, C. (2023). Collaboration and partnership in context. In Cree, V. E., & McCulloch, T. (Eds.), *Social Work* (pp. 240–246). Routledge. DOI: 10.4324/9781003178699-46

Wiener, J., & Daniels, L. (2016). School experiences of adolescents with Attention-Deficit/Hyperactivity Disorder. *Journal of Learning Disabilities*, *49*(6), 567–581. DOI: 10.1177/0022219415576973 PMID: 25795542

Williams, M., & Sharif, N. (2021). Racial allyship: Novel measurement and new insights. *New Ideas in Psychology*, *62*, 100865. DOI: 10.1016/j.newideapsych.2021.100865

Wilson, K., & Dallman, A. (2024). Strategies for promoting neurodiversity and autism acceptance in higher education. *Journal of Diversity in Higher Education*. Advance online publication. DOI: 10.1037/dhe0000550

Wlodkowski, R. J., & Ginsberg, M. B. (2017). *Enhancing adult motivation to learn: A comprehensive guide for teaching all adults* (4th ed.). Jossey-Bass.

Wolbring, G., & Lillywhite, A. (2023). Coverage of allies, allyship and disabled people: A scoping review. *Societies (Basel, Switzerland)*, *13*(11), 241. DOI: 10.3390/soc13110241

Woo, B., Fan, W., Tran, T. V., & Takeuchi, D. T. (2019). The role of racial/ethnic identity in the association between racial discrimination and psychiatric disorders: A buffer or exacerbator? *SSM - Population Health*, *7*, 100378. DOI: 10.1016/j.ssmph.2019.100378 PMID: 30923732

Woods, S. E. O. N., & Estes, A. (2023). Toward a more comprehensive autism assessment: The survey of autistic strengths, skills, and interests. *Frontiers in Psychiatry*, *14*, 1264516. DOI: 10.3389/fpsyt.2023.1264516 PMID: 37867767

Workforce Innovation & Opportunity Act 29 U.S.C. § 3101 et seq. (2014). https://www.govinfo.gov/app/details/USCODE-2023-title29/USCODE-2023-title29-chap32-sec3101

Wright, E., Smith, R., Vernon, M., Wall, R., & White, L. (2021). Inclusive, multi-partner co-creation for the teaching of special educational needs and disabilities in higher education. *Journal of University Teaching & Learning Practice*, *18*(7), 25–40. DOI: 10.53761/1.18.7.3

Youngblood, I. I. J.II, & Spencer, M. B. (2002). Integrating normative identity processes and academic support requirements for special needs adolescents: The application of an identity-focused cultural ecological (ICE) perspective. *Applied Developmental Science*, *6*(2), 95–108. DOI: 10.1207/S1532480XADS0602_5

Yu, L., Stronach, S., & Harrison, A. J. (2020). Public knowledge and stigma of Autism Spectrum Disorder: Comparing China with the United States. *Autism*, *24*(6), 1531–1545. DOI: 10.1177/1362361319900839 PMID: 32338539

Zastrow, C., Kirst-Ashman, K., & Hessenauer, S. (2019). *Understanding human behavior and the social environment* (11th ed.). Cengage.

Zeng, W., Ju, S., & Hord, C. (2023). Parental influences on student self-determination: Perspectives of college students with learning disabilities. *Learning Disability Quarterly*, *46*(3), 180–190. DOI: 10.1177/07319487221107890

Zhang, L., Carter, R. A.Jr, Greene, J. A., & Bernacki, M. L. (2024). Unraveling challenges with the implementation of Universal Design for Learning: A systematic literature review. *Educational Psychology Review*, *36*(1), 35. Advance online publication. DOI: 10.1007/s10648-024-09860-7

Zhou, C., Gao, M., Shi, X., & Zhang, Z. (2023). Suicidal behavior, depression and loneliness among college students: The role of school belonging. *Psychology Health and Medicine*, *28*(6), 1520–1526. DOI: 10.1080/13548506.2022.2113105 PMID: 35980293

Zirkel, P. A., & Gullo, G. (2024). Public school rates of Section 504-only students: The latest update. *West's Education Law Reporter*, 420, 1–13. https://perryzirkel.com/wp-content/uploads/2018/07/zirkel-and-huang-state-by-state-504-only-rates-article-061118.pdf

About the Contributors

Carol Rogers-Shaw, Ph. D., is an adjunct professor of Educational Administration at the University of Dayton. Dr. Rogers-Shaw earned a doctorate in Lifelong Learning and Adult Education from Pennsylvania State University. She is the co-editor of *Adult Learning*, an international, peer-reviewed, adult education practice-oriented journal. Carol taught secondary school English for over 30 years, she is the mother of a Neurodivergent adult, and her experiences with Neurodivergent adolescents led her to concentrate on work that highlights the strengths of all learners. Her research focuses on expanding adult educational inclusion for learners with disabilities, transition and support for Neurodivergent learners in postsecondary education, graduate and doctoral study, Universal Design for Learning, imposter phenomenon, profound learning, and spirituality. (carshaw33@gmail.com)

Tulare Williams Park, D. Ed. Candidate, ACSW, LSW, MSW, is an assistant professor of Social Work at Commonwealth University of Pennsylvania – Lock Haven. In addition to teaching and academic advising, she has practiced in student support roles and directed the Disability Resources Office. She also has professional experience in the corrections system and community-based mental health. Tulare is currently a doctoral candidate in Lifelong Learning and Adult Education at Penn State University. Her research interests include the emotional and relational experiences of adult learners, social work education, distance education, mental health, adult learner support, and disability studies. (tpark@commonwealthu.edu)

Kayla D. Mohney, Ed.D., is an associate professor within the department of exceptionality programs at Commonwealth University of Pennsylvania - Lock Haven. Dr. Mohney taught at a private school for students with exceptionality for seven years, working exclusively with students with extensive support needs prior to starting to work in higher education in 2014. She has taught a variety of courses including foundation and advanced special education teacher preparation courses which focus on supporting students with complex learning needs. Her research interests include test related anxiety reduction strategies, transition to post-secondary education for Neurodivergent learners, and disability inclusion and equity practices in higher education settings. (kayla.mohney@gmail.com)

Kari Sheward is the Vice President of Behavioral Health and Clinical Services for Tangram, Inc. She previously acted as Clinical Director for several autism clinics across Central Indiana. She worked in the mental health field as a crisis therapist for several years. When her youngest son received an autism diagnosis, she returned to school and earned her Board Certification in Behavior Analysis. Kari holds an undergraduate degree in psychology from Ball State University and a master's degree in psychology with a specialization in Applied Behavior Analysis from Purdue Global. Kari is currently a doctoral candidate in the University of Dayton's Leadership for Organizations program. Her research interests include transition programming for Autistic students and creating a sense of community on college campuses for Neurodivergent students. (shewardk1@udayton.edu)

***

Des Aston is Outreach Coordinator at the Trinity Centre for People with Intellectual Disabilities (TCPID), School of Education, Trinity College Dublin. He lectures on the Certificate in Arts, Science and Inclusive Applied Practice (ASIAP) and co-leads the Disability Rights module. Des is Chair of the Inclusive National Higher Education Forum (INHEF), a national group supporting inclusive education pathways for learners with intellectual disabilities. He was appointed by the Minister for Disability to the Disability Stakeholder Group (DSG 6) for 2022–2024, advising on the National Disability Inclusion Strategy. Des also sits on the TCPID Management Board and is a PhD candidate in the School of Education, researching the experiences of students with intellectual disabilities in higher education in Ireland.

Jennifer M. Banks is the Research Coordinator for the TCPID. She has responsibility for the coordination of research activities and development and implementation of TCPID's research strategy. As part of this Research Centre and Innovation Hub, Jenny chairs the Research Working Group and engages collaboratively with staff on a wide variety of research projects both within Trinity College and the European Union. Her research interests include co-research and inclusion of marginalized groups in the community.

Owen Barden is Assistant Professor in Intellectual Disability and Inclusion at Trinity College Dublin. Professor Barden has published extensively on learning disability, with interests in histories of learning disabilities and participatory methodologies.

Andrew Buck, Ph.D., is a research scientist at The Ohio State University, where he earned a doctorate in Educational Policy. Dr. Buck has dedicated his career to promoting positive outcomes for Neurodivergent students and individuals with disabilities. Andrew has authored publications and delivered presentations on topics such as evidence-based transition practices and community engaged research strategies. His work includes STEM mentorship initiatives for college students with disabilities and inclusive health projects that include partners with intellectual and developmental disabilities. (Andrew.Buck@osumc.edu)

Joellen E. Coryell, Ph.D., is Professor of Adult, Professional, and Community Education and Associate Dean for Academic Affairs and Educational Partnerships for the College of Education and at Texas State University. She has worked in academia and business organizations as an educational researcher, university administrator, faculty developer, English language educator, instructional designer and trainer, and program director in adult education and human resource development and training programs. Joellen's research focuses on the investment in the professional development of adult educators and leaders and on international, cross-cultural adult and higher education. (coryell@txstate.edu)

Eileen T. Crehan, Ph. D., is an Associate Professor at the Shriver Center at the University of Massachusetts T.H. Chan School of Medicine, affiliated faculty at the Eliot- Pearson Department of Child Study and Human Development at Tufts University and a licensed clinical psychologist. Dr. Crehan is interested in improving the accessibility of healthcare and education for Neurodivergent individuals using participatory methods and technologies. Specifically, Dr. Crehan focuses on adolescence and adults and affirming models of relationship education. Her own experience with OCD and executive functioning challenges have fueled her passion for the space where clinical science research and advocacy overlap. (Eileen.Crehan@umassmemorial.org)

Laura Dean, D. Ed., CPsychol, is President-Elect of the British Psychological Society, a Chartered Occupational Psychologist, and a Senior Lecturer at the University of Sheffield. Dr. Dean's work focuses on creating more inclusive workplaces, with a particular emphasis on neurodiversity. She collaborates directly with organizations to redesign and improve selection processes, ensuring they are accessible and equitable for Neurodivergent candidates. Laura's academic and applied work bridges research and practice to promote evidence-based, inclusive organizational development. (l.dean@sheffield.ac.uk)

Marie Devitt is the Business Partnerships Manager in the TCPID, School of Education, Trinity College Dublin. Marie is responsible for building the TCPID Business Partners Network and securing both financial and practical support from the business community for the TCPID. She works closely with the TCPID Business Partners to develop and nurture the partnerships and to source and support work placements, paid internships, and employment opportunities for students and graduates of the program.

Simone R. Dufresne, Ph. D., is a Lecturer in the Eliot-Pearson Department of Child Study and Human Development at Tufts University. Simone completed her Ph. D. at Tufts in 2024, with a dissertation titled Navigating Tufts for Neurodivergent Students: Developing, Implementing, and Evaluating a Workshop Series at a U.S. University. Her research focuses on how Autistic individuals understand themselves and their place in society and how interventions can support this development. Dr. Dufresne has been working in the autism field supporting youth and families for almost 15 years. (simone.dufresne@tufts.edu)

Sadbh Feehan is an Executive Officer in the Trinity Centre for People with Intellectual Disabilities. A graduate of the ASIAP program, she provides administrative support for the TCPID Business Partners program along with support to students on courses. Part of Sadbh's role is to assist TCPID students with orientation and help them integrate into student life on campus by getting involved with clubs and societies.

Steven Granich, Ph.D., is a full professor of social work at Commonwealth University of Pennsylvania – Lock Haven. Dr. Granich has published extensively in international social work. He has an interest in mental health, substance abuse, and family therapy. He has been a visiting professor in Pakistan. (sgranich@commonwealthu.edu)

Steven Granich, Ph.D., is a full professor of social work at Commonwealth University of Pennsylvania – Lock Haven. Dr. Granich has published extensively in international social work. He has an interest in mental health, substance abuse, and family therapy. He has been a visiting professor in Pakistan. (sgranich@commonwealthu.edu)

Jessie Green, Ph.D., is a research assistant professor and the LEND special education faculty member at The Ohio State University Nisonger Center. She oversees four community programs serving youth and adults with autism and intellectual disability to access their communities and postsecondary education. Jessie has research interests in community integrated employment, transition age youth, inclusive postsecondary education, and social integration. She brings leadership to both the Ohio Statewide Consortia and the Great Lakes Inclusive Postsecondary Alliance, supporting inclusive postsecondary education for students with intellectual disability. Previously, Jessie was an intervention specialist and job training coordinator in several public-school districts in Arizona and Ohio. Dr. Green has a B.S. and M.Ed. in special education from Ohio State and completed her Ph.D. in educational policy. Weaving her experience in the classroom as an intervention specialist and now in research, Jessie strives to always expand opportunities for those with disabilities and their families. (jessie.green@osumc.edu)

Margo Izzo, Ph. D., Professor of Psychiatry Emerita, The Ohio State University, is the previous Program Director of Special Education and Transition Services and Associate Director of The Ohio State University Nisonger Center. She has extensive experience designing and directing projects that improve the transition from high school to college and careers with funding from the U.S. Department of Education, National Science Foundation, and numerous state and local agencies. Dr. Izzo received the Mary E. Switzer Fellow from the National Institute of Disability Rehabilitation Research in 1996. She directed projects that included creating college programs for students with intellectual disabilities and improving digital curricula in high schools that increase reading achievement, IT literacy, and self-determination skills. Dr. Izzo co-authored a book with LeDerick Horne entitled: Empowering Students with Hidden Disabilities: A Path to Pride and Success. (margo.izzo@osumc.edu)

John Kubiak lectures at the School of Education, TCD and is based in the Trinity Centre for People with Intellectual Disabilities. Dr. Kubiak is program coordinator of the Certificate in Contemporary Living and the certificate in Arts, Science and Inclusive Applied Practice (ASIAP), an inclusive tertiary education program for people with intellectual disabilities. John's doctoral research - which was conducted with the input of co-researchers with intellectual disabilities - has led to the development of a model of how people with intellectual disabilities experience learning while in tertiary education.

Aoife M. Lynam, Ph. D., is an Assistant Professor in the Psychology of Education at Trinity College Dublin. Dr. Lynam earned her Ph.D. by exploring the experiences of bereaved young people in Irish schools. She has contributed to funded research projects with Trinity College Dublin, Stranmillis University, ESRI, Hibernia College, and DCU. She is an Advisory Board Member of the Irish Childhood Bereavement Network, sits on the Management Board of Trinity Research in Childhood Centre (TRiCC), and is a member of the Trinity Centre for

People with Intellectual Disabilities (TCPID) management board. Her research has been published and presented nationally and internationally. (AOLYNAM@tcd.ie)

Munawar Malik, Ph. D., serves as an Assistant Professor in the Institute of Special Education at the University of the Punjab. Besides being Ph. D. in special education, Dr. Malik also is a practitioner in Speech Language Therapy. His areas of interest include reading, writing, speech, language and exceptionalities. He enjoys teaching and is fond of writing. To his credit, he holds numerous research articles published in leading journals of Pakistan. On social fronts Munawar has contributed through his writings in magazines and newspapers. He remains hopeful for humanity and believes in cooperation and hard work. (munawar.dse@pu.edu.pk)

Angela Mazzocco is the Teaching and Learning Assistant in TCPID at Trinity College Dublin. She works closely with the teaching team and occupational therapists to support students academically during lectures and with independent study. Angela provides crucial and beneficial feedback to both the teaching and wider team on the challenges and successes of our students which allows for constant improvements in how we deliver content to our students.

Conor Mc Guckin, Ph. D., is the Director of TCPID, a Chartered Psychologist, and Associate Professor in Psychology of Education at Trinity College Dublin. Dr. Mc Guckin graduated from the University of Ulster with a B.Sc. in Psychology and Organizational Science and from the Open University with a B.Sc. degree. He earned his Ph.D. in Psychology for his research exploring bully/victim problems among school pupils across Northern Ireland. Conor has a long history of involvement in, and leadership of, national and international research and applied practice projects. (mcguckic@tcd.ie)

Carly McMorris is an Associate Professor in the School and Applied Child Psychology program at University of Calgary's Werklund School of Education. She is the director of the ENHANCE Lab and a registered child clinical psychologist. Dr. McMorris' research and clinical practice focuses on advancing mental health outcomes for Neurodivergent youth and young adults, such as those with autism, intellectual disability, and fetal alcohol spectrum disorder. (camcmorr@ucalgary.ca).

Emer Murphy is an Occupational Therapist working in the Trinity Centre for People with Intellectual Disabilities in the School of Education, Trinity College Dublin. The primary aim of Occupational Therapy is to facilitate people to participate in meaningful occupations. These are the daily activities that people want and need to do. Emer supports students and graduates to participate in college life and internships by supporting them to learn and develop skills, by adapting activities or materials, or by adapting environments. Emer works primarily with graduates and employers who participate in the internship program. Emer has an Honors Degree and a Master's Degree in Occupational Therapy. She is registered with Coru and is a member of the Association of Occupational Therapists of Ireland (AOTI). Emer has extensive clinical experience both in Ireland and abroad, primarily working with people with intellectual disabilities.

Sonia Omer is currently working as Associate Professor in the Department of Social Work, University of the Punjab, Lahore, Pakistan and Director of Sughra Begum Centre for Education Policy and Development in the same university. Dr. Omer is a sound researcher and likes to write on gender issues, social policy and entrepreneurship, socio-economic development, population and demography, child rights, and community development. She is also a motivational speaker and talks on national television on different social issues. Sonia has a number of research publications in higher education commission of Pakistan recognized journals and in impact factor international journals. She has also produced articles in the leading newspapers of Pakistan. Her interest in research led her to visit numerous developed regions of the world including universities in Nairobi, United Kingdom, United States of America and Germany where she participated in international conferences and presented her work. She is a board member and director of many renowned non-Government organizations including Agahi and Agahi Pakistan. (soniaomer78@gmail.com)

Vivian Rath is a Research Fellow in TCPID within the School of Education where he has co-coordinated the Disability Rights module and supervises masters students. He has a background and expertise in human rights, student leadership, success and in creating inclusive environments where everyone belongs. Vivian is a Government of Ireland Ministerial appointee to the Board of the National Disability Authority, and the Irish Human Rights and Equality Commission Disability Advisory Committee. He is founder and Chair of the Trinity College Dublin Forum for Disabled Staff. An award- winning equality and civil rights advocate, he has spoken in the EU Parliament and in the Oireachtas (Irish Parliament), national television and radio.

Barbara Ringwood is a Senior Occupational Therapist working in the Trinity Centre for People with Intellectual Disabilities (TCPID), School of Education, Trinity College Dublin.

Roxanne Ross is currently the Director, Student Success Centre at the University of Calgary. Her role involves working collaboratively within the institution to support the development and delivery of learning, writing, and advising services for undergraduate and graduate students. Roxanne's previous professional work includes the Coordinator of Writing Support Services at Carleton University as well as teaching within the field of post-secondary English for Academic Purposes (EAP). Her current research interests include post-secondary teaching and learning strategies that support student wellbeing and universal design for learning (UDL). (rossr@ucalgary.ca)

Michael Shevlin is a Professor in Inclusive Education at TCD and Patron of TCPID. Professor Shevlin is a former Director of the Trinity Centre for People with Intellectual Disabilities. He has moved into a policy development, strategy and advocacy role during this critical time for program provision for students with an intellectual disability in Ireland as the Path4 funded pilot program progressed.

Adrienne Taylor is a doctoral student in adult, professional, and community education at Texas State University, where their research investigates innovative workplace learning and development opportunities for individuals with disabilities. They are actively involved in the graduate student government and serves as a member of the Gold Star Society, the university's elite student ambassador group. They work as a graduate assistant for the Faculty Development department. With a robust background in instructional design, content strategy, and universal design, Adrienne also leverages their expertise as a consultant in the private sector, where they focus on enhancing user experience and accessibility. (amt259@txstate.edu)

Heather Thompson is an Academic Development Specialist at the University of Calgary, Student Success Centre. She works with students to develop learning strategies that are personalized to their individualized needs. Heather partners with students to deliver sessions to faculty and staff focused on creating a neuroinclusive environment by sharing best practices in Universal Design for Learning (UDL). (heather.thompson1@ucalgary.ca)

Emily Van Gaasbeek, Ph. D., received her doctorate in Intellectual and Developmental Disabilities Psychology from The Ohio State University. Dr. Van Gaasbeek's research interests include belongingness and mental health (anxiety, depression) among young adults with intellectual and developmental disabilities in college and the community. (emily.vangaasbeek@osumc.edu)

Jill Woodnutt is the INCLUDE-ID network Coordinator based in TCPID. The INCLUDE-ID network is a consortium of higher education institutions who are participating in the PATH 4 Phase 2 pilot project which funds the development and delivery of third level courses for people with intellectual disabilities across Ireland. The INCLUDE-ID Network focuses on advancing the development, delivery and long-term sustainability of program at a national level through collaborative research, workshops, and the creation of training materials.

Index

P

R

S

T

U

W

www.ingramcontent.com/pod-product-compliance
Ingram Content Group UK Ltd.
Pitfield, Milton Keynes, MK11 3LW, UK
UKHW050948290926
15470UKWH00005B/1716

9 798369 389201